AIDS in Europe

Major changes in the nature and dynamics of the AIDS epidemic over the last few years are reflected in changing epidemiological trends as well as in the progress made by biomedical research and treatment. *AIDS in Europe* brings together papers from leading social science researchers to look at the opportunities and challenges these changes bring in their wake and the different ways in which they are being responded to in both Western and Eastern Europe. Four main topics are covered:

- living with HIV and therapeutic advances
- new perspectives on sexuality
- drug use – user and policy perspectives
- accounting for the epidemic

AIDS in Europe provides a comprehensive overview of current social and behavioural research on HIV and AIDS for all health professionals.

Jean-Paul Moatti, Université d'Aix-Marseille II, France; **Yves Souteyrand**, Agence Nationale de Recherches sur le Sida, France; **Annick Prieur**, University of Oslo, Norway; **Theo Sandfort**, University of Utrecht, The Netherlands; **Peter Aggleton**, Institute of Education, London.

Social Aspects of AIDS
Series Editor: Peter Aggleton
Institute of Education, University of London

AIDS is not simply a concern for scientists, doctors and medical researchers, it has important social dimensions as well. These include individual, cultural and media responses to the epidemic, stigmatisation and discrimination, counselling, care and health promotion. This series of books brings together work from many disciplines including psychology, sociology, cultural and media studies, anthropology, education and history. The titles will be of interest to the general reader, those involved in education and social research, and scientific researchers who want to examine the social aspects of AIDS.

Recent titles include:

Mental Health and HIV Infection
Edited by José Catalán

Families and Communities Responding to AIDS
Edited by Peter Aggleton, Graham Hart and Peter Davies

Dying to Care?
David Miller

Power and Community: Organizational and Cultural Responses to AIDS
Dennis Altman

Moral Threats and Dangerous Desires: AIDS in the News Media
Deborah Lupton

Last Served? Gendering the HIV Pandemic
Cindy Patton

Crossing Borders: Migration, Ethnicity and AIDS
Edited by Mary Haour-Knipe

Bisexualities and AIDS: International Perspectives
Edited by Peter Aggleton

Sexual Interactions and HIV Risk: New Conceptual Perspectives in European Research

Edited by Luc Van Campenhoudt, Mitchell Cohen, Gustavo Guizzardi and Dominique Hausser

AIDS: Activism and Alliances
Edited by Peter Aggleton, Peter Davies and Graham Hart

AIDS as a Gender Issue
Edited by Lorraine Sherr, Catherine Hankins and Lydia Bennett

Drug Injecting and HIV Infection: Global Dimensions and Local Responses
Edited by Gerry Stimson, Don C. Des Jarlais and Andrew Ball

Sexual Behaviour and HIV/AIDS in Europe: Comparisons of National Surveys
Edited by Michel Hubert, Nathalie Bajos and Theo Sandfort

Men Who Sell Sex: International Perspectives on Male Prostitution and AIDS
Edited by Peter Aggleton

The Dutch Response to HIV: Pragmatism and Consensus
Edited by Theo Sandfort

Social Aspects of AIDS
Series Editor: Peter Aggleton
Institute of Education, University of London

Editorial Advisory Board:

AIDS in Europe

New challenges for the social sciences

Edited by
Jean-Paul Moatti, Yves Souteyrand,
Annick Prieur, Theo Sandfort and
Peter Aggleton

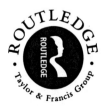

London and New York

First published 2000
by Routledge
11 New Fetter Lane, London EC4P 4EE

Simultaneously published in the USA and Canada
by Routledge
29 West 35th Street, New York, NY 10001

Routledge is an imprint of the Taylor & Francis Group

Transferred to Digital Printing 2004

Typeset in Times by Taylor & Francis Books Ltd

British Library Cataloguing-in-Publication Data
A catalogue record for this book is available from the British Library

Library of Congress Cataloging in Publication Data
AIDS in Europe: New challenges for the social sciences / Jean-Paul
Moatti ... [et al.].
(Social Aspects of AIDS)
Includes bibliographical references and index.
1. AIDS (disease) – social aspects – Europe.
I. Moatti, J.-P. (Jean-Paul) II. Series.
RA644.A25   A36354117   2000
362.1'969792'0094–dc21   99-048728

ISBN 1–857–28507–7 (hbk)
ISBN 1–857–28508–5 (pbk)

Contents

Illustrations

Contributors

Peter Aggleton is Professor in Education and Director of the Thomas Coram Research Unit at the Institute of Education, University of London. He has worked internationally in HIV/AIDS health promotion since the mid 1980s. His publications include *Health* (Routledge, 1990), *AIDS: Activism and Alliances* (ed. with Peter Davies and Graham Hart, Taylor and Francis, 1997), *Success in HIV Prevention* (AVERT, 1997) and *Men who Sell Sex* (ed., UCL Press, 1998).

Demosthenes Agrafiotis is Professor of Sociology at the National School of Public Health in Athens, Greece. He has conducted research on the socio-cultural and psychological aspects of AIDS and sexuality, as well as on the empowerment of people living with HIV/AIDS. Published articles in Greek on the social perception of AIDS and AIDS as a socio-cultural phenomenon include *Cultural Unfoldings* (1983), *Cultural Discontinuities* (1987), *Health and Illness, Sociocultural Dimensions* (1988), *Mobile Image* (1992), and *AIDS. Transversal Shade* (1998).

Eddy Beck is a senior lecturer in epidemiology and public health at Imperial College School of Medicine, St Mary's Campus. His main interests are in assessing the acceptability and cost-effectiveness of health care provision. His recent work on this has been in the field of HIV infection where he was instrumental in setting up the National Prospective Monitoring System on the Use, Cost and Outcomes of HIV Service Provision in English Hospitals.

Michael Bochow is a research fellow at Intersofia (Institute for Applied Interdisciplinary Research in Social Problems), Berlin. Since 1987, he has been commissioned by the Ministry of Health in Germany to conduct nationwide studies of HIV risk behaviour among gay and bisexual men. His publications include *Gay Men in Rural Areas and Smaller Cities: Lower Saxony as an Example* (Edition Sigma, 1998) and *The Particular Vulnerability of Working Class Gay Men to HIV Infection and AIDS* (AIDS-Forum DAH, 1997).

Mary Boulton is a Professor of Sociology at Oxford Brookes University. She has been involved in a wide range of research in relation to HIV infection and AIDS, including work on changing sexual behaviour amongst gay men, bisexual men and families of children with HIV/AIDS. She is also interested in research methods and edited *Challenge and Innovation: Methodological Advances in Social Research on HIV/AIDS* (Taylor and Francis, 1994).

José Catalán is a reader in psychiatry at Imperial College School of Medicine, Chelsea & Westminster Campus. His main clinical and research interests are in the area of mental health in general hospital settings, with particular interest in HIV infection and also in suicidal behaviour. He has published extensively in peer-reviewed journals and his books include (with Keith Hawton) *Attempted Suicide* (Oxford University Press, 2nd edn 1997) and (with Adrian Burgess and Ivana Klimes) *The Psychological Medicine of HIV Infection* (Oxford University Press, 1995). He has recently edited *Mental Health and HIV Infection: Psychological and Psychiatric Aspects* (UCL Press, 1999).

Valeriy Chervyakov is a sociologist and Director of the Transnational Family Research Institute in Moscow. He has conducted several surveys of young people's sexual behaviour in Russia and also works on problems of reproductive health.

François Delor is a researcher at Centre d'Etudes Sociologiques, Facultés Universitaires Saint-Louis, Brussels, where he is engaged in qualitative research on the sexuality of people living with HIV/AIDS and ways of adapting to different risks. He is also a psychoanalyst and an adviser to several NGOs involved in HIV/AIDS prevention in Belgium.

Owen Noel Gill is a consultant epidemiologist at the Communicable Disease Surveillance Centre, Public Health Laboratory Service, in London. He has been involved with national surveillance of HIV and AIDS in the UK since 1987 and has a special interest in the design and use of surveillance systems, both national and international.

Dominique Hausser is a physician with qualifications in prevention and public health. He is currently a senior researcher in the field of health-related problems in the urban context at the Swiss Federal Institute of Technology. Since 1985, he has conducted several research projects in the field of HIV/AIDS and drug use and has been director of the Swiss national programme of research on the psychosocial aspects of AIDS.

Dominique Joye is currently a senior researcher in the field of urban studies at the Swiss Federal Institute of Technology. Since 1983, he has conducted several research projects on local government, local participation and urban transformation, in particular in the field of drugs policy as well as social inequalities. His publications include (with Therese Huissoud and Martin Schuler) *Habitants des quartiers, citoyens de la ville*

(Seismo, Zurich, 1995); (with Jean-Philippe Leresche and Michel Bassand) *Métropolisations: Interdépendances mondiales et implication lémaniques* (Georg, Geneva, 1995); (with René Levy, Olivier Guye and Vincent Kaufmann) *Tous égaux? De la stratification aux représentations* (Seismo, Zurich, 1997).

Milena Komarova is a part-time social survey research consultant at the UNAIDS office in Sofia. Her work is focused on the social aspects of HIV/AIDS. She gained her professional experience working for social and market research companies.

Igor Kon is a sociologist and psychologist. He is a principal researcher at the Institute of Ethnology and Anthropology, Russian Academy of Sciences, and Head of the Advisory Board for the Transnational Family Research Institute in Moscow. His most recent books are *Sex and Russian Society* (ed. with James Riordan, Indiana University Press, 1993) and *The Sexual Revolution in Russia* (Free Press, 1995).

Mirjam Kretzschmar is a senior research scientist in the Department of Infectious Diseases Epidemiology at the National Institute of Public Health and the Environment (RIVM) in Bilthoven, The Netherlands. She is developing mathematical models for the spread and prevention of infectious diseases. The focus of her recent research has been on the influence of sexual network structure on the transmission and prevention of STDs and HIV/AIDS.

Daniel Kübler is a political scientist and researcher at the Swiss Federal Institute of Technology in Lausanne. He has worked on local and national drug policy in Western Europe, as well as on the epidemiology of drug use in Switzerland. His publications include *Politique de la drogue dans les villes suisses entre ordre et santé* (Paris, L'Harmattan, 1999).

Hugues Lagrange is a senior researcher at the Observatoire Sociologique du Changement (National Centre for Scientific Research) in Paris. He is engaged in qualitative and quantitative research on sexuality and deviance in France. His publications include (with Brigitte Lhomond, eds) *L'Entrée dans la sexualité á le comportement des 15–18 ans dans le contexte du sida* (Paris, La Découverte, 1997) and *Les Adolescents, le sexe, l'amour* (Paris, Syros, 1999).

France Lert is a senior fellow at INSERM, Saint-Maurice, France. She has carried out research on the evaluation of public health policy relating to drug use and HIV infection. She was commissioned by INSERM to define the framework for the evaluation of new substitution treatment programmes for injecting drug users implemented in 1996.

Brigitte Lhomond is a sociologist and researcher at the National Centre for Scientific Research (CNRS) in Lyons, France. She has worked for many years on the social construction of sexuality. With Hugues Lagrange, she was co-director of the national survey on sexual behaviour of youth in France.

Christine Ann McGarrigle is a senior scientist at the Communicable Disease Surveillance Centre, Public Health Laboratory Service, in London. She co-ordinates an unlinked anonymous survey which monitors HIV prevalence and associated risk behaviours among attenders of genitourinary medicine clinics in England and Wales. She has been involved in a number of European collaborative HIV projects, and has a particular interest in HIV testing and related risk behaviours.

Dominique Malatesta is a researcher in sociology at the Swiss Federal Institute of Technology in Lausanne. She has worked on drug policies in different Swiss cities and on urban services for drug users. She is currently working on new social movements and on the evolution of social housing.

Olga Metallinou has a specialist background in psychology and health. She worked for three years as a researcher in the Department of Sociology at the National School of Public Health in Athens, Greece. She is now working as a psychologist at the Counselling Centre of MERIMNA – a Society for the Care of Children and Families facing Illness and Death.

David Miller is Emeritus Professor of Public Health Medicine at Imperial College School of Medicine and Honorary Senior Research Fellow in the Department of Public Health at UMDS in London. His main interests have been in the epidemiology of infectious diseases, in particular acute respiratory infections in children, immunisation, HIV/AIDS and related health services.

Jean-Paul Moatti is Professor of Economics at the University of the Mediterranean and Director of the INSERM Research Unit on Social Sciences Applied to Medical Innovation in Marseilles, France. He has been a member of the Scientific Council of ANRS (the French Agency for Aids Research) and was the President of the Scientific Committee responsible for the 2nd European Conference on the Methods and Results of Social and Behavioural Research on AIDS in Paris (January 1998). His recent publications in the field of AIDS concern the impact of drug maintenance treatment on the reduction of HIV-related risk behaviours among injecting drug users, and the behavioural factors associated with optimisation of antiretroviral treatment. He is currently involved in an assessment of the UNAIDS Drug Access Initiative in developing countries.

Joanne Neale is a research fellow in the Centre for Drug Misuse Research, University of Glasgow. She is currently the principal investigator on a qualitative study of drug users' risk behaviour in relation to non-fatal overdose. Her research interests include drug misuse, housing and home-lessness, social work and social care issues.

Geneviève Paicheler is Director of Research at the National Centre for Scientific Research (CNRS) in France. She specialises in different aspects of health prevention, especially issues related to HIV and AIDS, and participated in a committee of the Ministry of Health involved in the implementation of the mass education campaigns. Her publications include *The Psychology of Social Influence* (Cambridge University Press, 1988) and (with M. Pollak and Janine Pierret) *AIDS, A Problem for Sociological Research* (Sage, 1992).

Pauline Pantzou is a psychologist and scientific collaborator at the Department of Sociology at the National School of Public Health in Athens, Greece. Her interests are in the psychological dimensions of health and illness and on methodological issues of social research. She has participated in studies on HIV/AIDS using quantitative and qualita-tive techniques, as well as more generally in the health promotion field.

Annick Prieur is a researcher at the NOVA Institute for Social Research in Oslo where she is engaged in a study of young immigrants. In Norway, she has carried out research on the clients of prostitutes, homosexual men and HIV/AIDS, as well as an evaluation of cultural changes among injecting drug users, homosexual men and female prostitutes due to HIV/AIDS. In Mexico, she has carried out work on gender constructions among men who have sex with men. Her publications include *Mema's House, On Transvestites, Queens, and Machos* (University of Chicago Press, 1998).

Michel Rotily is Director of Studies at the Regional Health Watch (ORS-PACA), Marseilles, France. He is also an associate researcher in socio-behavioural epidemiology at the INSERM U379 where he conducts studies on HIV and viral hepatitis, especially in the context of prisons. He co-ordinates the European Network on HIV and Hepatitis in Prisons.

Theo Sandfort is a social psychologist in the Research School of Psychology and Health at Utrecht University and at The Netherlands Institute for Social Sexological Research (NISSO, Utrecht). The research he directs focuses on HIV-preventive behaviour in gay men as well as in the general population, and on small and large scale interventions aimed at promoting safer sex. Beyond HIV/AIDS-related issues he studies aspects of gay and lesbian lives, including coming-out processes, lifestyles, rela-tionships and discrimination. He is editor of *The Dutch Response to HIV: Pragmatism and Consensus* (UCL Press, 1998) and co-editor of *Sexual Behaviour and HIV/AIDS in Europe: Comparisons of National Surveys* (UCL Press, 1998).

Yves Souteyrand is a health economist at INSERM (the French National

Institute for Health and Medical Research). He is currently Chief of the Office of Public Health and Socio-Behavioural Research at the National Agency for AIDS Research (ANRS). He organised the 2nd European Conference on the Methods and Results of Social and Behavioural Research on AIDS in Paris (January 1998) and is a co-editor of the ANRS series entitled *Sciences Sociales et Sida*. He is currently involved in an assessment of the UNAIDS Drug Access Initiative in developing countries.

Bruno Spire is a virologist who recently joined the INSERM Research Unit on Social Sciences Applied to Medical Innovation in Marseilles. He has been a member of *AIDES*, a community organisation of people affected or infected by HIV, since 1988, where he developed training programmes on compliance for health care workers and HIV patients.

Monika Steffen is a researcher in the French National Centre for Scientific Research (CNRS) and is an affiliate of the Institute of Political Studies at the University of Grenoble. Her work focuses on health policies, including European comparisons. She has edited (with B. Jobert) *Les Politiques de la santé en France et en Allemagne* (Espace Social Européen, Observatoire des Politiques Sociales et Européennes, Paris, 1994) and is the author of *The Fight against AIDS. A Public Policy Comparison: France, Great Britain, Germany, Italy* (Presses Universitaires de Grenoble, 1996). Her most recent publications concern the management of the HIV/blood crisis in France.

Chryssa Tselepi is a sociologist of health. For the last ten years, she has worked as a researcher in the Department of Sociology at the National School of Public Health in Athens, Greece. Her interests are in the methodological issues in social research, the sociological dimensions of health and illness, as well as on the implementation of health education programmes on schools.

Biliana Vassileva is a programme assistant at the UNAIDS office in Sofia. One focus of her work is qualitative research on the behaviour of vulnerable groups as a basis for the development of STD/HIV/AIDS prevention activities in Bulgaria.

Sam Walters is a senior lecturer in paediatric infectious disease at Imperial College School of Medicine, St Mary's Campus. He trained in paediatrics at Great Ormond Street Hospital and spent five years working as a paediatrician in Papua New Guinea. Since 1990 he has been primarily involved in providing care to children with HIV infection. He was a founder member of the Multi-disciplinary Paediatric HIV Team at St Mary's which has pioneered the development of family care for HIV infection.

Caren Weilandt is a psychologist and psychotherapist who has worked for the Scientific Institute of the German Medical Association (WIAD) since

1988. She is Co-ordinator of the WHO Collaborative Centre for Migration and Mental Health and Head of the WIAD Department of Migration and International Health Research. Since 1988, she has been involved in several studies on HIV prevention. Earlier research includes work on coping and psychoneuroimmunologic factors in HIV infection.

Jeffrey J. Weiss is a clinical psychologist who has been involved in HIV mental health treatment and research since 1988. He is the project leader of a randomised clinical trial to examine the effects of group psychotherapy on psychological, clinical and immunological outcomes in HIV-positive gay men at the Helen Dowling Institute for Biopsychosocial Medicine in Rotterdam, The Netherlands.

Acknowledgements

The articles published in this book were presented at the 2nd European Conference on the Methods and Results of Social and Behavioural Research on AIDS (New Challenges for Social and Behavioural Science), organised by the National Agency on AIDS Research (ANRS), in Paris in January 1998. ANRS also provided financial support for the preparation and distribution of this book, especially in Central and Eastern European countries. The editors would like to thank the European Commission (DGV), UNAIDS, UNESCO and the French Ministries of Health and Culture for their financial support for the Conference. The editors would also like to express their thanks to Helen Thomas (London) and Névada Mendes (Paris) for their kind assistance in preparing the manuscript for publication.

Introduction

Jean-Paul Moatti, Yves Souteyrand, Annick Prieur, Theo Sandfort, Peter Aggleton

The epidemiological profile of HIV infection in Europe has changed dramatically in the course of the last few years. For the first time since the beginning of the epidemic, and in three consecutive years between 1996 and 1998, the incidence of new AIDS cases decreased in Western Europe. This positive trend is associated with progress in prevention, most especially with respect to sexual transmission and transmission through injecting drug use. But it is also related to recent advances in our understanding of the natural history of HIV disease and, above all, the diagnostic and therapeutic means available for treating infection. Quantitative viral load measurement has offered a new and powerful biological marker for prognosis and for monitoring the impact of treatment. Furthermore, with the advent of highly active antiretroviral therapy (HAART), the course of HIV infection has been greatly modified. This more aggressive therapy has shown clear success in bringing about substantial and sustained suppression of HIV viral replication and in reducing the incidence of opportunistic disease among HIV-infected individuals in short-term studies at least. It has also provided a rationale for the earlier initiation of antiretroviral treatment.

However, these therapeutic advances are not the 'magic bullets' that can solve all the questions raised by the AIDS epidemic. In spite of medical progress, HIV is still spreading rapidly among marginalised and socially deprived groups in the richer Western European countries. A dramatic growth in the epidemic can also be observed in the Eastern part of Europe where higher rates of HIV infection seem to be part of the price to be paid for the liberalisation that has accompanied the end of the communist era.

Such clinical changes are creating new space for dialogue between social scientists, biomedical scientists, public health authorities and community organisations in the field of AIDS. However, interdisciplinary debate is not restricted to controversial issues associated with geographical and social inequities of access to therapy. It also links to divergent interpretations about the intrinsic nature of this advance itself, as well as to its sometimes negative consequences. Major uncertainties remain about the long-term consequences of currently available antiretroviral regimens and their impact on prevention, care and other features of the epidemic. The fact that prevention as well as treatment guidelines differ substantially between European countries, and sometimes within each country, is a clear indicator of how these uncertainties affect AIDS public policy and above all the lives of people with HIV/AIDS.

The contributions in this volume represent some of the most important attempts by European social scientists to engage with recent changes in the epidemic. Some revisit issues already extensively studied by previous research but whose context has been significantly modified over the course of the last three years. Others offer insight into new areas of enquiry so as to address new challenges raised by these changes. All the papers in this book were initially presented at the 2nd European Conference on the Methods and Results of Social and Behavioural Research on AIDS (New Challenges for Social and Behavioural Science) organised in January 1998, in Paris, by the French Agency for AIDS Research (ANRS) with the support of the European Commission, UNAIDS, UNESCO and the French Ministries of Health and of Culture. This conference was the second of its kind, and more than 500 social scientists came together from all over Europe to identify and debate new challenges that social and behavioural research on HIV and AIDS has to face.

While much earlier HIV and AIDS-related social and behavioural research focused on issues related to prevention and collective and individual behaviour change, recent developments have made studies of the impact of new treatments on HIV care, and of the experience of people living with HIV, a priority. Innovative studies linked to the themes of 'Living with HIV and therapeutic advances' are therefore presented in the first part of the book.

Qualitative studies involving in-depth interviews with HIV-infected individuals in Greece (Chryssa Tselepi *et al.*) and the parents of HIV-infected children in the UK (Mary Boulton *et al.*) provide insight into the behavioural strategies used by affected persons to cope with their disease and the responses and reactions of those who are close to them. Both chapters show how stigma and discrimination distinguish the experience of HIV infection from that of most other diseases and create specific difficulties for the disclosure of HIV serostatus. Cultural beliefs and expectations can add to these difficulties in the case of migrant families such as those interviewed by Boulton and her colleagues: parents often choose to conceal the HIV serostatus of their child, even from their closest relatives, and are therefore deprived of an important source of social support. Both chapters offer strong arguments against any attempt to breach the confidentiality of medical records and an HIV/AIDS diagnosis despite public health concerns over transmissibility. These chapters also highlight the continuing psychological burden associated with HIV and AIDS.

This last point is at the core of José Catalán's contribution which reviews the now substantial literature on the impact of the disease on the psychological status and well-being of people living with HIV. Catalán also discusses recent controversial evidence about the impact of psychological state on the natural history of HIV disease. Although current therapeutic advances clearly improve the quality of life of a significant number of HIV-infected individuals, they also raise new difficulties to the extent that they confront such persons with unresolved problems in the field of life goals, affective relationships and work. As Catalán points out, therapeutic progress may even have a negative effect on HIV-infected persons' psychological status by inducing feelings of guilt and self-blame if they are not able to remain healthy or improve their virological and immunological status.

In such a context, the issue of adherence (compliance) to antiretroviral treatment has become one where social scientific research may have a special role to play. As was earlier the case with respect to the promotion of condom use and protective behaviours, social scientific enquiry is now asked to help identify individual barriers to 'good' adherence and to design psychological and social interventions to improve patients' acceptance of prescribed regimens.

Jeffrey Weiss presents the results of one of the first in-depth socio-behavioural studies at the European and international level of the attitudinal determinants of adherence to protease inhibitor combination therapies. Jean-Paul Moatti and Bruno Spire review the existing evidence concerning access and adherence to HAART, including reports from work in progress in France among cohorts of HIV-infected patients. This latter review is carried out in reference to earlier research on attitudes and behaviours linked to medical treatments for disease. Both chapters are critical of the conventional biomedical approach which tends to consider any departure from complete compliance to physicians' prescriptions as an indicator of 'non-rational' behaviour. On the contrary, they show how apparently paradoxical outcomes (such as Weiss's finding that the less patients are optimistic about the effectiveness of HAART, the more likely they are to be adherent) may be understood as logical consequences of past and present experiences. Both contributions emphasise the value of social scientific research in which the subjective experience of illness is a central concern.

Fearing possible diffusion of untreatable drug-resistant HIV strains, some public health experts have advocated withholding treatment from certain groups such as injecting drug users or homeless people where the risks of patients' non-adherence are anticipated to be high. By demonstrating that adherence is not a black or white phenomenon, and that no *a priori* criteria can readily distinguish between non-adherent patients and others, recent social scientific research directly opposes these attempts to legitimate new coercive policies in the field of HIV care. Instead, it encourages approaches based on the active participation of HIV-positive persons in their own treatment.

Since the 1970s, research on the psychology and sociology of illness has drawn attention to the chronic illnesses that have become the major health problems in European societies, and to the difficulties the ill have to cope with as they manage their everyday activities. The extent to which current therapeutic advances are transforming HIV infection into such a chronic illness, and to which the analytic frameworks used for the long-term management of chronic pathologies can be applied to HIV/AIDS, remains a matter of debate and requires further research.

The second part of the book entitled 'New perspectives on sexuality' focuses on the sexual risk of HIV transmission. The AIDS epidemic has provided an extraordinary opportunity to develop our understanding of human sexuality and its cultural and social determinants. Large-scale quantitative data on sexual behaviour have become available for the general population in many European countries,[1] including adolescents and young adults at an early stage in their sexual life. Hugues Lagrange and Brigitte Lhomond report in this part on the results of the French national survey of sexual behaviour among 15 to 18 year-olds. In-depth quantitative and qualitative data have been collected about sexual behaviours that are often denied or socially stigmatised. Michael Bochow reports on comparative data on homosexual men in Germany, France and the UK.

Both reports confirm what has been already established by a huge body of AIDS-related social research, namely that HIV prevention efforts have been effective in promoting condom use among some of the groups most exposed to the risk of sexual transmission. But both chapters, as well as other contributions in this part, stress persistent and even growing difficulties for HIV prevention. A first difficulty concerns the long-term sustainability of HIV preventive behaviour. While the young French people studied by Lagrange and Lhomond tend to use condoms at first sexual intercourse and at the start of a new sexual partnership, they tend also to abandon their use as soon as they consider that a relationship has become stable. François Delor's chapter deals with the often neglected issue of HIV-related sexual risk behaviours among individuals who are already HIV infected. This research offers a good example of how qualitative approaches can highlight issues and problems unlikely to be captured by quantitative questionnaires. Delor's research shows that in serodiscordant couples, not using a condom may be one way of maintaining a steady relationship by symbolising love and affection, while not using a condom with an occasional partner may be seen as a way of avoiding disclosure.

The AIDS epidemic does not seem to have brought about major changes in the secular trends detectable in the evolution of Western European sexuality. As shown by Lagrange and Lhomond, age at first sexual intercourse in France has not been changed by the introduction of HIV/AIDS prevention programmes. On the contrary, social changes exogenous to the epidemic itself more likely affect sexual behaviour and impede HIV prevention efforts.

The contributions of researchers from Eastern Europe, from Bulgaria by Biliana Vassileva and Milena Komarova and from Russia by Valeriy Chervyakov and Igor Kon, are some of the most original features of this volume. They show how the rapid transition from totalitarian to pluralistic societies and the sudden freedom of access to international information networks have been associated with a rapid increase in sexual activity among young people. These political and societal changes create a difficult context for HIV prevention. Traditional intergenerational conflict between young people and their parents is exacerbated by the persistence of values, norms and rules that prevailed in the former political system. Preventive measures, such as the introduction of sex education in schools, become occasions for ideological conflict between conservative forces and proponents of liberalisation. These Eastern European contributions also demonstrate how AIDS research contributes to the current revived interest in social scientific research in countries where ideological manipulations have dominated the field for more than fifty years.

The spread of HIV in population groups already subject to socio-economic inequality raises a third major difficulty for HIV sexual prevention. Lagrange and Lhomond show that condom use remains lower among apprenticeship trainees than among regular high school students. Bochow shows that gay men from the lower social classes, unlike their middle-class counterparts, often need to leave their hometown to live out their homosexuality. However, the former have less capacity to adapt to their chosen new social environment and are more likely to be exposed to HIV-related sexual risk. Consequently, HIV prevalence is higher among homosexual men of low socio-economic status. These contributions, as well as those on drug users in the following part, illustrate strongly how HIV prevention cannot escape the effects of the social inequality that structures advanced industrial societies.

As a consequence of current therapeutic advances, more and more HIV-infected persons are living longer and better lives. This raises a fourth difficulty for HIV prevention. The extent to which advances in HIV-related care may promote false reassurance and denial among both HIV-positive and HIV-negative sectors of the population needs urgently to be assessed by social scientific research.

The third part of the book is devoted to the issue of drug use: user and policy perspectives. It is a well-established fact that HIV-infected injecting drug users tend to have poorer access to medical care, and especially to antiretroviral treatment, than other groups, even in European countries where free or low-cost public sector care is available. It is also clear that drug users are especially vulnerable to the cumulative effects of various sources of inequality. This vulnerability is of course exacerbated by the illegal character of drug use in all European countries which exposes active drug users to a high risk of imprisonment. The potential contribution of the prison environment to the spread of HIV infection has long been underestimated. Michel Rotily and Caren Weilandt's chapter presents findings from multi-centre surveys carried out by the European Network for HIV/Hepatitis Prevention in Prisons supported by the European Commission. These surveys are the first co-ordinated attempt at European level to measure the prevalence of HIV and associated infectious diseases and related risk behaviour during incarceration.

Epidemiological approaches, while clearly important for understanding the extent of HIV transmission among drug users, are not sufficient when it comes to explaining the why of human behaviour, and understanding how HIV-related risk behaviour is influenced by social context. Only social scientific research can provide the means of minimising biases due to social desirability when illegal and highly stigmatised behaviours are investigated.[2] Surveys carried out independently of prison administration and staff, such as those described by Rotily and Weilandt, are able to provide an objective approximation of the frequency of heterosexual and homosexual intercourse and drug injection inside prisons. Semi-structured interviews with illicit drug users in various areas of Scotland reported in Joanne Neale's chapter, provide a unique opportunity for understanding the real problems encountered by users when they enter into drug abuse treatment or when they try to obtain sterile injecting equipment.

Throughout Europe, the AIDS epidemic has brought about major changes in public policy with respect to drug use. Social scientific research has actively contributed to the assessment, and consequently the political legitimisation, of innovative harm reduction policies. France Lert's case study of the history of French drug policy tries to identify the reasons for that country's long delay in implementing harm reduction policies. Structural factors such as the dominance of psychoanalysis within the drug treatment community, and the inadequacy of the French tradition of social welfare, played a major role in the HIV/AIDS catastrophe among French injecting drug users until 1994. Although such policies remain highly controversial in many countries, the European Network findings presented by Rotily and Weilandt provide strong evidence to support the introduction of harm reduction programmes in prison including needle exchange, drug maintenance treatment, and the availability of bleach and condoms.

As described by Lert, interventions targeted towards drug users have been substantially strengthened and renewed in recent years by attempts to increase community approach and peer participation. While evaluation of drug service provision is nearly always limited to the views of providers, policy makers and sometimes the general population, Neale's chapter demonstrates that drug users' views should be taken into account when evaluating services in order to ensure a better fit with their need. Dominique Malatesta and colleagues report on research about the introduction of harm reduction facilities for IDUs in twelve Swiss cities and the conflicts such introduction may induce because of the unavoidable tensions between public health and public safety goals. Borrowing the concept of 'urban compatibility' from the sociology of urban studies, and combining surveys among the actors involved and the population in the neighbourhood of the facilities, the authors highlight various forms of mediation to increase social and political acceptability of these services.

In the future, cross-country comparative policy research will determine whether the AIDS epidemic and related changes in drug policy have brought about major changes in the characteristics of European welfare states by giving new emphasis to principles of 'social exclusion'. The hypothesis discussed in Lert's chapter is that future public health programmes will have to deal with more problems linked to social exclusion, and will need to broaden their scope so as to enhance the social integration of the most vulnerable segments of society.

The last part of this volume, 'Accounting for the epidemic', deals with analyses of recent trends in European HIV/AIDS public policy and theoretical debates among social scientists in relation to the evolution of the epidemic itself. The first two contributions tackle debates about AIDS public policy that were central during the Paris conference, as well as in many other arenas. In all Western European countries, the AIDS epidemic has caused a shift away from traditional public health policies for controlling infectious diseases based on compulsory measures and rigid interventions. Political scientists have characterised as 'AIDS exceptionalism' the profound innovations in the fields of prevention, patient care, health policy based on non-coercion and respect for privacy and human rights that have been associated with the epidemic.

Monika Steffen's chapter about the patterns of AIDS policies in Europe raises the possibility that an end to this exceptionalism may be nigh, with a normalisation of policy following therapeutic advances and the slowing of the AIDS epidemic in the more developed countries. She discusses how current changes in the epidemiological and political context call into question some of the innovations previously achieved through AIDS policies, while other changes are integrated into the agendas, priorities and networks of existing health care and welfare policies.

On the basis of the UK experience, where routine offering of HIV testing has been limited to pregnant women in high-prevalence geographical areas or those belonging to behaviourally vulnerable minorities, Christine McGarrigle and Noel Gill discuss the potentially deleterious effects for HIV prevention of normalising HIV testing within medical practice. Their provocative contribution highlights how the normalisation of HIV testing may be associated with a diminished role of preventive counselling and with reduced targeted efforts to reach those at higher risk of HIV infection.

More conceptual clarification is needed in current passionate debates about the normalisation of AIDS policy. The tendency to integrate HIV/AIDS programmes into the normal course of politics, administration, prevention and health care is an obvious ongoing trend in most European countries that needs to be documented by social scientific research. But the relevance and adequacy of these policy choices for the fight against AIDS and for solutions to other public health problems need critically to be assessed. Because of remaining uncertainties about the consequences of this process, it is not surprising that conflicts of interpretation still exist between social scientists and, more generally, between all actors in the AIDS field. The comparative effectiveness of programmes specifically targeted for HIV prevention and care, versus integration in the existing prevention and health care systems, must be established on the basis of rigorous assessment rather than on ideological *a priori* judgements.

Since the earlier days of the AIDS epidemic, traditional tensions between quantitative and qualitative research methods, between individualistic and holistic models, as well as between various disciplines, have given fuel for controversy as to the proper field of the social and behavioural sciences. Inevitably, the authors in this volume adopt different, and sometimes contradictory, stances with respect to these important debates.

Geneviève Paicheler's chapter presents a synthesis of the objections often raised against individualistic models of health and risk behaviour. Linked to the world-wide use of Knowledge, Attitudes, Beliefs and Practices (KABP) surveys, models of this kind, especially the Health Belief Model (HBM) and its various derivatives, have been predominant in the international social sciences literature. They still tend to dominate the growing field of research concerning patients' attitudes and behaviours with respect to HIV-related treatment and care. Deeply rooted in the holistic tradition of French social sciences, Paicheler makes a plea for the development of alternative risk management models based on phenomenological approaches. She argues that such dynamic and non-linear models are more able to capture both the impact of perceptive and cognitive elements on risk behaviour and vice versa. Other social scientists, including some represented in this same volume, may not agree with this theoretical perspective. The latter may not consider that any attempt to identify the determinants of behaviour through the statistical aggregation of individual self-reports and/or observed behaviours is doomed to oversimplification and exaggeratedly narrow conceptions of rationality. They may even argue that holistic approaches also encounter major difficulties in analysing the mechanisms by which the social environment influences individual behaviour and are not very fruitful in designing intervention strategies.

To a large extent, these differences of approach and interpretation between social scientists reflect the complexity of the changes in the AIDS epidemic and the difficulty of accounting for them. Beyond these tensions, the Paris conference as well as the contributions in this volume reveal a common interest in methodological developments, especially those whose aim it is to better understand individual and group interaction. A growing body of AIDS research has now been devoted to various forms of social network analysis. Mirjam Kretzschmar's chapter offers an extensive review of research using network analysis to build models of HIV transmission. It illustrates how such modelling can provide important insights for prevention.

Social and behavioural research has always had to confront difficult trade-offs between the urgent need to provide answers and the necessity for rigorous methodologies that often necessitate quite long time horizons for collecting and analysing data. The different chapters in this volume show that, contrary to popular belief, biomedical progress and the associated new challenges it creates for HIV/AIDS prevention and care, increase rather than diminish the need for social scientists to be actively involved in AIDS research.

Notes

1   See Hubert, M., Bajos, N. and Sandfort, T. (1998) *Sexual Behaviour and HIV/AIDS in Europe. Comparisons of National Surveys*, London: UCL Press.
2   See Stimson, G., Des Jarlais, D.C. and Ball, A. (1998) *Drug Injecting and HIV Infection*, London: UCL Press.

Part I

Living with HIV and therapeutic advances

1 Coping with a chronic illness

The experience of families of HIV-infected children

Mary Boulton, Sam Walters, David Miller and Eddy Beck

In the UK, as in other parts of Europe, the slow but steady increase in the number of children infected with HIV is beginning to pose new challenges for health care providers. The development of appropriate and effective services for children will require a sensitive understanding of the effect of HIV infection on their daily lives and of the needs to which this gives rise. As HIV infection affects not only the infected child but also those with whom he or she has close ties, understanding the impact of HIV infection on the family as a whole will also be important (Gibb *et al.*, 1991; Barratt and Victor, 1994).

Until recently, however, very little attention had been given to the experience of families with HIV-infected children (Bor *et al.*, 1993; Cohen, 1994; Sherwen and Boland, 1994). Most research on the psychosocial aspects of HIV and AIDS has concentrated on individuals, and what little work has looked at families has largely explored the impact of adults with HIV infection (Cates *et al.*, 1990; Rait, 1991). As more women of child-bearing age have become infected, interest has begun to turn to young families, but most publications have been concerned with clinical features of the condition (Van Dyke, 1991), the development of services (Mok, 1993) or the needs of children affected (but not infected) by HIV (Honigsbaum, 1994). Much of this literature also relates to a US context.

The study reported in this chapter was undertaken to provide a more detailed account, in an English context, of the concerns important to families caring for an HIV-infected child and of the ways they coped with them. A secondary aim was to consider the differences in experience amongst families according to their ethnic background, parental HIV status and family structure. As the intention was to explore these issues from the perspective of the families themselves, the research was designed as a small-scale qualitative study.

Sample and methods

The study was carried out in collaboration with a paediatric clinic in a London teaching hospital which is a regional centre for the care of children with HIV infection. Open-ended, loosely structured interviews were carried out with the parents or guardians of twenty-two HIV-infected children who were patients at the clinic (73 per cent of those eligible for inclusion in the study). Topics discussed included day-to-day coping; relationships within the family and household; relationships with schools, friends and community; managing symptoms and promoting health; medicines and treatments; and concerns for the future. Where the mother or grandmother was looking after the child, interviews were generally carried out with her. However, in one two-parent family, interviews were conducted with the father, and in another, both father and mother took part in interviews.

A total of sixty-three interviews were carried out between September 1994 and December 1995 with the twenty-two families. Where possible, these were tape-recorded and later transcribed; detailed field notes were kept where tape-recording was not possible. Transcripts and field notes were analysed according to the methods of inductive analysis used in qualitative research.

Characteristics of the sample

The HIV-infected children in the study were predominantly female (thirteen girls, nine boys), and very young: half were of pre-school age (eleven under 5 years old, including four children under 3 years old); eight children were 5 or 6 years old, two children were 7 or 8 years old and only one child was over 8 (she was 12 years old). All but one had been infected through vertical transmission; one child had been adopted from a Romanian orphanage and the route of transmission was unknown. Eleven (50 per cent) had been diagnosed as symptomatic non-AIDS, eleven (50 per cent) as AIDS.

The characteristics of the families are given in Table 1.1. For the sake of simplicity, fathers, mothers, stepmothers, adoptive mothers, adoptive fathers and grandmothers will all be referred to as 'parents'. In almost three-quarters of the families, at least one parent in the household was also HIV infected; in at least six others, a parent had already died from an AIDS-related illness. In reporting the parents' accounts, all names have been changed to maintain confidentiality.

Findings: the concerns of families of HIV-infected children

In talking about their families and describing their lives, parents raised a wide range of issues and concerns. Many of these were not directly related to HIV infection but reflected the problems commonly experienced by immigrants, minority ethnic groups and the more disadvantaged sectors of society. Their concerns specifically in relation to caring for an HIV-infected child were also diverse but could be grouped into three main areas, as in the following subsections.

Table 1.1 Characteristics of the families

Family composition

Single parent	Number	Two parents	Number
Single mother	7	Natural parents	8
Single father	2	Stepmother and father	2
Single grandmother	2	Adoptive parents	1
Total	11	Total	11

Ethnic background of parents

Nationality	Single parents	Two parents	Total	(%)
British/Irish	2	2	4	(18)
Other European	1	0	1	(5)
African	6	7	13	(59)
Mixed	2*	2	4	(18)

HIV status of parents

HIV status	Single parents	Two parents	Total (%)
Positive	8	3	11 (50)
Mixed	–	5	5 (23)
Negative	3	2	5 (23)
Not tested	0	1	1 (5)

* Includes one British father and one African mother.

Health and physical well-being

A fundamental concern to all the families in the study was the physical health of their children. All the children had progressed to the later stages of HIV disease and most had at some time been seriously ill. Their parents, in turn, were very sensitive to their current health status and very anxious about their underlying HIV infection. All made positive efforts to try to promote their children's health, drawing on one or more of three main strategies.

Adjusting prescribed drugs

The first strategy entailed experimenting with the way they gave their children the antibacterial and antiretroviral drugs prescribed by the hospital paediatricians, to find the regimen best suited to them. Parents saw drugs such as AZT and the antibiotic Septrin as very powerful and pointed out that this meant that they could do their children considerable harm as well as good. For this reason, some refused to give them to their children altogether. The majority, however, accepted the value of drugs but altered the way they administered them. The following father is typical of the way many parents in the sample had observed the effects of the drugs, adjusted the regimen and evaluated the results:

> She is really only on Septrin at the moment. She was on AZT but she had problems with it and we dropped it. She has been more healthier since. She has put on weight and she did have quite bad diarrhoea with it as well and that has stopped now. So it obviously didn't agree with her.
>
> (Derek Forsyth, father of Louise, aged 5)

What seemed important to this and other parents was the sense of at least partial control they gained by adjusting their children's treatment. While such adjustments were generally discussed with the doctors in the hospital, this was not always the case.

Complementary or alternative medicine

Another way in which parents tried to gain a sense of control over their child's health was to look outside orthodox medicine to complementary or alternative medicine. The most popular form of alternative therapy appeared to be herbal medicines, often described as traditional medicine or Chinese herbs. Its use was described at length by four parents, all from Africa, but was mentioned by other parents and is likely to have been widespread amongst the families. Complementary therapies were popular amongst parents because they gave them the hope of a 'cure' that orthodox medicine did not offer:

> I chose this because when he had PCP they told me 'We will try to keep him well but the truth is, because he has had PCP, he can become ill again soon', plus, 'It may happen in the next few months'. I believed them and I accepted that when I first heard that. But I am not going to sit down and wait. I will do everything I can. Because to them he is just another patient, and if he dies they say, well we told you. But the homeopathy gives you hope.
>
> (Deborah Storey, mother of Geoff, aged 1)

While never completely giving up on orthodox medicine, a number of families turned to complementary therapies to enhance its effects, to give their children a 'break' from powerful drugs or to establish a 'second front' in the battle with HIV disease.

Faith and prayer

Finally, some families turned to faith and prayer in their efforts to find a cure for their own and their child's illness. Several families mentioned their Church and the support they received from being part of a community of believers. However, two mothers looked to their religious beliefs as their primary source of hope and help. Both were originally from Africa and both were themselves HIV positive:

> I just trust in the Lord. Ever since I got saved, I don't feel it any more. I am not scared now, I am just looking to God. I have heard of some people in my country and they have prayed and prayed and prayed and they became negative. So I am praying to God. I'm just studying the words in the Bible because all the prophesies are in the Bible, so just with my Bible I pray. I am now waiting for God. So I am not scared any more. Actually, there is an improvement now, because I used to be so tired, weak, depressed but now I do everything. I don't even get ill at all.
> (Diana Gardner, mother of Margaret, aged 6)

As with alternative therapies, looking to God did not mean giving up on medical treatment but rather enhancing and explaining its effectiveness:

> It is God that is keeping him well. If the AZT is to work, it is God that will make it work. Nothing else.
> (Daphne West, mother of Edmund, aged 1)

Stigma and 'leading a normal life'

Alongside the families' concern for their children's physical health was their concern for their quality of life more generally. This was usually described in terms of leading a 'normal life' with regard to childhood activities and social relationships and being treated the same as other children.

The main threat to a normal life that parents were concerned about derived from the stigma of HIV infection. None of the families had themselves been persecuted because of their HIV infection, although one described the way another family had been forced to leave the neighbourhood when their child's HIV status had become known. Many others described instances of more limited social exclusion or ostracism and virtually all anticipated a response of fear, hostility and discrimination against their children if the diagnosis were more widely known. For this reason, parents wanted to maintain tight control over information about their child's condition and were very judicious about disclosing it to others.

Disclosure to outside institutions

With regard to outside institutions, parents wanted as few people as possible to know about the diagnosis. They accepted that those directly involved in the medical care of their children would have to be told, but were reluctant to tell anyone else, even their general practitioner. Their preference for secrecy was even more clear in relation to schools, where parents were concerned that disclosure would mean that their child would be treated differently. Of the eighteen families who sent their children to school or nursery, only three had informed it of the diagnosis and in two cases this was because they had been required to do so in order to secure a place. Mothers who were themselves HIV infected were particularly reluctant to inform the school, since disclosing the child's diagnosis also revealed their own HIV infection and their role in infecting their child. The distress this caused is evident in the comments of the following mother:

> How can I go to that school and sit in front of them, the Head Mistress, and start telling them 'I am like this, I am like that?' And what are they going to think of Susan? They won't like her at the school probably, or maybe the Head Mistress will keep watch on the child and say she mustn't mix with other children.
>
> (Agnes Oates, mother of Susan, aged 3)

In the longer term, concealing the diagnosis from the school could become difficult as long bouts of illness, frequent hospital visits or the need for regular medication attracted attention. Parents worried about these potential clues to their child's condition and took great pains to provide acceptable explanations for anything that might arouse suspicion:

> I told them that she had quite bad lungs because she had got problems with her lungs. So I wasn't actually telling a lie, although that was not telling the complete truth.
>
> (Jennifer Nichols, mother of Sarah, aged 4)

Such accounts appeared to provide successful 'cover' for indications of the children's illness and none of the parents had yet been forced to disclose the diagnosis to the school.

Disclosure to friends and family

With regard to friends and family, the situation was more complex. Parents were anxious that their children be accepted by those close to them and for this reason tended to favour a policy of non-disclosure. However, concealing the diagnosis also entailed many drawbacks including a sense of isolation, the strains of keeping a secret and the loss of practical help. The benefits of concealment thus had to be weighed constantly against the benefits of disclosure. The particular balances reached by families gave rise to different approaches to disclosure.

Families of African origin overwhelmingly favoured a strategy of secrecy, concealing their diagnosis from virtually everyone else, including their close family and friends. Typical of the families in this group is the following mother who had told none of her relations, not even her sister or sister-in-law who lived with her family:

> The other people in this house don't know. No one knows except me and my husband. People talk too much. I have seen this with other relatives and friends, the way that they are treated ... I have a sister, same dad, same mum. She lives across the road. She is positive. When she was in Africa, she lost her husband with AIDS ... My sister doesn't know about us. None of my family know. None of my husband's family know.
>
> (Naomi Bond, mother of Grace, aged 6)

Underpinning this imperative to conceal the diagnosis was a strong sense of their own shame about being infected, guilt at infecting their child and a fear that others would blame them if they knew. This sense of shame was felt most acutely – though not exclusively – in relation to the parents' own family members. Concealing the diagnosis and keeping it secret enabled parents to escape the censure of their extended family and to be accepted as 'normal' and 'respectable'. It also saved others from worry and distress. However, the burden of the diagnosis and the difficulties surrounding it were too much for most parents to bear on their own and many had eventually confided in at least one other person.

In contrast to the families of African background, European families tended to adopt a strategy of selective disclosure. While they were anxious to keep the diagnosis secret from people in general, they had shown only little hesitation in telling their closest relatives. The following grandmother was typical in the clear distinction she made between her immediate family and others:

> I keep it to myself. I don't want everyone knowing, do I? No one knows around here, I don't want them to know. You know what people are like ... So no one knows really. They might guess, I don't know, but I haven't told anyone. All my family knows and all her [the child's mother] brothers and sisters. They all help me, they all do. They all love her. Look at all the toys they have brought her. So really she gets it all.
>
> (Victoria Watkins, grandmother of Ruth, aged 7)

As this quote implies, underlying their willingness to disclose the diagnosis was an assumption that their own immediate family would accept and stand by them and provide the kind of practical help and support they needed. All the families who had disclosed their diagnosis to other relatives felt they had derived great benefit from doing so, in terms of both emotional support and practical help. None had reported problems with rejection or censure by their families, although this may reflect their own careful judgement as to whom to tell as much as the inherent compassion of their relatives.

Not all couples agreed on how information should be managed and the diagnosis concealed or disclosed to others. This was the case for three couples including both those of mixed ethnic background. In these families, differences in attitudes to disclosure had become the focus of considerable tension and conflict. In two families, the parents eventually separated.

Facing the future

The last theme which emerged from the parents' accounts was their concern about death and dying and their anxieties about the future. A third of the families had already endured the pain and disruption of a parental death from an AIDS-related illness. Of the remaining families, all but two had this prospect still in store. For all the families in the study, the future threatened separation and loss although the nature of these losses varied according to the family's circumstances.

HIV-infected parents

Concern about the future was most acute amongst families where the parents were themselves HIV infected and particularly where they were also single parents. In these families, parents had to face not only the prospect of their own death but also the realisation that this would leave their children as orphans. Their anguish was intensified by feelings of guilt and regret at not being there to care for their children when they were dying:

> I think about dying itself, I think I am beginning to come to terms with it and accept that before long I will have to die. But I feel sad for my son because, like maybe he will live longer than me, but I won't be there to look after him. And the way I think is, who is going to have the patience to look after him? I know other people can look after him but sometimes I can't help, maybe it is selfish, but I still can't help thinking that no one else can look after him and give him that love the way that I try to give him.
>
> (Alice Elliott, mother of Michael, aged 6)

Feelings of guilt were no less evident in relation to uninfected children. Where there were other children who would be orphaned by AIDS, parents worried about what would happen to them as well:

I used to be so scared. I used to think that I was going to die and leave Mary [her older daughter] behind. But I wasn't so sorry about Margaret because I knew she was going to die too. I was worried about Mary because she would be on her own.

(Diana Gardner, mother of Margaret, aged 6)

Because of the obvious vulnerability of their children, single HIV-infected parents were under great pressure to make contingency plans for the care of their children and, at the suggestion of their social workers, three of the seven single HIV-infected parents had discussed fostering arrangements for respite or emergency care. However, planning permanent placements for their children was extremely distressing and none of the parents had been able to face it directly. All wanted their children to stay with their family and be looked after by relatives, and most had given some thought as to which of their relatives they would like to take them in. But none had tried to arrange this nor even raised the issue with their kin.

Couples discordant in HIV status

Where one parent in the family was not HIV infected, the child's future appeared more secure: the assumption was that, should the HIV-infected parent die, the child would continue to be cared for by the surviving parent. However, while this arrangement was seen as appropriate or even inevitable, it was not always seen as entirely desirable. Differences in HIV status between parents more often than not gave rise to feelings of guilt, anger and resentment within the family and these could be projected into the future. The following mother, for example, was worried and angry at the way she thought her children might come to regard her when she had gone:

The one thing that worries me is that if I did leave my kids, I know that his mother would come and live here and look after them. It really scares me ... Because she is going to take over control and probably move in. She would make them forget me and poison them against me ... I have a feeling that grandma will try and make them forget me. It is just the way she thinks about me. I just get the feeling that if I was going to die today, they are not going to be allowed to remember me.

(Patricia Lennon, mother of Jill, aged 4)

While she accepted the advantages for her children of staying with their father's family, she bridled at the injustice of the imagined scenario and grieved in anticipation at losing them twice over.

Parents not HIV infected

In five families, none of the parents were themselves HIV infected. In two, the children's mothers had died of AIDS-related illnesses and their unin-fected fathers had continued to look after them; in one of the families, the father had remarried. In a third family, both parents had died of AIDS-related illnesses and the child was living with her grandmother; in a fourth, the child's HIV-infected mother had left her with her grandmother and was no longer in touch with the family. The fifth was an English family who had adopted an orphaned Romanian child.

In none of these families was the long-term care of the children an issue. Instead, the stress these families faced was the eventual loss of their chil-dren. Parents found this very hard to accept and all clung to the hope that it might never happen. Since they were not themselves ill, there was little to remind them of the long-term prognosis for their child and it was often easier to overlook it:

> It's a very hard thing to come to terms with and accept. When she is keeping well, you can wipe it away. When something comes up, you have to relive it all again. One of the things about this is that she looks so well and has so much energy that you can't believe that there is some-thing there. It is easy to push it aside. Because you just think that it will never happen. Which the doctor says it might never happen. Because there are some people that are pure carriers and so far as they know, as yet they don't actually get ill and die. They have talked about those people from abroad who have had it for years and years and they have only just found out. We did think that perhaps she is one of them.
> (Jennifer Nichols, mother of Sarah, aged 4, adopted)

All of the parents in this category expressed an attitude of optimistic denial and all could point to evidence to support their hope that their children could be amongst the rare survivors or could live long enough for doctors to find a cure. While this view might prove to be unfounded, it was important to the families in helping them face the future and find the present mean-ingful and rewarding.

Discussion

As more women of child-bearing age become infected, HIV is developing into an illness of children and young families. This chapter has described the findings of one of a small number of studies which have begun to explore the nature of the experience of these families. In contrast to previous studies, a substantial proportion of the families recruited included individ-uals who had emigrated from East and sub-Saharan African countries where heterosexual transmission of HIV infection is common. Like previous studies, however, it is limited by a small sample size and a poorly developed theoretical framework within which to interpret the findings.

The areas of concern identified in the parents' accounts are broadly similar to the problems identified in other studies (Cohen *et al.*, 1995; Goldie *et al.*, 1994; Mellins and Ehrhardt, 1994; Melvin and Sherr, 1995), although distinctive features have also emerged. With regard to health-related concerns, the US literature has put a greater emphasis on the practical problems that parents face in managing their children's illness, dealing with in-patient admissions and orchestrating appointments with the competing agencies which provide health care to parents and children. At least one study has also pointed to tensions between parents and the providers of health and social care who may disregard their experience and treat parents in a demeaning fashion (Mellins and Ehrhardt, 1994). While practical problems such as these had featured in earlier research in London (Barratt and Victor, 1994), they were not frequently raised by families in this study. This may be because, in the majority of families, the children themselves were not acutely ill and did not require frequent attendance at health care facilities. It may also reflect differences in the health care systems in the USA and UK and in developments in services for families in London in particular, which have gone a long way towards addressing the problems they faced.

Stigma has been universally identified as a major concern to families and one which distinguishes the experience of paediatric HIV infection from that of any other disease of childhood. In both the USA and Europe, studies have shown that families fear rejection and discrimination because of their HIV infection and hence keep the diagnosis to themselves. What is distinctive about the findings of the present study is the attitude of families from an African background to disclosing the diagnosis to their closest relatives. The very high degree of stigma associated with HIV infection and the notions of shame within the extended family made it virtually impossible for parents to confide even in their own immediate family. This contrasts with the position of the majority of families reported in other studies who generally distinguish between 'family' and 'others' in disclosing their diagnosis (Cohen *et al.*, 1995; Goldie *et al.*, 1994; Mellins and Ehrhardt, 1994). These differences highlight the way culture shapes responses to illness and the unexpected variations that are found in different social groups. They also point to the importance of extending this kind of research to other population groups and examining the response of families in different social and cultural contexts.

Concerns about the future were more diverse amongst the study families, reflecting their varying circumstances with regard to HIV infection (and its consequences) amongst other members of the family. This is consistent with the findings of at least one US study which has compared the responses of 'natural' parents (who were generally infected themselves) and foster parents (who were generally unrelated to the children) (Cohen *et al.*, 1995). Natural parents were described as finding the future difficult to face, feeling isolated and alienated from others and as particularly concerned about not being present at the severe illness and death of their HIV-infected child. Similar feelings were described by parents in this study. However, instead of the optimistic denial and hopes for the future described by uninfected parents in the present study, Cohen and her colleagues described foster parents as appreciating the present and as feeling better prepared to deal with the eventual death of their HIV-infected child.

Finally, it is important to point out that the findings presented in this chapter derive from the accounts given by the parents in the family. No attempt was made to interview children nor to elicit their perspective on living with HIV infection, in part because of the very young age of the children in the study. The range of issues of concern to children may well differ from those of their parents, although in one study where the views of older children were sought, the issues they raised were at least consistent with those of their parents (Mellins and Ehrhardt, 1994). While perspectives may differ, for all members of the family, living with HIV infection is a difficult and demanding experience.

Acknowledgements

The study was carried out as part of a study funded by a grant from the Department of Health. We would like to thank Katy Pepper for recruiting families and for carrying out and transcribing the interviews.

References

Barratt, G. and Victor, C. (1994) ' "We just want to be a normal family ...". Paediatric HIV/AIDS services at an inner London teaching hospital', *AIDS Care* 6: 423–430.

Bor, R., Miller, R. and Goldman, E. (1993) 'HIV/AIDS and the family: a review of research in the first decade', *Journal of Family Therapy* 15: 187–204.

Cates, J., Graham, L., Boeglin, D. and Tiekler, S. (1990) 'The effect of AIDS on the family system', *Families in Society* April: 195–201.

Cohen, R. (1994) 'Research on families and pediatric human immunodeficiency virus disease: a review and needed directions', *Developmental and Behavioral Pediatrics* 15: S34–S42.

Cohen, F., Nehring, W., Malm, K. and Harris, D. (1995) 'Family experiences when a child is HIV positive: reports of natural and foster parents', *Pediatric Nursing* 21: 248–254.

Gibb, D., Duggan, C. and Lwin, R. (1991) 'The family and HIV', *Genitourinary Medicine* 67: 363–366.

Goldie, R., King, S., DeMateo, D., Bergman, A., Weir, N. and Reinhart, T. (1994) *Children Born to Mothers with HIV/AIDS: Family Psychosocial Issues*, Toronto: The Hospital for Sick Children.

Honigsbaum, N. (1994) *Children and Families Affected by HIV in Europe: The Way Forward*, London: National Children's Bureau.

Mellins, C. and Ehrhardt, A. (1994) 'Families affected by pediatric acquired immun-odeficiency syndrome: sources of stress and coping', *Developmental and Behavioral Pediatrics* 15: S54–S60.

Melvin, D. and Sherr, L. (1995) 'HIV infection in London children – psychosocial complexity and emotional burden', *Child: Care, Health and Development* 21: 405–412.

Mok, J. (1993) 'HIV seropositive babies: implications for planning for the future', in D. Batty (ed.) *HIV Infection and Children in Need*, London: British Agencies for Adoption and Fostering.

Rait, D. (1991) 'The family context of AIDS', *Psychiatric Medicine* 9: 423–439.

Sherwen, L. and Boland, M. (1994) 'Overview of psychosocial research concerning pediatric human immunodeficiency virus infection', *Developmental and Behavioral Pediatrics* 15: S5–S11.

Van Dyke, R. (1991) 'Pediatric human immunodeficiency virus infection and the acquired immunodeficiency syndrome: a health care crisis of children and fami-lies', *American Journal of Diseases of Children* 145: 529–532.

2 HIV seropositivity, adaptation and everyday life in Greece[1]

Chryssa Tselepi, Pauline Pantzou, Olga Metallinou and Demosthenes Agrafiotis

Although AIDS shares many of the characteristics of chronic disease, it also has some specific features. It is, for example, a condition for which no cure has been found despite significant treatment advance in recent years. Its chronic nature derives from its debilitating characteristics, the fact that no effective treatment is available, and uncertainty over its course of development.

When people try to make sense of the onset of illness, they locate it within the wider context of their lives. Chronic illness can be understood as a biographical disruption in that it disturbs not only the physical body, but the life trajectory (Bury, 1982). Some individuals find that such biographical disruption has negative consequences, while others find it provides new opportunities and/or new insights into the self. Regardless of the outcome, however, from the time that someone knows they are infected, they have to face considerable uncertainty concerning life expectancy and disease progression.

While numerous studies (e.g. Pierret and Carricaburu, 1993; Lazarus and Folkman, 1984; Paternaude *et al.*, 1990) internationally have examined how people with AIDS cope with their illness, that described here is the first Greek investigation that has attempted to understand the difficulties that people with AIDS face in the management of their everyday lives. The fieldwork was undertaken between February 1995 and July 1995 prior to the widespread availability of triple combination therapy including the use of protease inhibitors.

Aims of the study

The aim of the study, which was funded by the Commission of the European Communities, was to identify the difficulties that people living with AIDS and HIV (PLWA/HIV) in Greece face in everyday life. More specifically, our goals were to examine (a) the main needs of PLWA/HIV, (b) the ways in which HIV and AIDS are experienced, and (c) the changes people make in everyday life in order to cope with the disease. We also hoped to compare Greece with two other European countries (France and

Belgium) through a 'parallel reading' of research experience with the emphasis on methodological issues.

Any approach to understanding the management of everyday life by people with HIV/AIDS needs to be sensitive to the multifaceted nature of the syndrome (Agrafiotis, 1995). Much existing European research on HIV and AIDS has therefore focused on self-management in relation to specific parameters such as stress, fears, depression, coping mechanisms and adaptation to the disease (Leiberich *et al.*, 1993; Cohen *et al.*, 1995). Previous work in Greece is no exception in this respect (Agrafiotis, 1988, 1991, 1993, 1995). In the present study, a holistic approach was taken to an analysis of the problems facing PLWA/HIV in the management of everyday life. Of particular interest was the interface between people with HIV/AIDS and NGOs, therapeutic and medical services, and the social environment (family, friends, work colleagues). Also of concern was sexuality, experiences of 'therapy' and information management in relation to seropositivity as a quality of the self that needs to be kept 'secret'. These experiences and responses were analysed in relation to time since learning of an HIV/AIDS diagnosis, health status (symptomatic or asymptomatic), socio-demographic characteristics (age, family, educational level, profession) and possible cause of infection.

Fieldwork

Data were collected between February and July 1995 by means of semi-structured interviews. In order to access potential respondents, the Department of Sociology at the National School of Public Health in Athens prepared a pamphlet describing the aims of the study, and inviting infected people to participate. The leaflet was distributed to collaborating hospitals and organisations, not only to promote awareness about the project, but also to enlist the co-operation of both PLWA/HIV and professionals such as doctors and social workers. Personal letters of invitation to participate in the project were also sent to PLWA/HIV through private and state hospitals in the Athens area, a state hospital in Thessaloniki, the National AIDS Reference Centre in the National School of Public Health, Athens, a hostel for psychosocial support in Piraeus, and voluntary organisations involved in work with PLWA/HIV.

The interview schedule was developed from our previous research (Agrafiotis *et al.*, 1994) and other relevant studies (e.g. Pierret and Carricaburu, 1993). The schedule had four principal sections:

1   Initial discovery of serostatus. This section included questions on reasons for testing, receiving the results (circumstances, place, time), first reactions to the news, and possible causes of infection.

2   Management of HIV/AIDS. This section included questions about feelings and emotions, understanding about AIDS and breaking the news to others.
3   Management of everyday life. This section elicited a description of a typical day, changes in health status, experiences of hospitalisation, relationships with family and friends, sexuality, relationships with NGOs and professionals offering support, religion and thoughts about the future.
4   Socio-demographic characteristics.

Interview data were subjected to thematic content analysis. Interviews were first analysed individually, isolating those parts of the narrative applicable to each section of the interview guide (vertical mode of analysis). The data were then analysed comparatively across all forty interviews (horizontal mode of analysis).

A number of difficulties were encountered in the course of the fieldwork. The special nature of the illness (anonymity, social stigma, special psychological significance, the protection of confidentiality) encouraged us to approach people with HIV/AIDS indirectly. Doctors treating patients, those in charge of the voluntary support associations for people with HIV/AIDS and state social institutions therefore acted as intermediaries. Given the unknown dimensions of the overall HIV-positive population in Greece, it is unclear if the sample differed in any significant way from this wider group.

Another difficulty derived from the fact that respondents frequently requested counselling and psychological support during the interview, since for some of them this was their first opportunity to talk about their HIV/AIDS status and their life as a whole. The interview procedure encouraged self-reflection and having to confront new thoughts. A balance had therefore to be struck between the demands of research and the need to satisfy counselling needs.

Socio-demographic characteristics

Forty PLWA/HIV (thirty-four males and six females) participated in the study (Table 2.1). Their age range was 21–63 years, with the length of time that they had known of their HIV status varying between fifteen days and ten years. The age distribution of respondents was relatively analogous to those of AIDS cases in Greece with the majority of respondents being between 26 and 40 years of age. With respect to educational level, there was a relatively equal distribution of respondents of different educational levels. The majority of respondents (thirty) were single, nine lived alone, seven lived with at least one member of their family, five lived with their parents, four lived in a hostel for psychosocial support in Piraeus, while the remaining four lived with a roommate, and one with a sexual partner. Seven individuals were married and living with their spouse and children. One was married but lived alone. The final two respondents were widows whose husbands had died from AIDS; one was divorced.

As health status had brought about changes in respondents' professional activities, perhaps even forcing them to leave their employment, there was considerable difficulty in allocating individuals to occupational categories. Participants were, however, required to state their main occupation although some were not working at the time of the study, or had taken extended leave from their employment or retired because of HIV/AIDS.

According to their own accounts, thirty-seven subjects had been infected through sexual contact. Two of these reported being drug users. One person had haemophilia and reported having been infected through a blood transfusion. The remaining two individuals refused to provide information about

Table 2.1 Socio-demographic characteristics of study participants

Characteristic	No. of participants
Age groups:	
20–25 years	2
26–30 years	7
31–35 years	12
36–40 years	4
41–45 years	5
46–50 years	7
51–60 years	2
61+ years	1
Educational level:	
primary education	11
secondary education	12
technical diploma	7
university degree	10
Profession:	
self-employed	8
business staff	2
state officials	8
skilled workers–technicians	5
lower- and middle-level office workers	4
manual workers	4
retired	1
farmers	1
housewives	5
unemployed	2
Family status:	
unmarried	30
married	7
divorced	1
widow/widower	2

the cause of infection. Of the thirty respondents, twenty self-identified as heterosexual, fifteen as homosexual and three as bisexual.

Six persons had known of their HIV status for less than a year, twenty for between one and five years and nine for more than five years.

Findings

Learning about an HIV-positive serostatus was a critical point in the life trajectory of people with HIV/AIDS. Knowledge of being seropositive usually brought discontinuity and change to the life course. Preparation for receiving a positive test result was reported as having been minimal, both by those who discovered their seropositivity in the course of examinations for health problems, and by those who, worried about being infected, took a test in order to discover whether this was true. The circumstances of the announcement together with the lack of systematic counselling and psychological support mean that at this crucial point of their lives many people with HIV/AIDS found it difficult to accept and deal with a positive result. After an initial phase of grief and anger, each tried to find support from different resources such as family, friends, employment, religion and NGOs, in an effort to adjust and survive.

In Greece, the treatment given to people with HIV/AIDS is hospital oriented. For this reason, the role, organisation, available equipment and service provision of the hospital are crucial for the management of the disease and the psychological status of people with HIV/AIDS. The doctor's role is vital. On the one hand doctors have to deal with the uncertainties of the disease itself; on the other they have to meet patients' expectations for emotional, psychological and moral support. There are significant differences in the way doctors develop their therapeutic relationships with patients. Many factors affect this: the doctor's personality, mood, his or her ability to communicate, workload, time pressures, etc. Relationships between patients and doctors were generally reported as being positive, in contrast to relationships with nurses and paramedical staff. With respect to the latter, patients expressed either strongly positive or strongly negative opinions. The latter were particularly prevalent when they received positive test results or were being nursed by nursing and paramedical staff who were untrained, and who reacted without any sensitivity to the situation. Respondents expressed the need to have regular personal contact with nursing staff in what are termed the Special Infection Units where people with HIV and AIDS are treated. Finally, lack of provision for the systematic support and counselling of both patients and medical and nursing staff in hospitals was commented on.

Managing 'the secret' of HIV seropositivity constituted a central axis around which problems relating to the management of everyday life revolved. Usually people who decided to reveal their serostatus did so to a small number of people whom they trusted, mainly their family and friends.

The leak of information about serostatus to the workplace or to the family was usually connected with the violation of medical confidentiality, and brought undesirable changes in the life of people with HIV/AIDS.

In order to manage the problems of everyday life, people with HIV/AIDS look for and mobilise sources of support, either pre-existing ones such as family, friends and colleagues, or new ones such as the support provided by voluntary associations and statutory bodies, or creativity through art. Despite any initial shock, the family still remained the most important source of support, offering moral, psychological and financial care and encouragement for those who could be open about their HIV status.

Sexual life after learning of seropositivity varied significantly according to the evolution of the disease. Asymptomatic persons usually reported having an active sex life in contrast to persons who manifested serious symptoms, most of whom abstained from sex. Generally, respondents with an active sex life used condoms either to protect their sexual partners against HIV infection or to protect themselves against a possible reinfection, although there were cases where condoms were not used. In general, respondents who did not use condoms before learning of their seropositivity changed their behaviour and attitudes towards condoms afterwards and attempted to use them systematically.

Thoughts about the future were defined both by the limits imposed by seropositivity and by the self-restrictions people with HIV and AIDS placed upon themselves. Much of the uncertainty and insecurity which characterised their thoughts derived from uncertainty about the future. The way in which this uncertainty was managed, however, was dependent upon resources provided by respondents' socio-cultural ambience. A preliminary analysis of findings from this study highlight the existence of major profiles of response. First, and most important, there were those respondents who held the perception that AIDS comes to interrupt and destroy a life course. As two interviewees put it:

> My life finished after AIDS.
>
> (Male, aged 34, homosexually infected)

> AIDS destroyed my life.
>
> (Male, aged 32, heterosexually infected)

More than 50 per cent did not feel that their lifestyle justified the infection. They usually spoke about having had bad luck and blamed others for their infection (sexual partner, infected blood). They perceived themselves as 'victims'. Such people had usually learned about their seropositivity by accident, in the course of other medical examinations. They tended not to tell others about their condition, be they family, friends or colleagues at work. When they had to announce it, they chose one or two people whom they trusted. Thus, the whole management of everyday life is interwoven with, and takes meaning from, the keeping of the 'secret':

> I feel so bad, someone may learn about it and treat me differently ... I keep it to myself ... I am afraid it may be announced.
>
> (Female, aged 41, heterosexually infected)

Typically, such individuals did not look for new sources of support, but utilised pre-existing sources, or even rejected these. Seropositivity was thereby experienced as a dramatic isolation fed by fears of rejection, stigmatisation and uncertainty. Not infrequently, members of this group of respondents reported experiencing depressive symptoms:

> You stop dreaming, planning, not knowing what to expect from one day to another ... you only live for the moment.
>
> (Female, aged 29, heterosexually infected, drug user)

> I live for the next moment, I have no future prospects and this is terrible. Thus I often think ... what is the meaning of my life?
>
> (Male, aged 33, heterosexually infected)

The difficulties and constraints individuals encountered in the management of everyday life caused them considerable distress. Members of this same group reported not having an active sex life, or, when they did, were acutely anxious about precautionary measures, fearing the transmission of the disease to their sexual partner:

> Since I learned that I am a carrier, I have no relationships at all. Sexually, I am dead.
>
> (Male, aged 38, homosexually infected)

> I don't want someone to be infected by me, for me to be the cause of infection, I'd rather be shot dead with a gun.
>
> (Male, aged 34, heterosexually infected)

The main characteristic of a second group of respondents was their more positive approach to coping. This was linked to the belief that AIDS had come to interrupt, change and sometimes improve a way of life:

> AIDS changed my life, I became a teacher ... I am a new person ... I started to read ... it taught me to love and to understand life.
>
> (Male, aged 36, homosexually infected)

This more positive perception and attitude to life was also reflected in perceptions of the disease:

For me, my mind is my medicine, my thoughts, that I see everything positively ... that is, I don't just live with the virus for seven years, but I offer hospitality to it ... I have personalised the virus in visions.

(Male, aged 36, homosexually infected)

Individuals in this group usually felt more responsible for their infection, described having an intense sex life, and were conscious of their risky behaviour:

I haven't counted how many partners I had, I didn't have a permanent sexual partner ... I am aware of the means of protection, but I haven't used condoms ... love with condoms is not love.

(Male, aged 29, homosexually infected)

Seropositivity and disease were not kept a secret by such individuals; they shared the news with some individuals in their immediate social surroundings. They looked for new sources of support (voluntary associations, artistic activities, alternative treatment, religion) or mobilised existing sources:

It's been a positive change in my life because I sat and wrote two books about art and aesthetics, things that I had inside me for years and I had postponed.

(Male, aged 41, homosexually infected)

AIDS has changed everything, I am grateful to it.

(Male, aged 50, homosexually infected)

Individuals in this group also reported having set new objectives and aims, and having made new plans for the future:

I make future plans ... this helps me a lot ... all this keeps me alive ... I arrange my life and my emotions according to the plan, like a diary ... a documentation of life.

(Male, aged 32, homosexually infected)

Sexual and emotional life constituted important sources of support; sexual life was not interrupted by AIDS, but simply adapted to the restrictions imposed by the disease. With a few exceptions (see above) people in this group reported taking precautionary measures:

I am now stable in my sexual life. I have been involved with a girl for 5–6 months and we have no problem ... we use condoms.

(Male, aged 20, heterosexually infected)

A third and final group was characterised neither by the negative thoughts typical of the first group, nor the positive attitudes of the second. Its major characteristic was the belief that life just goes on:

> Nothing changed, I went to work, I walked, I travelled, all the things I do every day ... nothing changed and I don't think it will.
>
> (Male, aged 42, heterosexually infected)

Some members of this group felt they were responsible for their infection, which they explained as having occurred through their way of life, while others attributed responsibility to their sexual partner or to bad luck. News of seropositivity was usually shared with a small number of trusted individuals, most usually friends and family members. Members of this group continued to use pre-existing sources of support such as family, friends and work colleagues, and made little effort to look for new sources. Constraints on everyday life did not cause undue distress; on the contrary individuals made efforts to solve their problems or overcome them. Having an active sex life was not seen as a major source of support:

> In the beginning, I had my ups and downs, my fears, but I overcame them ... and now I have a normal sexual life.
>
> (Male, aged 36, bisexually infected)

It needs to be emphasised that the above categories identified general trends observable in the data and do not constitute a clearly defined typology. There were individuals whose views cut across the boundaries between different categories. Moreover, an important factor influencing individuals' orientation to everyday life was the phase of life in which people found themselves in relation to the stage of the disease. If we exclude the six persons who were still in the first year of knowing about their seropositivity, a stage characterised by uncertainty and efforts at adjustment, the remaining respondents had already developed adjustment strategies and had organised their life taking into account their seropositivity.

The typologies presented here also need confirmation and verification by further research both in Greece and in the rest of Europe. Additionally, they need to be made more specific and linked to social variables such as age, gender, socio-economic status, civil support and psychological variables such as the ability to cope with anxiety.

Conclusions

Overall, there is evidence from this study that HIV infection can function as a turning point in people's life careers as, entering into the 'world of the epidemic', they are obliged to revise and reorganise their relationships, their abilities and sources of support. In the Greek socio-cultural environment, people with HIV/AIDS confront specific challenges which they perceive, evaluate and face in different ways. Three strategies are especially prevalent:

1   what may be termed a 'universal' strategy similar to that employed when confronting any infectious condition and involving close ties with medical and other personnel;
2   a 'Greek' strategy utilising the ties and support of family; and
3   a 'personal' strategy reliant on personal psychological forces and living positively.

It remains an open question as to how the three strategies articulate with the first typology which has been elaborated and based on the findings in the field. This open question needs more research in the light of new diagnostic therapeutic possibilities.

Notes

1   This study was supported financially by the Wellcome Foundation Ltd through Positive Action, the company's international programme for HIV education, care and community support.

References

Agrafiotis, D. (1988) *Health and Illness. Sociocultural Dimensions*, Athens: Litsas.
——(1991) 'Greek society and AIDS', *Third PanHellenic Congress on AIDS* (Abstracts), Athens: Vita.
——(1993) 'AIDS as a social reformer', *AIDS Economics and Management in Greece*. Athens: Centre for Health Social Sciences (in Greek).
——(1995) 'Trends in social research for AIDS', *7th PanHellenic Congress on AIDS, Athens, November*.
Agrafiotis, D., Avgeridis, K., Pantzou, P., Papastamou, S. and Tselepi, Ch. (1994) *Sexuality and Social Representation. A Contribution to AIDS Prevention*, General Secretariat of Research and Technology, Athens: National School of Public Health.
Bury, M. (1982) 'Chronic illness as biographical disruption', *Sociology of Health and Illness* 4(2): 167–182.
Cohen, R., Mount, B., Strobel, M. and Bui, F. (1995) 'The McGill Quality of Life Questionnaire (MQOL); acceptability and psychomeric properties', *2nd International Conference on Home and Community Care for Persons living with HIV/AIDS*, Abstract 12 (B36).
Lazarus, R. S. and Folkman, S. (1984) *Stress Appraisal, and Coping*, New York: Springer.
Leiberich, P. *et al.* (1993) *Psychische Situation von HIV-Infizierten und AIDS-Kranken* Nr 80, Universitat Erlangen-Nurnberg: Institut fur Psychologie Lehrstuhl III.
Paternaude, A. F. *et al.* (1990) 'Psychosocial effects of transfusion-related HIV infection in paediatric cancer patients', *Journal of Psychosocial Oncology* 8(49): 41–58.
Pierret, J. and Carricaburu, D. (1993) 'HIV infected men, daily life and biographical reconstructions', *IXth International Conference on AIDS, Berlin, June*, Abstract No. F42.

3 Psychological and behavioural factors and the natural history of HIV infection

José Catalán

It is a truism to say that psychological and behavioural factors and physical disease are intimately associated, although it is less easy to agree on what the direction of this association is – do psychological factors cause physical disease or vice versa? Earlier this century the concept of 'psychosomatic disease' was developed, suggesting that some physical diseases had a primary psychological aetiology, resulting from a particular personality type, or perhaps developing in response to outside psychological stressors. More recently, this conceptual model has been widened, so that the idea of a limited group of 'psychosomatic' disorders has been modified to suggest that states of mind, attitudes and behaviour can play a part in the development of physical diseases, their subsequent progress and their nature of the response to treatment. All physical disorders should therefore be regarded as having a psychosocial component which in some disorders may be more important than others (Engel, 1977).

HIV infection offers a good example of the usefulness of this model. The infection is usually acquired through behaviours which can be influenced by psychological and social factors; HIV infection has in addition to its medical aspects significant psychological and social consequences; disease progression can lead to important neuropsychiatric syndromes; and comprehensive treatment of HIV infection needs to include attention to its psychosocial aspects. Is there, however, another level at which psychological factors play a part in HIV infection? Can attitudes and behaviour influence the progression of the disease, and thus slow down or speed up the development of symptoms and complications?

Psychological and behavioural factors include a range of variables which could be understood as 'endogenous' or 'exogenous' (Fox, 1981). The endogenous psychological component includes such things as thoughts and feelings, attitudes and expectations, as well as personality traits and possibly their behavioural correlates. The 'exogenous' dimension refers mostly to behaviours that may have an effect on disease progression. Obvious examples of these would be such things as whether to take prophylactic or antiretroviral treatment, or avoidance of sexually transmitted disease. Psychological and behavioural factors as concepts are easy to grasp, but much harder to define and measure in a reliable and valid way. There are many methodological problems in attempting to make sense of what is loosely known as 'psycho-immunology', and one of them is the measurement of the psychological and behavioural variables that are thought to be relevant.

There is another important methodological problem when attempting to study the role of psychological and behavioural factors in relation to the natural history of HIV infection: there is no such thing as 'natural history of HIV' any more, except possibly in the case of asymptomatic individuals in the earlier stages of infection. In practice, few people with symptomatic disease living in developed countries will have failed to have some form of treatment, either in the form of antiretrovirals or else as prophylaxis against secondary complications, such as opportunistic infections. The clinical course of HIV infection has changed over the years, leading to longer survival and lower rates of disease progression as a result of antiretroviral and other treatments. Research into the contribution of psychological and behavioural factors to disease progression therefore needs to take into account the range of treatments that patients are receiving, and to attempt to evaluate the relative contribution of psychological and behavioural factors and medical treatments.

In this chapter, the association between psychological and behavioural factors and HIV infection will be discussed under three headings. First, by reviewing the evidence for an association between HIV disease progression and psychological and neuropsychiatric problems; second, by considering whether psychological status and other factors may affect immune function and disease progression; and finally, by examining whether behaviour may have an effect on disease progression.

HIV disease progression and risk of psychological and neuropsychiatric problems

There is very good evidence, and not just from the field of HIV infection but from research into the psychological aspects of cancer and other serious or disabling physical disorders, which shows that the iller or the more symptomatic the person is the greater will be the likelihood of developing psychological problems (Catalán et al., 1995). Surveys have found high levels of anxiety, depression and other psychological symptoms in HIV symptomatic individuals compared with negative controls or people with HIV who are asymptomatic. In some studies, non-AIDS symptomatic disease is reported to be associated with worse psychological status than AIDS itself (Perry and Markowitz, 1986; Tross et al., 1987). Studies involving gay and bisexual men and men with haemophilia have tended to find worse psychological status in those who are symptomatic, but studies involving injecting drug users or mixed populations are less likely to find such differences (Lyketsos et al., 1996). HIV symptomatic individuals represent the vast majority of people referred to specialist mental health services, some studies indicating that as many as 30 per cent of medical in-patients with AIDS were referred for psychiatric care (Dilley *et al.*, 1985). Common problems in symptomatic people with HIV referred to mental health services include organic brain syndromes (dementia and delirium), major depression, substance-misuse-related problems, and problems adjusting to declining health.

It is easy to understand why psychological problems are more prominent in symptomatic, advanced HIV infection. Asymptomatic individuals, especially those who remain well for many years, are able to find ways of adjusting to their HIV status and to continue maintaining a normal life, even if some have concerns about the possibility of becoming ill at some stage in the future. In contrast, the development of symptoms, in particular if they are severe, disabling or with marked effects on the person's appearance, such as molluscum or facial Kaposi's sarcoma, will be likely to cause alarm and distress, fears about the future, and difficulties in social interaction and social functioning. Similarly, the administration of medical treatments with adverse side effects, complex treatment regimes, hospitalisation or multiple hospital appointments will be likely to add to the psychological impact and social disturbance. HIV brain dysfunction tends to occur in advanced HIV disease and, even in the absence of HIV-associated dementia, the severe form of brain impairment caused by HIV, memory problems, fatigue and loss of interest may become apparent.

It is too early to be clear about the full impact of new antiretroviral treatment regimes and combinations on the mental health consequences of HIV infection. While there is no doubt about the beneficial effects of the new treatments in terms of reduction in mortality and morbidity in people with HIV (for a recent review and discussion see Gazzard, 1999), mental health responses are mixed: for many individuals health improvement has led to an increase in confidence and a normalisation of their lives, with a resumption of employment, social life and formulation of longer-term plans, but for others the possibility of a real future has opened up unresolved problems in the field of life goals, relationships and employment, amongst others (Catalán, 1999).

The effects of psychological status and personality on immune status and HIV disease progression

This is a much more controversial and disputed area and one where methodological difficulties are paramount. Good research in this area of 'psycho-immunology' will need to be able to define and measure in a reliable and valid way thoughts, feelings, moods, attitudes and personality traits, and ideally do so over a period of time, so as to be able to compare long-term and persistent patterns of, for example, depression, with brief periods of sadness, and then in turn examine their relationship with immune parameters, disease progression and survival. Evaluation of immune response can also be very complex, going well beyond the study of CD4 and CD8 levels, the choice of measures being in itself a subject of debate. Similarly, indicators of disease progression will need to be standardised and measured reliably. Plasma viral load has not yet been included in many investigations.

Psycho-immunological investigations in HIV can be of three kinds: cross-sectional studies, longitudinal studies and intervention studies. Recent reviews are available (Catalán *et al.*, 1995; Dupont and Burgess, 1999), and here a summary will be given of the main findings.

Cross-sectional studies

Cross-sectional investigations are those in which subjects are studied once, when information is collected simultaneously about psychological and social variables, immune function disease state, and then statistical analyses are carried out to establish, for example, whether individuals with good immune function have particular psychological profiles, personality traits or levels of depression.

Cross-sectional studies have given mixed results. Sahs *et al.* (1994) compared HIV-positive and HIV-negative gay men in terms of psychological distress and natural killer cell numbers. Studying seropositive and seronegative men together, they found no association between natural killer cells and psychological variables. HIV-positive men showed a decrease in natural killer cell numbers, but no association was found between psychological distress and immune function. On the other hand, Evans *et al.* (1995) showed a link between severe stress and reductions in natural killer cells in the HIV-positive group. This association was not due to greater levels of depression or to more advanced disease in those with more stress. In the HIV-negative group no consistent associations were found. Moreover, Goodkin *et al.* (1992) report having found a possible association between coping actively with the situations and natural killer cell activity.

Longitudinal studies

Longitudinal studies involve following up individuals for some period of time, and obtaining information about their psychological status and other variables at baseline and at regular intervals thereafter. Longitudinal studies can provide better information than that obtained from cross-sectional investigations, as they begin to explore systematically the direction of associations between variables.

A number of investigators have found interesting links using longitudinal study designs. For example, Burack *et al.* (1993) found that individuals who were depressed at baseline were more likely to show greater decline in CD4 levels over a four-year period, when compared with individuals without depression. Similarly Vedhara *et al.* (1997) found that the emotional impact of stress affected adversely CD4 levels over a twelve-month period. In contrast with the above studies, other researchers using much larger samples followed for up to eight years have failed to find any significant associations (Lyketsos *et al.*, 1993; Mayne *et al.*, 1996). Similarly, Zorrilla *et al.* (1996) in a meta-analysis of nineteen published studies concluded that stressors did not affect the cause of HIV disease.

A more complex association has been described by Kemeny *et al.* (1995) who studied the impact of the death of a partner as a result of AIDS on HIV-positive individuals, and compared it with HIV-positive men who were not bereaved. Bereaved individuals showed a decline in immune function following bereavement while this did not happen in the control group. Interestingly, levels of depression in the bereaved group were not correlated with immune function, suggesting that the impact of bereavement on immune function was not mediated by depression but by other factors.

Our research group in the UK has carried out a prospective investigation of a cohort of HIV-positive gay men followed up for up to nine years, studying the contribution of psychological state and neuropsychological function to survival and disease progression (Catalán *et al.*, 1998). In addition, this study also involved looking at individuals' antiretroviral use. When psychological status, neuropsychological function and antiretroviral use were included in the analysis, three variables predicted survival: higher CD4 count at baseline, antiretroviral use, and high scores on one of the neuropsychological tests (the age-scaled digit-symbol test). However when psychological variables, immune function at baseline and antiretroviral use were entered into the analysis but neuropsychological function variables were excluded, the results show that in addition to CD4 count and antiretroviral use, low levels of psychological distress also predicted survival. When neuropsychological function variables were included in the analysis but psychological ones were taken out, the neuropsychological tests, in addition to the CD4 count and antiretroviral use, were found to predict survival. The study therefore suggests, first, that results obtained in this kind of investigation will depend to some extent on the nature of the variables studied; second, that neuropsychological function appears to be a more powerful predictor of survival than levels of psychological distress; and third, the importance of antiretroviral treatment use as a factor in survival.

Ways of coping have also been studied longitudinally and here again the results have been inconsistent. Mulder *et al.* (1995) have reported finding no association, while Ironson *et al.* (1994) and Antoni *et al.* (1995) found that denial and behavioural disengagement had a short and adverse effect on CD4 levels.

Intervention studies

In this kind of design, efforts are made to alter a particular psychological variable which is thought to play a role in modulating immune function, and then the impact of this change is studied by identifying changes in immune function, disease progression or other variables. This kind of investigation is methodologically complex, but has advantages over observational techniques in cross-sectional and longitudinal studies, in that it allows to test experimentally the possible role of selected variables. There are only a small number of published studies of this kind, and again the results are somewhat mixed.

LaPerriere *et al.* (1991) found that a five-week aerobic training period following notification of HIV status had a protective effect in terms of immune function, compared with a no-intervention control group, while Antoni *et al.* (1991) reported that cognitive behavioural stress management over five weeks following notification of HIV status also had a protective effect compared with a non-intervention control group.

In contrast with these two studies, three other investigations have failed to find any effects from cognitive behavioural stress management, stress reduction or training to increase active coping skills (Lutgendorf *et al.*, 1997; Coates *et al.*, 1989; Auerbach *et al.*, 1992).

The effects of behaviour on HIV disease progression

It is fairly uncontroversial to state that behaviour can have an effect on HIV disease progression. For example, using antiretroviral medication and other treatments can have powerful effects in modifying disease progression. Furthermore, attitudes, thoughts and beliefs have an important role in determining whether individuals take medication regularly or not. Treatment adherence will be a very important factor in disease progression and psychological and behavioural factors play a crucial role here (Chesney and Ickovics, 1997; Hecht *et al.*, 1998; see also Weiss in this volume).

Another way in which behaviour can affect disease progression in HIV is through the acquisition of other infections, in particular other sexually transmitted diseases the presence of which may worsen the outcome of HIV infection. Finally, individuals who adhere to illicit drug use treatment programmes such as methadone maintenance, compared with those not in treatment, are more likely to show greater compliance with antiretrovirals and to have better disease progression (Hawkins, 1999).

Conclusions

While it is acknowledged that the relationship between psychological and behavioural factors and HIV disease progression is an important one, it is also clear that there are complex methodological problems that make it hard to establish clear and definite causal links, in particular in the area that is known as 'psycho-immunology'. Even if it could be established conclusively that psychological status, attitudes and ways of coping can have an important effect on disease progression, it is also relevant to establish the strength of their contribution, in particular by comparison with the role of antiretro-viral medication or prophylactic treatment, or indeed to neuropsychological function.

It is nevertheless important to continue encouraging individuals with HIV infection to maintain a positive outlook and an active coping style, so that they develop control over their lives and avoid depressed mood or undue stress levels. These are all good things in themselves, whether or not they translate into a better immune function and subsequent improved prognosis. We should, however be cautious about giving the message that disease progression depends solely on attitudes, mood and coping skills. What has been described as 'the tyranny of positive thinking' may well lead individuals with HIV infection to feel guilty and blame themselves should their HIV infection progress and their immune function decline. If we are to help people with HIV to remain healthy, it will be more important to help them gain control of the kind of behaviours that will definitely arrest disease progression, such as ensuring that treatment adherence is high.

References

Antoni, M. *et al.* (1991) 'Cognitive-behavioural stress management intervention buffers the stress responses and immunological changes following notification of HIV-1 seropositivity', *Journal of Consulting and Clinical Psychology* 59: 906–915.

Antoni, M., Goldstein, D., Ironson, G., LaPerriere, A., Fletcher, M. and Schneiderman, N. (1995) 'Coping responses to HIV-1 serostatus notification predict comparant and prospective immunologic status', *Clinical Psychology and Psychotherapy* 2: 234–248.

Auerbach, J., Oleson, T. and Solomon, G. (1992) 'Behavioral medicine intervention as an adjuvant treatment for HIV-related illness', *Psychology and Health* 6: 325–334.

Burack, J. *et al.* (1993) 'Depressive symptoms and CD4 lymphocyte decline among HIV infected men', *Journal of the American Medical Association* 270: 2568–2573.

Catalán, J. (1999) 'Psychological problems in people with HIV infection', in J. Catalán (ed.) *Mental Health and HIV Infection – Psychological and Psychiatric Aspects*, London: UCL Press/Taylor and Francis.

Catalán, J., Burgess, A. and Klimes, I. (1995) *Psychological Medicine of HIV Infection*, Oxford: Oxford University Press.

Catalán, J., Champion, A., Baldeweg, T. and Gazzard, B. (1998) 'Psychological and neuropsychological predictors of mortality in disease progression and HIV infection', *Abstracts of the 12th International AIDS Conference, Geneva*.

Chesney, M. and Ickovics, J. (1997) 'Adherence to combination therapy in AIDS clinical trials', Paper developed for the Recruitment, Adherence and Retention Committee of the ACTG, Annual Meeting of the AIDS Clinical Trials Group, July, Washington, DC.

Coates, T., McKusick, L., Quno, R. and Stites, D. (1989) 'Stress reduction training changed number of sexual partners but not immune function in men with HIV', *American Journal of Public Health* 79: 885–887.

Dilley, J., Ochitill, H., Pearl, M. and Volberding, P. (1985) 'Findings in psychiatric consultation with patients with AIDS', *American Journal of Psychiatry* 142: 82–86.

Dupont, S. and Burgess, A. (1999) 'Psychoneuroimmunology and HIV infection', in J. Catalán (ed.) *Mental Health and HIV Infection – Psychological and Psychiatric Aspects*, London: UCL Press/Taylor and Francis.

Engel, G. (1977) 'The need for a new medical model: a challenge for biomedicine', *Science* 196: 129–136.

Evans, D. *et al.* (1995) 'Stress-associated reduction in cytotoxic T lymphocytes and natural killer cells in asymptomatic HIV action', *American Journal of Psychiatry* 152: 543–550.

Fox, R. (1981) 'Psychosocial factors and immune system in human cancer', in R. Ader (ed.) *Psychoneuroimmunology*, Orlando, FL: Academic Press.

Gazzard, B. (1999) (ed.) *Chelsea and Westminster Hospital AIDS Care Handbook*, London: Mediscript.

Goodkin, K. *et al.* (1992) 'Active coping style is associated with natural cell cytotoxicity in asymptomatic HIV-1 seropositive homosexual men', *Journal of Psychosomatic Research* 36: 635–650.

Hawkins, D. (1999) 'Drug users and HIV', in B. Gazzard (ed.) *Chelsea and Westminster Hospital AIDS Care Handbook*, London: Mediscript.

Hecht, F. M. *et al.* (1998) 'Adherence and effectiveness of protease inhibitors in clinical practice', Paper presented at the Vth Conference on Retroviruses and Opportunistic Infections, 2–6 February, Chicago.

Ironson, G. *et al.* (1994) 'Distress, denial and low adherence to behavioral interventions predict faster disease progression in gay men infected with HIV', *International Journal of Behavioral Medicine* 1: 90–105.

Kemeny, M. *et al.* (1995) 'Immune system changes following the death of a partner in HIV positive gay men', *Psychosomatic Medicine* 56: 547–554.

LaPerriere, A., Fletcher, M., Antoni, M., Kleimas, N. and Ironson, G. (1991) 'Aerobic exercise training in an AIDS risk group', *International Journal of Sports Medicine* 12 (Supplement): S53–S57.

Lutgendorf, S. *et al.* (1997) 'Cognitive-behavioral stress management decreases dysphoric mood and Herpes Simplex Virus-Type 2 antibody titers in symptomatic HIV seropositive gay men', *Journal of Consulting and Clinical Psychology* 65: 31–43.

Lyketsos, C. *et al.* (1993) 'Depressive symptoms as predictors of medical outcomes in HIV infection', *Journal of the American Medical Association* 270: 2563–2567.

Lyketsos, C. *et al.* (1996) 'Psychiatric morbidity on entry to a HIV primary care clinic', *AIDS* 10: 1033–1039.

Mayne, T., Vittinghoff, E., Chesney, M., Barratt, D. and Coates, T. (1996) 'Depressive affect and survival among gay and bisexual men infected with HIV', *Archives of Internal Medicine* 156: 2233–2238.

Mulder, C., Antoni, M., Duivenvoorden, H., Kauffmann, R. and Goodkin, K. (1995) 'Active confrontational coping predicts decreased clinical progression over a one year period in HIV infected homosexual men', *Journal of Psychosomatic Research* 39: 957–965.

Perry, S. and Markowitz, J. (1986) 'Psychiatric interventions for AIDS-Spectrum disorder', *Hospital and Community Psychology* 37: 1001–1006.

Sahs, J., Goetz, R., Reddy, M., Rabkin, J., Williams, J., Kertzner, R. and Gorman, J. (1994) 'Psychological distress and natural killer cells in gay men with and without HIV infection', *American Journal of Psychiatry* 151: 1479–1484.

Tross, H. *et al.* (1987) 'Determinants of current psychiatric disorder in AIDS-Spectrum patients', Paper presented at the 3rd International Conference on AIDS, Washington, DC.

Vedhara, K. *et al.* (1997) 'Greater emotional distress is associated with accelerated CD4 cell decline in HIV infection', *Journal of Psychosomatic Research* 42: 379–390.

Zorrilla, E., McKay, J., Luborsky, L. and Schmidt, K. (1996) 'Relation of stressors and depressive symptoms to clinical progression of viral illness', *American Journal of Psychiatry* 153: 626–635.

4   Attitudinal factors and adherence to protease inhibitor combination therapy

Jeffrey J. Weiss

The medical management of HIV disease in the developed world has changed markedly in recent years. Highly active antiretroviral therapy (HAART) is able effectively to bring the plasma HIV-1 RNA concentrations (viral load) to below detectable limits (50 copies/ml) in large percentages of treated individuals (rates reported vary from 60 to 90 per cent). The suppression of viral replication can be sustained for at least two years in HIV-1-positive people who are able to adhere to the complex HAART regimes. Sustained suppression of HIV-1 has been shown to be related to better quality of life, slower clinical disease progression, lower hospitalisation rates and longer survival. Viral load has become an important parameter used in clinical decision making and in predicting long-term clinical outcome. International medical treatment guidelines for HIV-1-positive individuals (Carpenter *et al.*, 1998) recommend HAART for all HIV-1-positive people with a viral load greater than 5000 to 10,000 copies/ml regardless of CD4 cell count, and who are 'committed to the complex, long-term therapy'.

HAART has brought new hope to many people with HIV-1 infection. It does, however, make many demands on the daily life of the HIV-1-positive person. It usually involves taking at least three different medications at specific times of the day and in co-ordination with meals, and it may prohibit the use of some medications being taken for other medical or psychiatric conditions. HAART does not work for all HIV-1-positive people; it is expensive; and it can result in toxicity (metabolic abnormalities and alterations in body fat distribution) that may require treatment to be discontinued. The long-term medical effects of HAART are not yet known; the therapy fails to work for a considerable number of HIV antiretroviral-experienced people, and the extent to which functional immunity can be restored despite rises in absolute CD4 cell counts is still unclear.

Perfect adherence to HAART requires individuals always to take their medication on time, in the right amounts, and in the prescribed relationship to diet. Carpenter *et al.* (1997) report that 'less than excellent adherence' to HAART 'may result in virus breakthrough and emergence of drug-resistant (HIV-1) strains'. Even short-term (less than two weeks) non-adherence to

HAART 'may result in rapid virus re-population in lymph nodes. Given the potential for cross-resistance among the available protease inhibitors, the efficacy of future treatment options can also be severely compromised by less than excellent adherence' (Carpenter et al., 1997: 1964).

Data presented in September 1997, at the 37th Interscience Conference on Antimicrobial Agents and Chemotherapy, provide an indication that the success of treatment is strongly dependent on adherence. A report from the large public AIDS clinic at San Francisco General Hospital on 136 HIV-1-positive individuals who started on protease inhibitor-containing combination regimens in March 1996, found that HIV-1 load had returned to detectable levels in 54 per cent of the sample (Deeks et al., 1997). In comparison, a report from a carefully controlled clinical trial of indinavir, zidovudine and lamivudine found that after almost two years HIV-1 was still undetectable in peripheral blood of 79 per cent of the sample (Gulick et al., 1997). One plausible explanation for this difference in rates of continued viral suppression is that subjects in drug trials were more adherent than those given the same treatments in a clinic setting.

Behavioural scientists have an important role to play in the context of medical advances in the treatment of HIV-1 infection. There is a need for research into the determinants of adherence in HIV-1-positive people using HAART. Moreover, information gained from determinant studies of adherence can be used to develop innovative interventions to increase medication adherence. In the absence of these interventions, some physicians are hesitant to prescribe HAART to individuals whom they feel are likely to have poor adherence (e.g. people with a substance abuse disorder, the severely and persistently mentally ill, and the homeless).

The factors which are most strongly related to adherence can be categorised as characteristics of the (a) individual, (b) patient–provider relationship, (c) treatment regimen, (d) disease and (e) clinical setting (Ickovics and Meisler, 1997). Review studies have shown that there is little or no association between adherence, in general, and individual characteristics – such as age, gender, social class, race and religion (Cluss and Epstein, 1985; Haynes, 1976).

Research investigating individual determinants of adherence to medication in HIV-1-positive people has primarily focused on adherence to nucleoside reverse transcriptase inhibitor (NRTI) monotherapy. These studies have identified the following individual factors as predictive of poor adherence: a high amount of psychological stress and poor coping skills (Singh et al., 1996); poorly developed social support networks (Morse et al., 1991); low belief in the efficacy of treatment (Muma et al., 1995; Samet et al., 1992; Smith et al., 1997); and few perceived benefits and many perceived barriers (Aversa and Kimberlin, 1996).

Adherence is a behaviour, and success in achieving this behaviour requires an intention to adhere. This is a necessary, but not a sufficient, condition. In addition to the intention to adhere, the skills to adhere (e.g. the ability to impose structure on one's self) must be present and the skills to counteract factors leading to non-adherence (e.g. creatively finding a way to take one's pills while in the company of those to whom one does not want to reveal one's HIV serostatus) must also be present.

In developed countries, where HAART is available, HIV disease is in transition from being a life-threatening illness to a chronic illness. This confronts those who have known they are HIV-1 positive for several years and already once revised their life goals accordingly, with the need yet again to reassess these goals to realign them with the changing health expectations brought about by HAART. HIV-1-positive people must make decisions regarding when to begin HAART in the absence of definitive data regarding the long-term implications of doing so. In many cases, individuals who are asymptomatic and have just been notified of their HIV-1 serostatus are beginning intensive medication therapy in the absence of any visible signs of being ill.

Several questionnaires have been developed to assess attitudes and beliefs in relation to zidovudine (AZT) (Catt *et al.*, 1995; Muma *et al.*, 1995; Smith *et al.*, 1997). More favourable attitudes towards AZT have been found to be related to deciding to begin AZT treatment (Catt *et al.*, 1995), better adherence to AZT treatment (Muma *et al.*, 1995), and the decision to remain on AZT treatment (Smith *et al.*, 1997).

The introduction of the protease inhibitors and HAART to the medical treatment of HIV-1-positive people has largely been responded to with great enthusiasm and optimism by the media and the medical community. The response of HIV-1-positive individuals is more ambivalent and varied, however. Clinical experience with HIV-1-positive gay men at the time that the protease inhibitors became available in The Netherlands strongly indicated that attitudinal factors were among the important determinants in their decision of whether or not to begin on HAART and in their adherence to HAART once it was begun. Given that there was no existing attitudinal questionnaire focusing on combination regimens, we decided to develop one: the Protease Inhibitor Attitudinal Questionnaire (PIAQ).

In the following two sections, the PIAQ will be discussed in terms of its adequacy as an attitude scale, including how it relates to other relevant variables; and several variables, including the PIAQ, will be cross-sectionally related to adherence in a sample of those using HAART.

PIAQ development

The larger study in which these data were collected is a randomised clinical trial in which the effect of a group psychotherapy programme on psychological, immunological and clinical outcome measures is being investigated. In this study, which began in 1994 in The Netherlands, HIV-1-positive gay men are followed over a period of thirty-three months. Many of these men began to use HAART in the period March 1996 to April 1997. This research cohort therefore provided an opportunity to investigate attitudes towards HAART in a group of HIV-1-positive gay men. The sample includes those who had already begun HAART, as well as those who had not.

The PIAQ consists of sixteen attitudinal statements which can be answered on a five-point rating scale (strongly agree, agree, neutral, disagree, strongly disagree). Eight of the items are positively worded, and eight are negatively worded. The items were formulated to measure a dimension of optimism (as well as scepticism) that protease inhibitor-containing combination regimens are leading/will lead to positive changes in the length and quality of life of HIV-1-positive people. The items were developed based on the dominant themes and concerns which were clinically observed in the context of group psychotherapy sessions and research interviews with HIV-1-positive gay men who were considering whether to begin HAART or had already done so. The PIAQ was distributed (in spring–summer 1997) to the ninety-seven HIV-1-positive gay men participating in our ongoing psychosocial intervention research study. Participants were informed that the purpose of the questionnaire was to learn more about how HIV-1-positive people view protease inhibitor-containing combination regimens. Eighty-six questionnaires (89 per cent) were returned, one of which was incompletely filled in.

At the time they entered the HIV psychosocial intervention study (recruitment from October 1994 to March 1997), these eighty-six participants had a mean age of 39.2 years (range 22.4–57.7): 77 per cent were Dutch, 19 per cent were Belgian and 4 per cent were of other nationalities; 13 per cent had a high level of education (university), 69 per cent had a middle level of education (high school) and 18 per cent had a low level of education (less than high school); 68 per cent were working, 19 per cent were unable to work due to illness and 13 per cent were unemployed; 56 per cent were in a steady relationship with another man; 59 per cent were asymptomatic (1993 CDC stage A), 34 per cent were early symptomatic (stage B) and 7 per cent were diagnosed with AIDS (stage C). The mean CD4 cell count was 415 cells/mm^3 (range from 26 to 960). These eighty-six men knew their HIV serostatus from six months to over thirteen years at the time of filling in the PIAQ in 1997 (mean = 61.2 months).

A factor analysis (principal components analysis – oblique) was carried out on the PIAQ items of the eighty-five participants with complete data. A scree plot indicated that there were two principal factors. These two factors accounted for 39 per cent of the variance. The first factor is made up of the eight positively worded items (those loading greater than 0.4). The second factor is made up of the eight negatively worded items. Cronbach's alphas of internal consistency were computed for the two factors. The first factor had an alpha value of 0.81, and the second factor had an alpha value of 0.63. The correlation between the two factors was significant ($r = -0.215$; $p = 0.024$). The decision was made, therefore, to combine the two factors into one scale, rather than to use them independently. This scale is labelled the Optimism/Scepticism (O/S) scale.

Reliability analysis resulted in acceptable internal consistency of the sixteen items comprising the O/S scale (Cronbach's alpha = 0.76). The O/S scale score is formed by summing the answers to the sixteen questions in the direction such that a higher score represents greater optimism. Answering neutral to all sixteen questions would produce an O/S score of 48. The O/S scores of the eighty-five participants are normally distributed with a mean of 43.8 and a standard deviation of 7.2. The potential range of scores is from 16 to 80; and the actual scores range from 28 to 59.

It is of note that on only two of the sixteen PIAQ items did more than 50 per cent of the sample endorse answers corresponding with an optimistic attitude towards protease inhibitor-containing combination regimens. The hesitancy on the part of this sample of HIV-1-positive gay men to be optimistic in regard to protease inhibitor therapy is reflected in its most extreme form in the answer to the final question of the PIAQ: 'We know too little about the long-term effects of protease inhibitor therapy to already be optimistic.' Ninety-three per cent of the sample indicated that they agreed or strongly agreed with this statement.

Relationship of PIAQ to medication status

Of the eighty-five PIAQ respondents, forty-five were currently on HAART; thirteen were on NRTI therapy (three on monotherapy; ten on double NRTI regimens); twenty-five were on no antiretroviral medication; and two had stopped HAART and were now on double NRTI therapy.

The various medication class combinations included in the category of HAART were as follows: one protease inhibitor and two NRTIs ($N = 36$); two protease inhibitors ($N = 3$); two protease inhibitors and one NRTI ($N = 2$); two NRTIs and one non-nucleoside reverse transcriptase inhibitor NNRTI ($N = 2$); two protease inhibitors and two NRTIs ($N = 1$); one protease inhibitor, two NRTIs and one NNRTI ($N = 1$).

A t test was used to compare those currently using HAART ($N = 45$) with those who had never used HAART ($N = 38$) on the O/S scale of the PIAQ. The attitudes towards protease inhibitor therapy of those on HAART were more optimistic (mean = 45.49, standard deviation = 7.56) than of those who had never used HAART (mean = 42.32, standard deviation = 6.33) ($t(81) = -2.049, p < 0.05$).

Subsequent information reported upon is only for those with HAART regimens which include at least one protease inhibitor ($N = 43$). The HAART group subsequently discussed therefore excludes the two individuals using two NRTIs and one NNRTI. Those using a combination with at least one protease inhibitor had been on this combination at the time of filling in the PIAQ from several days to thirteen months (mean = 6.3 months, standard deviation = 3.6).

To test the discriminant validity of the PIAQ, the HAART group was split in two: those who knew that since beginning HAART their viral load had declined (N = 26) and those who did not know whether HAART had affected their viral load (N = 17). It was expected that knowledge of the effect of HAART on viral load would influence attitudes towards protease inhibitor-containing combination regimens. This expectation was confirmed ($F(2,78)$ = 6.56, p < 0.01). The group who knew that their viral load had decreased was more positive in attitude (mean = 47.77, standard deviation = 7.07) than both the group who were on HAART but did not know their viral load result (mean = 41.59, standard deviation = 6.54) and the group who were not on HAART (mean = 42.32, standard deviation = 6.33). These latter two groups did not differ from one another in their attitudes.

The two primary reasons for not knowing whether one's viral load had decreased were that (a) HAART was quite recently begun and no post-treatment viral load measurement had yet been carried out, and (b) viral load measurements were not yet included in the standard of care at the participant's hospital. As would be expected based on the first reason, those who knew that their viral load had decreased had been on HAART on average longer (mean = 7.35 months, standard deviation = 3.01) than those who do not know their viral load results (mean = 4.59 months, standard deviation = 3.86) ($t(41)$= 2.62, p < 0.05). These two groups did not differ in the length of time they knew their HIV serostatus.

In the entire sample, no relationship was found between the O/S score and the amount of time the person had known his HIV serostatus. For those on HAART there was also no relationship between the O/S score and the amount of time since the person had begun the regimen. This relationship was also not significant within the two subgroups of those on protease inhibitor-containing therapies: those who knew that their viral load had decreased and those who did not know their viral load results.

Relationship of PIAQ to knowledge about HAART

Level of knowledge regarding HAART was assessed by one item of the PIAQ and was found to be quite high in this sample: 42 per cent of individuals reported being well informed, 46 per cent reported being somewhat informed, 11 per cent reported being minimally informed, and 1 per cent reported being uninformed. The level of knowledge did not relate to whether one was on HAART, nor to the amount of time one had known one's HIV serostatus. For the entire sample, self-reported level of knowledge did not relate to the O/S scale score. For those on HAART, the level of knowledge was not related to time on therapy, nor to whether they knew the effect of their therapy on viral load.

Relationship of PIAQ to HAART toxicity

When asked how the side effects of HAART compared with what was expected, 51.1 per cent reported that they were better than what was expected, 25.6 per cent reported that they were worse than expected, and 23.3 per cent reported that they were about what was expected. Contrary to what was predicted, the attitude towards HAART (O/S score) among those on HAART was not related to the self-reported experience of toxic side effects. In the group not on HAART, a lower (more sceptical) O/S scale score was significantly related to the fear that one would not benefit from, or have to stop taking, HAART due to toxicity ($F(3,37) = 3.33$, $p < 0.05$).

In summary, the most positive attitudes towards HAART were found in those who used HAART and knew that it had successfully reduced their viral load. Attitudes towards HAART were not found to be related to the amount of time individuals had known that they were HIV-1 positive, level of HAART knowledge, nor, in those who had begun HAART, to the experience of side effects nor the length of time using HAART.

Determinants of adherence

The following variables were theoretically posited to be related to HAART adherence: attitudes towards HAART (O/S scale), time on HAART, experience of HAART side effects, level of knowledge about HAART, HIV medication naïve or experienced status pre-HAART, and length of time known to be HIV-1 positive. The hypotheses were that better adherence would be related to a more optimistic attitude towards HAART, less time on HAART, experiencing less worse HAART side effects than had been anticipated, greater knowledge about HAART, HIV medication naïve status, and less time that one has known he is HIV-1 positive.

The PIAQ was administered a second time at subsequent follow-up assessments to participants in the HIV psychosocial intervention research project. For subsequent analyses, the first PIAQ was chosen for participants on protease inhibitor-containing HAART regimens for which we also had collected self-report adherence data within a three-week period of completion of the PIAQ ($N = 35$; all data collected between March and October 1997).

Bivariate relationships were first individually examined between the theoretical determinants and adherence, in order to choose which determinants to enter into a regression on adherence ($p < 0.10$ used as selection criteria).

The HAART regimens of the thirty-five participants include: one protease inhibitor and two NRTIs ($N = 26$); two protease inhibitors and two NRTIs ($N = 4$); two protease inhibitors ($N = 3$); one protease inhibitor, two NRTIs and one NNRTI ($N = 1$); and one NRTI and two protease inhibitors ($N = 1$).

The O/S score for those on HAART ranged from 34 to 58 (mean = 46.5). The men had been on HAART at the time of filling in the PIAQ an average of 7.85 months (standard deviation = 4.89 months). The self-reported adherence data collected came from a validated, four-item scale (Morisky *et al.*, 1986). The scale asked the participant for yes/no answers to (a) whether or not he missed taking a dose of his medication in the last week; (b) whether or not he had ever been careless in taking his medication; (c) whether or not he had ever stopped taking his medication if he felt better; and (d) whether or not he stopped taking the medication if he felt worse when he took it. Each question was scored 0 (yes) or 1 (no) producing a scale score from 0 (worst adherence) to 4 (best adherence).

Of the sample, 54 per cent ($N = 19$) reported a scale score of 4; 29 per cent ($N = 10$) reported a scale score of 3; and 17 per cent ($N = 6$) reported a scale score of 2. Given the uneven distribution, the group was divided into two groups based on this scale score: optimally adherent (scale score of 4) and suboptimally adherent (scale score less than 4).

In order to test whether there was a relationship between attitudinal factors and adherence, the O/S score was compared between the two adherence groups. There was a trend for the optimally adherent group to score lower on the O/S scale (mean = 44.8, standard deviation = 5.6) than the suboptimally adherent group (mean = 48.5, standard deviation = 5.9) ($t(33)= 1.91, p = 0.065$). In contrast to what was hypothesised, the trend was for better adherence to be related to a less optimistic attitude towards HAART.

Given the challenge involved in maintaining adherence after initially beginning to take HAART, it was expected that the level of self-reported adherence would decrease the longer the person had been on HAART. This hypothesis was confirmed. Those with optimal adherence had been on HAART on average less time (mean = 6.2 months, standard deviation = 4.6) than those with suboptimal adherence (mean = 9.8 months, standard deviation = 4.6) ($t(33)= 2.28, p = 0.030$).

As hypothesised, there was a tendency for adherence to be related to the experience of side effects such that reporting that the side effects were worse than what one had expected was related to poorer adherence ($x^2 = 5.67, p = 0.059$).

Self-reported level of knowledge regarding HAART was not related to adherence. Whether or not the person was HIV therapy naïve upon beginning HAART, and the length of time the person had been HIV-1 positive, were also not related to adherence.

To determine the relative importance of the three variables found to be related to adherence, a standard multiple regression was performed between adherence as the dependent variable and O/S score, side effects and time on HAART as independent variables. Table 4.1 displays the standardised regression coefficients (β), the standard error (SE), and the p value for each independent variable.

While R for regression was significantly different from zero ($R^2 = 0.32$, $F(3,31) = 4.9, p < 0.01$), only one of the independent variables (O/S score) contributed significantly to adherence in the regression.

In order to understand further which aspects of the PIAQ attitude scale were most relevant to adherence, *post-hoc* item correlations were carried out

Table 4.1   Multiple regression: adherence predicted by O/S score, time on HAART and side effects ($N = 35$)

Variable	β	SE	p
O/S score	−0.326	0.020	0.04
Time on HAART	−0.287	0.025	0.08
Side effects	0.255	0.074	0.11

between the sixteen PIAQ items and the adherence score. Three of the individual items were found to be highly correlated ($p < 0.05$) with adherence. Better adherence was correlated with *disagreeing* with the following statements:

> Knowing that protease inhibitor therapy is available, I expect to live as long as I would have had I not been HIV-positive.

> Before the news of the protease inhibitors, I thought of HIV as a fatal illness; now I think of it as a chronic illness.

> I believe that the combination therapies which are available make it possible to entirely eliminate the HIV virus from the body.

Discussion

It was originally hypothesised that an optimistic attitude towards HAART would provide the necessary motivation to adhere and the necessary stamina to overcome the many practical barriers along the path to perfect HAART adherence. This is widely held to be true and it is frequently reported in the literature that 'negative attitudes about medications or illness may also interfere with patient adherence' (Mehta *et al.* 1997: 1667). While this may have been the case regarding antiretroviral monotherapy, the findings of this study suggest that something quite different may be occurring with adherence to HAART, at least in this sample of individuals.

In the multiple regression analysis, attitudes toward HAART emerged as the most significant of the three variables in predicting adherence cross-sectionally. The O/S scale accounted for 11.5 per cent of the variance in adherence (adjusted R^2 in model with O/S scale as only independent variable). Having a less optimistic attitude towards HAART was found to be related to better adherence.

An examination of the specific attitudinal items which were found in *post-hoc* correlations to be most related to adherence points to a possible interpretation of this unexpected finding. It is those who were cautious in their optimism towards HAART who were most adherent. Awareness that these medications might not be 'the answer' is perhaps what was providing an increased motivation for adherence. The cautiousness is perhaps accompanied by the HIV-positive person seeing a greater role for himself in determining the outcome of HAART. Maintaining a high level of adherence is one way in which these individuals may be taking an active role in trying to impact the effectiveness of their treatment. Those who are rather more optimistic regarding HAART perhaps may feel less personal responsibility for the effectiveness of HAART. They have more of an attitude that the medication itself is 'the answer' and may more passively await receipt of the positive benefits that the medication has to offer.

The measurement of the attitudes of the HIV-1-positive men in our sample towards HAART was preceded by a period of on average 5.2 years (range: 1.4–12.6 years) of life as an HIV-1-positive person. During these pre-HAART years, these men had direct and indirect experiences with the development and clinical testing of new antiretroviral medications. Their experiences included several cycles of hopefulness followed by disappointment. Despite the continual development of new medications, many HIV-1-positive people continued to be diagnosed with AIDS and die.

Given this historical backdrop against which the attitudes of HIV-1-positive people towards HAART have developed, it is not surprising that participants in this study are more sceptical than optimistic in regard to HAART. Clinical experience indicates that people doing well on HAART quite often have fears of their viral load increasing and of toxicity. Scepticism towards HAART may serve as a form of psychological protection against these feared events. It may be that having this protection facilitates the process of making a difficult behavioural investment (strict adherence) in the presence of so much uncertainty and past disappointment.

Support was found in bivariate analyses for the hypothesised relationships between adherence and HAART side effects as well as time on HAART. Experiencing side effects that were less worse than expected was related to better adherence. Reactions to the initial side effects to HAART quite likely resonate with deeper fears of developing toxicity and having to discontinue treatment. Early attention by medical staff to the emotional impact of side effects and their relationship to adherence may help improve adherence. Being on HAART for a shorter period of time was related to better adherence. This argues for a focus not only on the initial attainment of adherence in those beginning on HAART, but also on the long-term maintenance of this behaviour. Different determinants may play a central role in initial vs. long-term adherence.

A limitation of the present study is in the measurement of adherence. Given that this investigation was carried out in the context of a larger study not focused on adherence, no measure of adherence was available other than self-report (e.g. electronic monitoring or judgement by a health care worker). It is known that patients tend to overestimate their level of adherence on self-report (Besch, 1995).

There are many factors related to the behavioural intention to adhere, having the skills to adhere, and having the skills to counteract factors leading to non-adherence which have not been investigated in these analyses, and which likely account for a large portion of the remaining variance in adherence. This chapter has only focused on a limited number of individual determinants of adherence. Aspects of the patient–provider relationship have not been studied at all. One such aspect which is possibly important to adherence is the HIV-1-positive person's feeling that beginning on HAART is a choice he or she has made jointly with medical staff, rather than an acquisition to pressure from the physician, AIDS nurse, partner, friends or family.

Conclusions

Initial data from this study indicate that the O/S scale of the PIAQ can be used to assess relevant attitudinal factors in research investigating adherence to HAART. A less optimistic attitude towards HAART was found to be related to better adherence. This finding differs from those of earlier studies that found a positive relationship between attitudes and adherence when studying antiretroviral monotherapy. This suggests that the determinants of adherence to HAART may differ from the determinants of adherence in the time of antiretroviral monotherapy and argues for the use of instruments specifically designed to assess the variables relevant to adherence to HAART in research investigating this topic.

Prospective studies are needed which assess determinants of adherence prior to the person beginning on HAART, as well as once HAART is begun, in order to identify these risk factors for low adherence (in the short and long term). These studies in turn can guide the development and subsequent evaluation of interventions to improve adherence.

Acknowledgements

The inspiration for this research comes from the participants of the Helen Dowling Institute HIV Study who have so openly and willingly shared with us their struggle to adapt to the rapidly changing face of HIV illness. The PIAQ was translated into Dutch by Roelinda Vording. Michael Antoni, Bert Garssen, Karl Goodkin, Niels Mulder and Theo Sandfort provided valuable critique and guidance. The funding for this research came from the Dutch Organization for Scientific Research (NW0), the Dutch Ministry of Health (VWS) and the Dutch AIDS Fund.

References

Aversa, S. L. and Kimberlin, C. (1996) 'Psychosocial aspects of antiretroviral medication use among HIV patients', *Patient Education and Counseling* 29: 207–219.
Besch, C. L. (1995) 'Compliance in clinical trials', *AIDS* 9: 1–10.

Carpenter, C. C. J., Fischl, M. A., Hammer, S. M., Hirsch, M. S., Jacobsen, D. M., and Katzenstein, D. A. (1997) 'Antiretroviral therapy for HIV infection in 1998: updated recommendations of the International AIDS Society – USA Panel', *Journal of the American Medical Association* 277: 1962–1969.

——(1998) 'Antiretroviral therapy for HIV infection in 1998: updated recommendations of the International AIDS Society – USA Panel', *Journal of the American Medical Association* 280: 78–86.

Catt, S., Stygall, J. and Catalan, J. (1995) 'Acceptance of zidovudine (AZT) in early HIV disease: the role of health beliefs', *AIDS Care* 7: 229–235.

Cluss, P. A. and Epstein, L. H. (1985) 'The measurement of medical compliance in the treatment of disease', in P. Karoly (ed.) *Measurement Strategies in Health Psychology*, New York: John Wiley.

Deeks, S., Loftus, R., Cohen, P., Chin, S., and Grant, R. M. (1997) 'Incidence and predictors of virologic failure to indinavir or/and ritonavir in an urban health clinic', *37th International Conference on Antimicrobial Agents and Chemotherapy, Toronto*, Abstract LB-2.

Gulick, R. *et al.* (1997) 'Indinavir, zidovudine, and lamivudine: concurrent or sequential therapy in ZDV-experienced patients', *37th International Conference on Antimicrobial Agents and Chemotherapy, Toronto*, Abstract I-89.

Haynes, R. B. (1976) 'A critical review of the "determinants" of patient compliance with therapeutic regimens', in D. L. Sackett and R. M. Haynes (eds) *Compliance with Therapeutic Regimens*, Baltimore, MD: Johns Hopkins University Press.

Ickovics, J. R. and Meisler, A. W. (1997) 'Adherence in AIDS clinical trials: a framework for clinical research and clinical care', *Journal of Clinical Epidemiology* 50: 385–391.

Mehta, S., Moore, R. D. and Graham, N. M. H. (1997) 'Potential factors affecting adherence with HIV therapy', *AIDS* 11: 1665–1670.

Morisky, D. E., Green, L. G. and Levine, D. M. (1986) 'Concurrent and predictive validity of a self-reported measure of medication adherence', *Medical Care* 24: 67–74.

Morse, E. V., Simon, P. M., Coburg, M., Hyssop, N., Greenspan, D. and Balson, P. M. (1991) 'Determinants of subject compliance within an experimental anti-HIV drug protocol', *Social Science and Medicine* 32: 1161–1167.

Muma, R. D., Ross, M. W., Parcel, G. S. and Pollard, R. M. (1995) 'Zidovudine adherence among individuals with HIV infection', *AIDS Care* 7: 439–447.

Samet, J. H., Libman, H., Steger, K. A., Dhawan, R. K., Chen, J. and Shevitz, A. H. (1992) 'Compliance with zidovudine therapy in patients infected with Human Immunodeficiency Virus, Type 1: a cross-sectional study in a municipal hospital clinic', *The American Journal of Medicine* 92: 495–502.

Singh, N., Squier, C., Sivek, C., Wagener, M., Hong Nguyen, M. and Yu, V. L. (1996) 'Determinants of compliance with antiretroviral therapy in patients with human immunodeficiency virus: prospective assessment with implications for enhancing compliance, *AIDS Care* 8: 261–269.

Smith, M. Y., Rapkin, B. D., Morrison, A. and Kammerman, S. (1997) 'Zidovudine adherence in persons with AIDS: the relationship of patient beliefs about medication to self-termination of therapy', *Journal of General Internal Medicine* 12: 216–223.

5 Living with HIV/AIDS and adherence to antiretroviral treatments

Jean-Paul Moatti and Bruno Spire

In this chapter, we will show how HIV and AIDS have renewed interest in patients' responses to medical treatment and, in particular, questions of adherence and compliance, the latter not being free of paternalistic (or even coercive) overtones. We will describe how issues of patient adherence came to the fore with the advent of highly active antiretroviral therapy (HAART), and will argue that two alternative and conflicting approaches persist. The first of these approaches aims to predict and correct non-adherent behaviour in patients, and sometimes suggests that such predictions may justify denying individuals treatment. The second, alternative, approach aims to offer support to all HIV-infected patients medically eligible for HAART through individualised plans to help facilitate the management of treatment in daily life. Both approaches encourage socio-behavioural researchers to increase their understanding of the determinants of adherence to treatment, but the demands they make on social science are quite different. The first 'predictive' approach mainly focuses on the identification of individual barriers to good adherence and calls for social interventions to help improve patients' acceptance of prescribed regimens. The alternative 'empathic' approach emphasises the value of social science research in which patients' subjective experience of illness is a central concern, and which aims to go beyond issues of adherence to promote a new type of physician/patient relationship based on shared decision making.

From compliance to adherence

An old issue

Long before the AIDS epidemic, social scientists described how lay people's beliefs and perceptions of ill health may differ from biomedical models of diseases, and how patients' behaviours often do not conform to the medical regimens prescribed by physicians (e.g. Becker, 1985; Myers and Midence, 1998). As highlighted in a 1984 review of sixteen studies on patients' attitudes and behaviours in response to medical prescriptions in various chronic diseases (hypertension, diabetes, chronic renal failure, asthma, etc.), non-compliance has always been a widespread and possibly universal phenomenon. In all of these studies, long-term compliance to medical prescriptions was observed in only 20 per cent to 40 per cent of patients, and with respect to keeping medical appointments in no more than 50 per cent to 80 per cent of cases (Janz and Becker, 1984). Some authors have gone so far as to argue that non-compliance is the most serious problem that modern medicine will have to face in the future (Dunbar, 1990; Miller, 1997).

It is fairly trivial for social scientists to observe that lay people do not always behave in the way experts think they should. Numerous studies have shown how cultural context and social representations (i.e. individual mental schemes influenced by group pressure and norms) have a direct effect on the physician/patient relationship (e.g. Herzlich, 1973). What may be less trivial is that a body of social science research has shown that non-compliance to medical care is not necessarily some kind of irrational behaviour, and is related not only to patients' individual responsibilities but also to their inter-actions with physicians, the health care system and the social environment. Studies have described how discriminatory stereotypes often interfere with health care professionals' attitudes towards patients with marginal lifestyles (Kelly *et al.*, 1987; Moatti *et al.*, 1997), while other work has analysed how medical decision making with respect to similar clinical conditions, including physician's descriptions of case presentations themselves, may vary according to patients' gender, ethnicity or social class (Conrad and Schneider, 1980; Anspach, 1988).

In the early years of the AIDS epidemic, when no effective antiretroviral drugs were available, compliance to treatment among HIV-infected patients was not a matter of much debate. The potential detrimental effects of delays in access to HIV testing in populations with a high frequency of HIV-related risk behaviours, as well as delays between first medical visit for HIV care after an initial HIV diagnosis, on the natural history of HIV infection were, however, commented upon (Katz *et al.*, 1992). Later, clinicians, epidemiologists and public health experts expressed concern that important biases might be introduced into randomised clinical trials of the first antiretroviral drugs (zidovudine – AZT – and the other nucleoside reverse transcriptase inhibitors) if a significant number of enrolled patients were lost for follow-up and/or failed to comply with the study protocols without medical staff knowing it. Consequently, eligibility criteria for clinical trials often included, in addition to clinical and immunological variables (CD4+ cell counts), a rather vague psychological assessment of the patient's ability to comply with the trial protocol. The application of these principles resulted in the limited participation and sometimes open exclusion of women, ethnic minorities and injecting drug users. Reports that in San Francisco HIV-infected asymptomatic patients enrolled in the most important US trial (ACTG 019) of zidovudine versus a placebo were developing sophisticated strategies, including the interpretation of biological assays, to unblind the trial and to guarantee access to the drug for all participants,[1] created alarm in the scientific and biomedical community (Chesney and Folkman, 1994).

A new major issue

Over the last three years, the clinical care of people with HIV has been substantially affected by the introduction of HAART (i.e. by multiple combination therapies involving the new HIV-specific protease inhibitors (PIs) and previously existing antiretroviral drugs). These new therapies can decrease viral loads to undetectable levels, significantly reduce the incidence of HIV-related opportunistic infections, and restore health and a decent quality of life among a large number of people with HIV and AIDS. Scientific evidence has offered a strong rationale for the earlier initiation of these more aggressive antiretroviral therapies, and for their long-term maintenance until other new, not yet discovered, drugs can guarantee the total eradication of HIV from the body (Deeks *et al.*, 1997).

Inadequate adherence has important implications both for the individual and the public heath effectiveness of these therapeutic advances (Mehta *et al.*, 1997). At the 12th World AIDS Conference in Geneva in July 1998, a total of 190 abstracts were devoted to this topic, consideration of which was nearly completely absent in the previous eleven meetings. Poor adherence can lead to a rapid rate of viral replication. This, together with a high rate of mutation, can in turn lead to the development of drug resistance, particularly in the presence of selective pressure by antiretroviral therapies. Although it may have other pharmacological and biological causes, resistance can develop if drug doses are inadequate or doses are missed, and the subsequent loss of drug activity may impede the long-term effectiveness of therapy. In early trials of HAART, patients receiving suboptimal dosages quickly developed resistance, which persisted even when higher doses were later administered. In more recent trials, non-adherence has been suspected as being the main explanatory factor for short-term 'therapeutic failure' (Descamps *et al.*, 1998; Hecht *et al.*, 1998a). Another unfortunate long-term consequence can be cross-resistance to alternative HIV treatments not yet tried – resistance to one agent being potentially able to limit sustained suppression of viral replication by other existing or future drugs (Moutouh *et al.*, 1996).

Last but not least, the prospect of resistance not only makes individual patients vulnerable to HIV strains that are unresponsive to available treatments, but also raises the spectre of a public health threat that could potentially neutralise the collective benefit of therapeutic advances (Wainberg and Friedland, 1998). If a new infection occurs with an HIV subtype which has already acquired genetic resistance against actual therapies, the newly infected individual will not only have contracted a deadly disease but have a reduced chance of survival due to the ineffectiveness of current (and maybe future) drugs. Outbreaks of multidrug-resistant tuberculosis have been observed among AIDS patients in the past (Edlin *et al.*, 1992), and the first cases of infection by strains of HIV which are already resistant to protease inhibitors have been reported (Hecht *et al.*, 1998b).

Fearing the possible diffusion of untreatable drug-resistant HIV strains, some physicians have advocated withholding HAART where the risks of patients' non-adherence are high (Senak, 1997; Stewart, 1997). Because AIDS is caused by an infectious transmissible agent, conflicts and heated controversies have often occurred over the tension between protecting individuals' rights and public health interests (Emanuel, 1988; Kirp and Bayer, 1992). Current concerns that individual non-adherence may, in the aggregate, have catastrophic consequences for public health have revived conflicts about the degree of coercive control that is needed in AIDS policy.

As is often the case in similar circumstances where social and ethical controversies imply fundamental value judgements in the context of major uncertainties about technical and scientific data (Fischhoff, 1983), debates about terminology that may seem unnecessarily subtle and even pathetic take on strong social meanings. This has clearly been the case with respect to the use of the term 'compliance' in the field of AIDS. Previous research addressing the extent to which a patient's behaviour towards care or preventive recommendations coincides with medical or health advice nearly always referred to patient 'compliance', and, initially, much HIV- and AIDS-related literature used the words 'compliance' and 'adherence' interchangeably.

As soon as the political and social implications of the issue became clearer, however, the term 'compliance' was criticised by many, including NGOs, as carrying judgemental and pejorative overtones, and for putting too great an emphasis on patient failings with respect to norms dictated by the medical profession. The now systematic replacement of the word 'compliance' by the notion of adherence,[2] which is thought to allow for a more balanced perspective between physicians and patients (Ley, 1988), may be understood as a political message sent to the world, and especially to people living with HIV. It is a way of suggesting that it is still necessary to oppose openly coercive AIDS policies, even if therapeutic advances provide some opportunity for coercive public health measures to be presented as overriding patients' own wishes. As will be shown below, it remains to be seen whether or not some approaches of adherence nevertheless carry subtle elements of blame and discrimination with respect to access to care for certain patients groups.

How adherent is adherent enough?

How much adherence is needed?

Several US public health researchers have recently proposed a less passionate approach to this debate (Mehta *et al.*, 1997). They have suggested that adherence, on the one hand, should relate to an objective measurement of the 'extent to which the patient follows a prescribed regimen'. Compliance, on the other hand, should be considered as 'an overall evaluation of adherence', from the point of view of medical effectiveness of treatment. This suggestion has the merit of pointing out that a key factor in the adherence/compliance debate is the minimum threshold of therapy necessary for effectiveness.

For the prophylaxis of HIV-related opportunistic infections such as *Pneumocysitis cariniii* pneumonia, the threshold had been shown to be fairly low. It has been shown that such treatments tend to be effective even where there is limited patient adherence (Ruskin and Larivière, 1991). What the threshold for clinical effectiveness is for HAART is still unclear. Preliminary data suggest that it is necessary to take a high proportion (90 per cent or more) of protease inhibitor doses to maintain the suppression of viral replication (Hecht *et al.*, 1998a). A recent study in a small sample of patients concluded that 'more than 95% adherence to protease inhibitor therapy is associated with virologic success and failure rates increase sharply with decreasing levels of adherence' (Paterson *et al.*, 1999). Limited scientific evidence exists for recommendations to patients about the 'acceptable' levels of adherence and about the behaviours that are most detrimental to the effectiveness of antiretroviral drugs and which therefore should be avoided.[3]

Because no rigorous assessments in large cohorts of patients with sufficient follow-up have as yet been undertaken, it is by pragmatic analogy with treatments of other infectious diseases such as tuberculosis (Mehta *et al.*, 1997) that experts consider that a minimum of 80 per cent ingestion of prescribed doses of HAART is required.

How much adherence is possible?

Maintaining such high levels of adherence for an indefinite period of time (and perhaps for life) may seem a quite unrealistic goal. Documented adherence to treatment drugs in other chronic diseases has always been lower than this in the past history of modern medicine. With respect to AZT monotherapy, less than half of HIV-infected patients were able to reach 80 per cent adherence once the period of observation was greater than a week (Muma *et al.*, 1995; Singh *et al.*, 1996).

The constraints that current HAART combinations impose on patients' daily lives make it difficult to anticipate that a medical norm of 80–100 per cent adherence can be reached and sustained by most individuals. The daily number of prescribed pills for antiretroviral treatments alone varies from ten to twenty, and daily intakes from three to four. Furthermore, the pharmacological properties of each drug often impose very specific modalities of intake in order to guarantee optimal delivery in the human body: some drugs have to be taken at regular time intervals; others have to be taken before or after meals; and some drugs can never be taken together at the same time. Prescribed regimens quickly become complex as soon as the combined drugs simultaneously necessitate different types of constraints.[4]

Moreover, all HAART combinations are associated with short-term painful or disturbing side effects that can affect patients' quality of life. In the French APROCO cohort,[5] for example, 85 per cent of patients reported at least one disturbing side effect during the first month after the initiation of HAART, mainly diarrhoea (50 per cent), nausea (48 per cent) and abdominal pain (42 per cent) (Souville *et al.*, 1999). In addition, there are growing concerns about possible long-term toxicity of HAART, as suggested by the observed high incidence of metabolic disorders among patients receiving this kind of treatment. The most common of these is lipodystrophy – an abnormal fat distribution which increases risk of cardio-vascular diseases, but also negatively affects body image.

It is therefore not surprising that in all current studies world-wide the reason most often cited by patients for skipping doses is that they 'simply forgot'. Clinical and pharmacological research to identify simpler and easier effective antiretroviral regimens will help reduce some of the practical constraints on patients' lives. However, contrary to the beliefs of some pharmaceutical company experts, modifications to the technical characteristics of drugs are not sufficient *per se* to solve the adherence problem, because these are not mechanistic determinants of patients' behaviours. For example, in a subsample (n = 164) of the French MANIF 2.000 cohort study of patients HIV infected through injecting drug use,[6] we found no correlation between the number of prescribed pills and self-reported adherence to HAART during the week prior to the first follow-up visit in the cohort after the initiation of these therapies.

Although some patients will have more difficulties than others with treatment, it can be expected that nearly all patients will not strictly adhere to the prescribed regimens at some point in time. Repeated measures in longitudinal studies reveal how cross-sectional assessments (on which most current evidence is based) globally classify as non-adherent patients who have very heterogeneous behaviours and face very different kinds of difficulties. In the APROCO cohort, for example, 61.9 per cent of patients report having been strictly adherent to protease inhibitors during the week prior to both the first- and fourth-month follow-up visits after the initiation of HAART, and only 17.0 per cent reported non-adherence at both visits. However, an additional 21.1 per cent were non-adherent at one of the two points of measurement (Souville *et al.*, 1999).

Adherence assessment itself raises complex methodological difficulties. Biomedical scientists often argue that an 'objective' assessment can only be obtained through technical means because self-reported measures of medication adherence are subject to social desirability and recall bias (Paterson *et al.*, 1999). They argue that pill counts obtained through electronic monitoring and bioassays measuring the plasma concentration of drugs should become the 'gold standards' of adherence assessment, implicitly suggesting that such technical assessments do not lie as human beings do. These arguments ignore the fact that such approaches, although they may help cross-validate individuals' self-reports, are also subject to bias and practical limitations. Current pharmacological techniques can only indicate the absorption of drugs over the last few hours (going back no more than forty-eight to seventy-two hours), and they cannot distinguish between suboptimal dosages due to non-adherence and biological interindividual variability.

Although self-reports may underestimate non-adherence, especially when data collection is part of the ongoing patient/medical staff relationship, when used in a controlled design and as part of a multimethod approach, patients' accounts do have good validity (Morisky *et al.*, 1986). Recent significant correlations between viral load and self-reports of adherence in patients treated with HAART tend to confirm this (Nieukwerk *et al.*, 1998 ; Weidle *et al.*, 1998). In the MANIF 2.000 cohort study mentioned above, at first visit after initiation of HAART, the fifty-seven patients (34.8 per cent) who reported having taken less than 80 per cent of the total dose prescribed in the previous week had significantly higher mean plasma viral values, as well as a lower decrease in viral load titres measured before and after initiation of HAART, than the 107 patients who reported 80–100 per cent adherence.

Adherence: from prediction to understanding

Methodological debates about the assessment of adherence reflect basic controversies between the two alternative approaches to defining and understanding adherence referred to earlier.

The limits of the 'predictive approach' to adherence

The standard approach of predicting non-adherent behaviours and identifying those patients most 'at risk' of exhibiting such behaviours is still predominant among health care givers. This approach can either lead to various interventions for 'correcting' non-adherent behaviours (Haynes *et al.*, 1996) or, in extreme cases, provide justification for denying treatment to certain patients. This 'predictive' approach faces many problems as health care professionals committed to the care of HIV/AIDS patients have progressively discovered.

Contrary to the beliefs of many clinicians, studies prior to AIDS never established stable and clear correlations between patient adherence, socio-demographic and cultural characteristics and personality traits (Becker, 1985; Dunbar, 1990). Social research instead highlighted the importance of positive interaction, adequate social support, quality of communication and physician trust, etc., as a means of increasing adherence. Because non-adherence cannot reliably be predicted on the basis of a few easy-to-identify patient characteristics, the 'predictive approach' is always prone to judgemental and pejorative assessments of patient behaviours, knowingly or unknowingly influenced by social stereotypes. This approach also ignores the dynamic character of patients' behaviours toward care by trying a priori to distinguish between intrinsically non-adherent patients and others. Longitudinal follow-up shows how adherence is not a black or white phenomenon but rather a continuously evolving set of behaviours.

Of course, some studies among HIV-infected patients have found that younger age, male gender, lower socio-economic status, alcohol and drug abuse, stress or depressed moods are statistically correlated with non-adherence (Mehta *et al.*, 1997), but other studies in similar populations are not consistent with these findings, or have even found correlations between the same factors, in the opposite direction (Broers *et al.*, 1994; Kissinger *et al.*, 1995; Singh *et al.*, 1996; Eldred *et al.*, 1997). From our point of view, these contradictory interpretations of study findings result from a misleading and basic flaw in the 'predictive' approach. By placing too much emphasis on unidirectional pseudo-causal relationships, this approach does not sufficiently take into account the possibility that the same individual or group characteristics may produce very different outcomes in terms of adherence, depending on their interactions with the social environment. As we will discuss in more depth below in relation to injecting drug users (IDUs), the 'predictive' approach tends to underestimate the conjoint responsibilities of the health care system itself in the 'social production of non-adherence'.[7]

The case of IDUs: supplier-induced non-adherence?

HIV-infected IDUs are a group that professionals often view as being at high risk for non-adherence. Official US guidelines recommend the prescription of HAART to medically eligible former IDUs, but suggest delaying such treatment until active drug use has ceased (CDC, 1998). It is also well established that HIV-infected IDUs tend to have poorer access to medical care than other transmission groups (Crystal *et al.*, 1995; Tramarin *et al.*, 1997). Lack of health care insurance coverage is of course related to unmet health care needs of people living with HIV/AIDS (Hu *et al.*, 1995), but important inequities in the utilisation of HIV health care services still exist when free or low-cost public sector care is available (Kissinger *et al.*, 1995), as is the case in the French context where financial barriers to care have been abolished for all HIV-infected individuals.[8] For example, among the 123 patients with less than 400 CD4+ cells/mm^3 enrolled in the first year of the MANIF 2.000 cohort (October 1995–1996, i.e. before diffusion of HAART), only a minority (43.9 per cent) had already received antiretroviral treatment, despite official guidelines strongly recommending the initiation of treatment at this level of immunosuppression (Carrieri *et al.*, 1999).

Moreover, with respect to former IDUs, and after adjustment for clinical stage and other medical characteristics, HIV-infected patients who were still active IDUs were three times less likely to receive treatment. Interestingly, while the proportions of active and ex-IDUs who self-reported that they are 'rarely' adherent with medications were similar in both groups (33.8 per cent vs. 38.2 per cent – not significant), prescribing physicians' perceptions of individual patients' adherence did differ. Physicians viewed only 23.1 per cent of their ex-IDU patients as being 'poorly' adherent, while they strongly associated active injectors with non-adherence (56.8 per cent).

Subjective judgements of doctors and anticipation of poor adherence influence decisions to withhold antiretroviral treatment to HIV-infected patients who continue to use drugs. These judgements are not the 'pure' products of preconceived ideological categories: physicians in the MANIF 2.000 study were part of hospital departments with long experience of HIV care, and it is well known that discriminatory biases decline as health professionals become familiar with treating people with HIV (Gerbert *et al.*, 1991). These professional judgements are all the more powerful because they were partly based on previous experience with these patients in clinical interaction and on the fact that active IDU patients, in our sample as in others (Bonuck and Arno, 1997), live in worse social and psychological conditions than ex-IDUs, which create additional difficulties for continuity of care.

The problem here, that as the emerging paradigm of 'social exclusion' discussed elsewhere in this volume[9] points out, is that these judgements, by taking for granted the mental representation of the fatally 'non-compliant' IDU, reinforce marginalisation which, in turn, may further compound IDUs' difficulties with adherence. These judgements also ignore the possibility that, when specific and appropriate efforts are made to encourage IDUs to accept treatment, they can be as adherent as other patient groups (Freeman *et al.*, 1996; Broers *et al.*, 1994).

A similar, but opposite, discordance between physicians' perceptions and patients' behaviours can be found elsewhere in the MANIF 2.000 study, after the advent of HAART. Among the 164 patients who have started HAART, physicians persist in claiming that ex-IDUs ($n = 113$) are more likely in their view to be 'always or often adherent' (82.3 per cent) than opiate-dependent patients receiving ambulatory buprenorphine drug maintenance treatment ($n = 30$) (64.5 per cent) ($p < 0.05$). Assessment, however, shows that the latter are at least as adherent (78.1 per cent) as the former (65.5 per cent).[10] Physicians *de facto* tend to underestimate the fact that through changes in the IDU's interactions with his or her environment associated with a reduced quest for illegal drugs, drug maintenance treatment may be a useful adjunct to antiretroviral treatment in this population. In this same study, and independently of current drug use, the number of reported stressful negative 'life-events' (such as loss of financial resources or confrontation with the police) in the prior six months was significantly higher among non-adherent patients than in the rest of the sample.

The alternative 'empathic' approach

The hope, but also some of the challenges, that HAART has brought to people living with HIV and AIDS and also to care givers has contributed to the emergence of an alternative approach. This new approach establishes a radical break with 'predictive' notions of adherence and paternalistic models of compliance. Rather than trying to 'predict' non-adherent behaviour, it urges physicians instead to 'focus on helping all patients to take their medications more successfully' and to 'encourage the active participation of HIV-positive persons in their own treatment' (Lerner *et al.*, 1998). In this approach, which derives from the positive heritage of AIDS 'exceptionalism' in the historical management of the epidemic, priority is given to the patient's autonomy of choice and the protection of individual rights. These principles are even seen as a more effective means of preventing the public health risk of the development of treatment resistance. From this perspective, psychosocial interventions are not conceived as a way of 'removing barriers' that are supposed to impede patients from behaving accordingly to medical norms. Rather, they are seen as a tool for encouraging all HIV-positive patients to devise individualised treatment plans that will enable them to obtain maximum benefit from treatment (Lerner *et al.*, 1998).

From adherence to shared decision making

Do we hear the furious echoes from the real world?[11]

Until HAART, the official involvement of social scientists in HIV- and AIDS-related clinical research projects had been fairly limited, especially in Europe. Key addresses to the 2nd European Conference on the Methods and Results of Social and Behavioural Research on AIDS (New Challenges for Social and Behavioural Science) by prominent clinical and biomedical experts were emblematic of a change. Social and behavioural scientists are currently sought by proponents of both 'predictive' and 'empathic' approaches to adherence, as well as by patients' self-help groups. But the essence of these demands emanating from the 'real world' are quite different, and have direct repercussions on scientific and methodological debates among social scientists.

The 'prescriptive' approach is more in line with studies that tend to analyse patients' reluctance to conform to medical prescriptions in terms of the 'social acceptability' of techniques and innovations. This idea of social acceptability has been (and to a certain extent still is) the dominant paradigm in social science work on technological hazards and risks (National Research Council, 1989). It establishes a clear-cut distinction between scientific knowledge and other forms of human experience, and sees technical expertise as the main source of instrumental rationality in modern societies (Fischhoff *et al.*, 1981). The lay public's attitudes and behaviours which diverge from technical 'rationality' can be understood as the product of misconceptions and misunderstandings resulting from individuals following their own self-interests. These conceptions do not necessarily mean a conservative defence of existing public policies and the dominant social order; they can sometimes express radical criticisms (as soon as they estimate that current policies are not a rational use of resources for maximising the collective 'good'). However, they assume that social scientists have a useful social function to play if their work helps increase the social acceptance of collectively beneficial technological innovations.

In our view, the 'prescriptive' approach to adherence shares an affinity with traditional health sociological concepts concerned with the 'sick role' and 'illness behaviour'. These concepts argue that in order to prevent the potentially disruptive consequences of illness on a group or society, there exists a set of shared cultural rules or norms (the sick role). These norms legitimate the deviations caused by illnesses, but at the same time channel sick people's illness behaviours into reintegrating the physician/patient relationship (Segall, 1976; Parsons, 1951). While these concepts have contributed to social scientific understanding of illness and medical care, they reinforce a 'doctor/centred' picture by making the receipt of medical care the centrepiece of attention, and by neglecting patients' subjective experience of illness. Therefore, in the context of current HIV-related debates about adherence, such concepts may insufficiently depart from normative biomedical models.

Alternative approaches such as Corbin and Strauss's (1986) concept of 'illness trajectories' focus more on insider accounts of what it is to be sick, interactions with others, effects of illness on identity and people's strategies for managing symptoms (Radley and Billig, 1996). Such approaches consider that the patient's actual experience of his or her disease and care must be placed at the centre of social scientists' investigations, and consequently are more closely allied to the new 'empathic' approach to adherence.

These debates should not, however, be confounded with the classical opposition between qualitative and quantitative methods. On the one hand, it is true that ethnological or anthropological methods may more easily capture the complex impact of recent therapeutic advances on the individual histories of people living with the HIV/AIDS disease. However, generalisation of qualitative findings necessarily implies going beyond anecdotal reports to look at regularities in patients' behaviours, and their determinants.

On the other hand, most quantitative surveys and analyses of adherence explicitly (or unconsciously) rely on methodologies derived from individualistic approaches.[12] The most common (and paradigmatic) of these psychosocial models is the Health Belief Model (HBM) (Janz and Becker, 1984). In the case of adherence, this model tries to explain variance of individual responses to medical prescriptions in terms of a set of belief-related factors (perceived 'barriers' to treatment, i.e. subjective expectations about material and psychological costs associated with seeking and consuming health care, perceived severity of disease, and perceived individual benefit of treatment) that are assumed to have multiplicative interactive effects. In our view, the criticism already addressed to the applications of this model to HIV prevention still holds in the field of HIV care. This model usually obtains 'a largely tautological set of results where what are taken to be the explanatory factors are in fact nothing but another way of expressing the dependent variable that the model is supposed to explain' (Moatti et al., 1997).

But, contrary to other critics of the HBM and of affiliated psychosocial theories,[13] we do not consider that any attempt to identify the determinants of adherence through the quantitative (statistical) aggregation of individual patients' self-reports and/or observed behaviours is doomed to oversimplification. On the contrary, appropriate quantitative data collection can help us better understand the social interactions that are key to promoting an 'empathic' approach to adherence. To go beyond old quarrels between quantitative and qualitative research, and to try to combine both methods so as to investigate the problems faced by patients in the course of their disease and treatment, not only is a matter of esoteric debate among social scientists, but may affect the impact of their work in the 'real world' of HIV care.

Shared decision making for managing uncertainties

Since the beginning of the AIDS epidemic, health sociologists have recognised that dealing with uncertainty is a central problem for people living with HIV (Weitz, 1989; Pierret, 1991). With the advent of HAART, the management of therapeutic uncertainty is an increasing burden for both patients and their care givers (Dormont, 1997; DHHS, 1998).

Current data, including variability among different biological assays, do not permit the determination of an absolute plasma HIV RNA threshold for initiation of HAART. Criteria for identification of treatment failure and clinical decisions to switch HAART regimens also remain a matter of debate. The biological plausibility of early intervention needs to be weighed against the potential toxicity of therapy and the restrictions placed on treatment options in later disease. On all these issues, clinical guidelines tend to differ between countries, and within countries, or offer rather ambiguous recommendations (Voelker, 1997). Thus HIV/AIDS physicians and patients must continually make choices based on data that are not fully mature, and have to face major uncertainties about choices which may jeopardise their future.

Experience with adherence to antiretroviral treatments of people living with HIV/AIDS has already profoundly challenged the conventional model of medical decision making, where patient involvement (if any) is limited to providing consent to the treatment advocated by the physician and doing their best to comply with it. In this 'paternalistic' model, the medical expert is supposed to act as the 'perfect agent' of the patient accordingly to the

Hippocratic oath (i.e. to take the decision that the patient would have taken if he or she had the same level of scientific knowledge (Mooney and Ryan, 1993)).

In most acute and chronic deadly diseases, therapeutic decisions imply difficult trade-offs between prolonging life and enhancing its quality. It is an established fact which contradicts conventional medical decision making that patients' perceptions and preferences towards such trade-offs may widely (and legitimately) differ from those of prescribing physicians (McNeil and Pauker, 1982). Shared decision making between the patient and his or her physician is therefore increasingly advocated as the ideal model in the choice of medical treatment (Emanuel and Emanuel, 1992).

Major uncertainties about the long-term effectiveness of HAART at the individual as well as the community level make these trade-offs even more complex in HIV-related care; people living with HIV/AIDS and their care givers will have to be pioneers of this new type of partnership between patients and biomedical experts. Social scientists should not restrict themselves to contemplating the course of this historical process of change in relationships between patients and professionals, which is likely to affect the future not only of the fight against AIDS but of the whole health care system. Rather, they should take an active part in it. They also have to take clear stands in the debates and conflicts that will certainly arise along the way between the alternative approaches of adherence that currently co-exist in the biomedical field of AIDS research and care.

Notes

1 Patients quickly knew that AZT increases MCV (mean corpuscular volume) values that are easily measured by a simple blood count. They used the result of the bioassay to identify whether or not they were in the placebo arm and started to share their AZT with patients in the experimental arm.
2 The term 'compliance' was *de facto* banned at the 12th World AIDS Conference. It is worth noting that the correct French word of reference (*observance*) takes a more neutral and intermediary stance between compliance and adherence.
3 The only recommendation over which there is a consensus in the current state of knowledge is that 'skipping doses' from time to time is worse that totally stopping treatment for a certain period of time.
4 To give one example, a patient taking a combination of stavudine, didanosine and indinavir will have a minimum of four different intakes per day. Some of them will have to be separated by eight hours and all of them must be taken outside meals. In practice, adherence to this regimen implies getting up every day at 7 a.m. and going to bed at 11 p.m. with very little flexibility in between, and strict planning of hours for meals.
5 The APROCO cohort is a multicentre cohort of unselected HIV-infected patients recruited at first medical visit in hospital departments where a protease inhibitor is prescribed. The protocol incorporates in-depth psychosocial assessment. Results presented here concern the first 362 patients included (May–November 1997). Adherence assessment is based on patients' reports on self-administered questionnaires about their behaviour during the week prior to the visit.

6 MANIF 2.000 is a prospective study started in October 1995 which enrols patients initially infected by HIV through injection drug use, aged 18 years or more, with CD4+ cell counts greater than $300/mm^3$ and no opportunistic infections at the last visit before enrolment. Enrolment is in hospital departments in south-eastern France and in the Paris inner suburbs. For patients receiving antiretroviral treatment, assessment of adherence takes place via a face-to-face questionnaire administered by a nurse at each visit. This asks for the daily number of doses prescribed and taken during the previous week. Patients' reports are cross-validated by their answers on the same issue in an additional self-administered questionnaire which they fill in alone during the same visit. In the data presented here, adherence assessment was carried out after a median duration of 5.3 months of protease inhibitor use (interquartile range = 3.0–9.3).

7 We use this expression as an analogy to the more global idea of the social production of disease and illness, a familiar concept in the sociology of health (Conrad and Schneider, 1980).

8 Since 1993 all medical care has been free of charge, paid for by the French social security system as soon as a patient has a diagnosis of HIV infection.

9 See France Lert's contribution in this volume.

10 This difference in favour of greater adherence for patients on DMT does not, however, reach statistical significance, even after adjustment for confounding factors, in multiple logistic regression. The mechanism we have just described can be viewed as a special case of 'achieved auto-prophecy' (Boudon et al., 1997).

11 The French-speaking reader may detect the analogy here with the emblematic song of anti-Nazi partisans during the Second World War.

12 Including Jeffrey Weiss's contribution in this volume, as well as our own research presented above with the APROCO and MANIF 2.000 cohort studies.

13 See, for example, Geneviève Paicheler's contribution in this volume.

References

Anspach, R. R. (1988) 'The language of case presentation', *Journal of Health Social Behaviour* 8(29): 319–338.

Becker, M. H. (1985) 'Patient adherence to prescribed therapies', *Medical Care* 23: 539–555.

Bonuck, K. A. and Arno, P. S. (1997) 'Social and medical factors affecting hospital discharge of persons with HIV/AIDS', *Journal of Epidemiology and Community Health* 22: 225–232.

Boudon, R., Bouvier, A. and Chazel, F. (1997) *Cognition et Sciences Sociales*, Paris: PUF.

Broers, B., Morabia, A. and Hirschel, B. (1994) 'A cohort study of drug users' compliance with zidovudine treatment', *Archives of International Medicine* 154: 1121–1127.

Carrieri, M. P. et al. (1999) 'Access to antiretroviral therapy among French HIV-infected injection drug users (IDUs): the influence of continued drug use', *Journal of Epidemiology and Community Health* 53: 4–8.

Centers for Disease Control and Prevention (CDC) (1998) 'Guidelines for the use of antiretroviral agents in HIV-infected adults and adolescents', *MMWR* 47(RR-5): 43–82.

Chesney, M. and Folkman, S. (1994) 'Psychological impact of HIV disease and implications for intervention', *Psychiatric Clinics of North America* 12: 259–268.

Conrad, P. and Schneider, J. W. C. (1980) *Deviance and Medicalization: From Badness to Sickness*, Saint Louis, MO: Mosby.

Corbin, J. and Strauss, A. (1986) 'Managing chronic illness at home: three lines of work', *Qualitative Sociology* 8: 224–247.

Crystal, S., Sambamoorthui, U. and Merzel, C. (1995) 'The diffusion of innovation in AIDS treatment: zidovudine use in two New Jersey cohorts', *Health Service Research* 30: 593–614.

Deeks, S. G., Smith, M., Holodniy, M. and Kahn, J. O. (1997) 'HIV-1 protease inhibitors. A review for clinicians', *Journal of the American Medical Association* 277: 145–153.

Department of Health and Human Services (DHHS) (1998) *Panel on Clinical Practices for Treatment of HIV Infection. Guidelines for the Use of Antiretroviral Agents in HIV-infected Adults and Adolescents*, Updated March, Washington, DC.

Descamps, D. *et al.* (1998) 'Analyse génotypique de la résistance chez les patients échappant au traitement de maintenance dans l'essai Trilège ANRS O72', *2ᵉ Séminaire annuel de la recherche clinique sur l'infection à VIH, ANRS, Paris, 10–11 December.*

Dormont, J. (ed.) (1997) 'Stratégies d'utilisation des antirétroviraux dans l'infection à VIH' (in French), Rapport 1997, Paris, Ministère de l'Emploi et de la Solidarité-Secrétariat d'Etat à la Santé, Médecine-Sciences: Flammarion.

Dunbar, J. (1990) 'Predictors of patient adherence: patient characteristics', in S. A. Shumaker *et al.* (eds) *The Handbook of Health Behavior Change*, New York: Springer.

Edlin, B. R. *et al.* (1992) 'An outbreak of multidrug-resistant tuberculosis among hospitalized patients with the acquired immunodeficiency syndrome', *New England Journal of Medicine* 326: 1514–1521.

Eldred, L. J., Wu, A., Chaisson, R. and Moore, R. D. (1997) 'Adherence to antiretroviral therapy in HIV disease', Paper presented at the Fourth Conference on Retroviruses and Opportunistic Infections, Chicago, January.

Emanuel, E. J. (1988) 'Do physicians have an obligation to treat patients with AIDS?', *New England Journal of Medicine* 318: 1686–1690.

Emanuel, E. J. and Emanuel, E. L. (1992) 'Four models of physician/patient relationship', *Journal of the American Medical Association* 267: 2221–2226.

Fischhoff, B. (1983) ' "Acceptable risk": the case of nuclear power', *Journal of Policy Analysis and Management* 2: 559–575.

Fischhoff, B., Lichtenstein, S., Slovic, P., Derby, S. L. and Keeney, R. L. (1981) *Acceptable Risk*, New York: Cambridge University Press.

Freeman, R. C., Rodriguez, G. M. and French, J. F. (1996) 'Compliance with AZT treatment regimen of HIV seropositive HIV injection drug users: a neglected issue', *Aids Education & Prevention* 8: 58–64.

Gerbert, B. *et al.* (1991) 'Primary care physicians and AIDS: attitudinal and structural barriers to care', *Journal of the American Medical Association* 266: 2837–2842.

Haynes, R. B., McKibbon, K. A. and Kanani, R. (1996) 'Systematic review of randomized trials of interventions to assist patients to follow prescriptions for medications', *Lancet* 100: 258–268.

Hecht, F. M., Colfax, G., Swanson, M. and Chesney, M. (1998a) 'Adherence and effectiveness of protease inhibitors in clinical practice', Paper presented at the 5th Conference on Retroviruses and Opportunistic Infections, Chicago, February.

Hecht, F. M., Kahn, J. O., Dillon, B., Chesney, M. and Grant, R. M. (1998b) 'Transmission of protease inhibitor resistant HIV-1 to a recently infected antiretroviral-naïve man: the UCSF-options primary HIV project', *12th International AIDS Conference, Geneva*, Abstract 32228.

Herzlich, C. (1973) *Health and Illness*, London: Academic Press.

Hu, D. J. *et al.* (1995) 'Characteristics of persons with late AIDS diagnosis in the United States', *American Journal of Prevention Medicine* 11: 114–119.

Janz, N. K. and Becker, M. H. (1984) 'The Health Belief Model: a decade later', *Health Education Quarterly* 11: 1–47.

Katz, M., Bindman, A. and Komaromy, M. (1992) 'Coping with HIV infection: why people delay care', *Annals of International Medicine* 117: 797–800.

Kelly, J. A., Lawrence, J. S., Smith, S., Hood, H. V. and Cook, D. J. (1987) 'Stigmatization of AIDS patients by physicians', *American Journal of Public Health* 77: 789–791.

Kirp, D. L. and Bayer, R. (1992) *AIDS in the Industrialized Democracies. Passions, Politics and Policies*, New Brunswick, NJ: Rutgers University Press.

Kissinger, P., Cohen, O., Brandon, W., Rice, J., Morse, A. and Clark, R. (1995) 'Compliance with public sector HIV medical care', *Journal of National Medical Association* 87: 19–34.

Lerner, B. H., Gulick, R. M. and Neveloff-Dubler, N. (1998) 'Rethinking nonadherence: historical perspectives in triple-drug therapy for HIV disease', *Annals of Internal Medicine* 129: 573–578.

Ley, P. (1988) *Communicating with Patients*, London: Croom Helm.

McNeil, B. J. and Pauker, S. G. (1982) 'On the elicitation of preferences toward alternative therapies', *New England Journal of Medicine* 306: 1259–1262.

Mehta, S., Moore, R. D. and Graham, N. M. H. (1997) 'Potential factors affecting adherence with HIV therapy', *AIDS* 11: 1665–1670.

Miller, N. H. (1997) 'Compliance with treatment regimens in chronic asymptomatic diseases', *American Journal of Medicine* 17: 43–49.

Moatti, J. P., Hausser, D. and Agrafiotis, D. (1997) 'Understanding HIV-risk related behaviour: a critical overview of current models', in L. Van Campenhoudt *et al.* (eds) *Sexual Interactions and HIV Risk: New Conceptual Perspectives in European Research*, London: Taylor and Francis.

Mooney, G. and Ryan, M. (1993) 'Agency in health care: getting beyond first principles', *Journal of Health Economics* 12: 125–135.

Morisky, D. E., Green, L. W. and Levine, D. M. (1986) 'Concurrent and predictive validity of a self-reported measure of medication adherence', *Medical Care* 24: 67–74.

Moutouh, L., Corbeil, J. and Richman, D. D. (1996) 'Recombination leads to the rapid emergence of HIV-1 dually resistant mutants under selective drug pressure', *Proceedings of the National Academy of Sciences USA* 93: 6106–6111.

Muma, R. D., Ross, M. W., Parcel, G. S. and Pollard, R. B. (1995) 'Zidovudine adherence among individuals with HIV infection', *Aids Care* 7: 439–447.

Myers, L. B. and Midence, K. (eds) (1998) *Adherence to Treatment in Medical Conditions*, Amsterdam: Harwood Academic.

National Research Council (1989) *Improving Risk Communication*, Washington, DC: National Academy Press.

Nieukwerk, P. T. *et al.* (1998) 'Self-reported adherence to ritonavir/saquinavir andritonavir/saquinavir/stavudine in a randomized clinical trial: preliminary results', *12th International Aids Conference, Geneva*, Abstract 32362.

Parsons, T. (1951) *The Social System*, Glencoe, IL: Free Press.

Paterson, D., Swindells, S. and Mohr, J. (1999) 'How much adherence is enough? A prospective study of adherence to protease inhibitor therapy using MEMScaps', Paper presented at the Sixth Conference on Retroviruses and Opportunistic Infections, Chicago, January–February.

Pierret, J. (1991) 'Coping with AIDS in everyday life', *Current Sociology* 40: 66–84.

Radley, A. and Billig, M. (1996) 'Accounts of health and lllness: dilemmas and representations', *Sociology of Health and Illness* 18: 220–240.

Ruskin, J. and Larivière, M. (1991) 'Low-dose cotrimoxazole for prevention of *Pneumocysitis Cariniii* pneumonia in human immunodeficiency virus disease', *Lancet* 337: 468–471.

Segall, A. (1976) 'The sick role concept: understanding illness behaviour', *Journal of Health and Social Behaviour* 17: 163–170.

Senak, M. (1997) 'Predicting antiviral compliance: physician's responsibilities vs. patients' rights', *Journal of International Association of Physicians in AIDS Care* 3: 45–48.

Singh, N., Squier, C., Sivek, C., Wagener, M., Nguyen, M. H. and Yu, V. L. (1996) 'Determinants of compliance with antiretroviral therapy in patients with human immunodeficiency virus: prospective assessment with implications for enhancing compliance', *AIDS Care* 8: 261–269.

Souville, M. *et al.* (1999) 'Factors associated with short-term adherence to protease inhibitors therapy in a French cohort', Paper presented at the 4th International Conference on AIDS Impact: Biopsychosocial aspects of HIV infection, Ottawa, July.

Stewart, G. (1997) 'Adherence to antiretroviral therapies', in E. Van Praag *et al.* (eds) *The Implications of Antiretroviral Treatments. Informal Consultation*, Geneva: WHO/UNAIDS.

Tramarin, A. *et al.* (1997) 'The influence of socio-economic status on health service utilisation by patients with AIDS in North Italy', *Social Science and Medicine* 45: 859–866.

Voelker, R. (1997) 'Debating dual AIDS guidelines', *Journal of the American Medical Association* 278: 613.

Wainberg, M. A. and Friedland, G. (1998) 'Public health implications of antiretroviral therapy and HIV drug resistance', *Journal of the American Medical Association* 279: 1977–1983.

Weidle, P. J., Ganea, C. E., Ernst, J., McGowan, J., Irwin, K. L. and Holberg, S. D. (1998) 'Multiple reasons for nonadherence to antiretroviral medications in an inner city minority population: need for a multifaceted approach to improve adherence', *12th International AIDS Conference, Geneva*, Abstract 32360.

Weitz, R. (1989) 'Uncertainty and the lives of persons with AIDS', *Journal of Health Social Behaviour* 30: 111–122.

Part II

New perspectives on sexuality

6   Seropositivity, risk and sexuality

François Delor

The topic of this chapter is sexuality and risk management strategies among people with HIV/AIDS (PWHAs). The aim is to shed light on the complexity of identity adjustment and relational processes in relation to events such as seropositivity and serodiscordance, whether known or unknown, inside an interaction. The chapter is based on findings from a recent survey of seropositive people conducted in the French-speaking community of Belgium (Delor, 1997).

Context

Generally speaking, research which aims to understand the risk-related behaviour of people with HIV or AIDS (PWHAs) can be divided into two major categories: (a) studies focusing on the individual determinants of risk behaviour including personality or temperament (Cloninger *et al.*, 1993), related research on self-esteem (Niklowitz, 1994), depression (Sandfort *et al.*, 1994), psychological state (Maasen, 1994) and the use of substances such as drugs and alcohol (Kennedy, 1993); and (b) research focusing on relational or interactional processes that allows one to understand risk as a social process (e.g. Bastard *et al.*, 1997; Van Campenhoudt and Cohen, 1997; Ingham and Van Zessen, 1997).

This first approach contains two major strands of work. First, there are studies influenced by the dominant model of the rational individual. These include KABP-type quantitative studies that strive for a kind of 'readaptation' of attitudes and practices by improving knowledge and 'correcting' certain beliefs, guided by a linear cause-and-effect logic (Franck, 1994). Then there are studies influenced by anthropology, sociology or phenomenology that strive to take account of behaviours or thoughts which, although seemingly irrational, may link to other motives of the person involved. Here, understanding is usually achieved by the use of qualitative methods including, among others, unconscious content analysis (Lisandre, 1995) and biographical analysis (Carricaburu and Pierret, 1992). A key US study (Remien *et al.*, 1995) doubtless blazed the trail in the second category of research by trying to envision the variety of factors likely to influence behaviour regardless of whether they are rooted in the individual, linked to the relational characteristics of situations, or within the broader social context.

Keogh *et al.*'s (1997) and Green's (1997) recent work offers examples of the concern to situate risk taking within a relational context by taking account of seropositive individuals' own perspectives on events. Our own qualitative enquiry also sheds light on how each person is likely to interpret the world and to assign particular meanings to its elements in line with his or her own intentions, ideals and fears at each moment. The ideal of protection takes on even more importance in that our aim here is to explore sexuality and emotions. In these areas more than any others, the individual is situated at the very crossroads between his or her desires and weaknesses, demands and deficiencies, while trying simultaneously to protect the many facets of his or her private life.

Research framework

Our research was carried out in 1995 and 1996 and involved an in-depth analysis of semi-structured interviews with forty seropositive individuals. The aim was not to obtain a representative picture of the population, but rather to pinpoint key processes at work. This was achieved by selecting interviewees so as to get as great a diversity of cases as possible. We talked with both men (twenty-five) and women (fifteen) who had been infected through heterosexual relations (thirteen), men infected by homosexual relations (seventeen), and male and female injecting drug use (seven). We also interviewed three self-defined bisexual men and one transsexual. Interviews were conducted in both urban and rural areas. A further fifteen interviews were conducted with health care workers, prevention workers, members of associations, and solidarity movements in Belgium and abroad (more specifically in France and Greece).

The analysis dealt with a wide range of topics, including social pathways, interactions or relationships, as well as the influence of social context in a broader sense. We tried to uncover both the objective or socio-structural significance of the elements we observed and their subjective or socio-symbolic significance. Finally, these elements were interpreted within the framework of identity construction or dynamics (Dubet, 1994).

Within the confines of this chapter it is not possible to describe in detail all the issues identified. Issues not addressed include the importance of social norms, notably those governing sexuality, on homosexually active men's life courses, the influence of sexual identity, gender and sexual preference on interactions, socio-economic factors, etc. A publication arising out of this research (Delor, 1997) offers a more detailed treatment of these and other factors. In this chapter we will focus on seropositivity or serodiscordance as potentially salient elements in sexual interaction.

Figure 6.1 shows how HIV-related social vulnerability may have at least

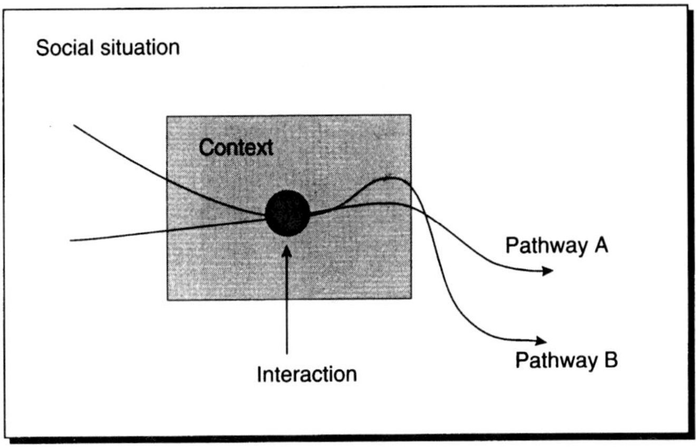

	Socio-structural or objective dimension	Socio-symbolic or subjective dimension
Pathway level	Life cycle, age, social mobility, social identity, etc.	Subjective time, plans for life, perception of the future, etc.
Interaction level	Partners' ages, setting of the interaction, serological status, etc.	Subjective representations of *alter*, perception of condoms according to serostatus, etc.
Context level	System of collective norms, institutions, instituted balances of power, inequalities, etc.	Subjective perception of norms, personal interpretation and expectation of punishment, etc.

Figure 6.1 The three levels of reading the social situation

three sources of origin, namely life courses (trajectories); specific types of interaction, which can be seen as the points of intersection between trajectories; and the social context in which trajectories and interactions occur. Elements at each of these three levels may be understood from two contrasting viewpoints. On the one hand, there is the tangible, observable or describable side of each element in line with an 'objective' or commonly accepted meaning. On the other hand, there is the special, more latent perspective developed by each individual in line with a particular meaning or the subjective purpose that he or she assigns to it.

Serodiscordance in steady relationships

One respondent, Ann, gave an enlightening account with regard to seropositivity and the process that revealing one's serostatus triggers within a recently formed relationship in which both partners are in love with each other.

It was very hard. He was close to me and took me in his arms. He wasn't angry. He supported me. At the same time, when I tried to tell him that maybe we should end our relationship because I didn't want him to stay in those circumstances. He didn't say 'yes' or ... Did he say no? We talked about it all the time in the beginning. He didn't want to share my fork, knife, plate, glass, kiss me ... We made an appointment to take a second test.

(Ann)

By announcing one's seropositivity, one is also telling the person – not always explicitly – that there is a possibility that the *couple* is serodiscordant. Finding out what one may and may not do, coping with the emotional fear of being abandoned, and reassuring oneself about the other partner's serological status appear to be the prime concerns. As long as the partner's test results are not known, the couple may enter into a phase of retreat.

He had to be tested to make sure he hadn't caught it. We no longer truly dared touch each other. We were supporting each other but at the same time we were very far apart all of a sudden. It stayed like that until the moment he knew he hadn't caught anything.

(Ann)

Giuseppe spells out the tension that followed from the announcement of his seropositivity:

I had to come to grips with reality at some time and I had to tell him and know if he also was positive, like me ... I didn't know if my friend was seropositive or negative. It was also possible that he might be positive too, just by chance.

(Giuseppe)

The onset of effective serodiscordance occurs when the partner learns and announces that he or she is seronegative, for at this point the two individuals know they are of different serostatus. As of that moment, a process of managing the difference is switched on, mixing emotions, interests and resistance in a climate of tension. For example, Ann sees her boyfriend's sadness. He can't hide it. After a first stage dominated by an emotional crisis, they attempt to adapt in a technical way to the risk of AIDS:

We learned to live together, to use a condom when making love, and everything. But actually, he's someone who doesn't like making love wearing a condom. He felt so ill at ease with it that he ended up by no longer really wanting to make love.

(Ann)

The technico-sensorial argument that Ann proposes to explain her partner's difficulties is superimposed on the emotional register, and as her story unfolds it becomes clear that this issue was just one of a number of problems.

> It was a little uncomfortable for him, 'cos he's rather big, and the condoms you can buy in Belgium are not big enough. He couldn't put them on. They hurt too much, they were too small, they burst too often. I had to go to Finland to get condoms, because you can buy different sizes there. And that worked.
>
> (Ann)

Solving this technical problem was not enough. Fear – which was not expressed at first – later proved to be an essential element in the relational process.

> He became so afraid that he started putting two on. Even though the doctor had explained how he could have oral sex, he almost no longer dared ... it was really when I asked ... For me, it's something that should be spontaneous in a relationship. It was no longer relaxed. In the beginning, with the condoms, it was fine. Then it started to get worse and worse.
>
> (Ann)

The condom and the possibility of its failure can be the legitimate argument that enables people to cope with an apparently irrational or inexpressible fear. Ann tried to understand why her partner refused vaginal penetration or oral sex despite the doctor's reassurances and the right size condom. She turned to the explanation that she found most plausible: 'he's no longer attracted to me'. This explanation was an extension of her long-standing lack of self-confidence, one of the key identity problems that lurk in Ann's story: 'I don't have much confidence in myself'. That is perhaps why penetration became such a crucial part of sex, which for Ann is a true place of self-validation:

> If he truly needed to make love he tried to make me make love with him without him doing anything with me. It was very hard for me to accept that as a woman, but also because I don't have much confidence in myself and I need that part of the relationship to prove to myself that he truly wants to be with me. I continued to be the one who had to ask.
>
> (Ann)

For Ann, seropositivity and her partner's adaptation to fear are events that are part of her biography and identity construction (Carricaburu and Pierret, 1992, 1995). More specifically, these events reiterate questions that she has not resolved. Another respondent, Martine, explained that once her partner, who was seropositive, learned that she, too, was infected, sex became difficult. Their seroconcordance triggered feelings of guilt or remorse in her partner. What is more, he imagined in Martine a hostility that she herself did not feel.

> The day he knew I was also HIV positive, it was over. The slightest overtures he had made toward me were things of the past. So, I was the one who had to take the initiative every time. It was hard for a while. Then it is no longer morally possible, at a certain point, you just can't do it anymore. You've had enough.
>
> (Martine)

The tensions generated by the onset of a real risk can lead to the break-up of a relationship. Adapting to serodiscordance in a couple can produce a divergence in interests ('It's in my interest not to leave him now to avoid feeling guilty, and at the same time it's in my interest to leave him quickly because I can't take the situation'); divergences between one's private thoughts and spoken words ('I'm afraid, but prefer to say that I have a headache'); tensions between various areas of legitimacy ('I have the legitimate right to protect myself, but she has a legitimate right to ask me to prove my love'); and so on. As Ann explained:

> And I started to destroy the relationship by asking him why he stayed out so late with friends. I told myself that, since he wasn't making love with me, he had to be looking for it elsewhere. We are the ones who destroyed the relationship. Actually, I don't think he stopped making love to me because he no longer wanted to be with me or because he didn't love me. I believe that he stopped making love because he was afraid.
>
> (Ann)

The absence of precautions can, in turn, take on a special meaning in serodiscordant couples. This is a way of dealing with the risk that threatens the relationship itself and the elements of identity that are at stake within it. Resus' remarks illustrate some of the issues involved here.

> If she had asked me, I would have taken some precautions, but she didn't want to and, well, I didn't always take precautions. I know, I sort of didn't bloody well care. It was monstrous of me, but ... well. From 1987 on, she no longer had the choice. I told her 'No', loud and clear, but nevertheless we played with fire a few times. But 'No'. She asked me, but 'No' ... She became pregnant in 1988.
>
> (Resus)

Here we see Resus wavering between different poles with respect to the significance of using condoms. He first sees the condom as something that his wife refuses and that he tries to force her to accept. The haphazard use of the condom opens up a relational area in which the couple 'play with fire'. Finally, not using the condom is equated with monstrous behaviour. Resus describes himself both as a responsible man who wishes to impose the use of protection, as a risk taker who 'plays with fire', and as a monster who does not 'bloody well care'. These three subjective positions are ways for Resus to cope with three socially constructed risks within relational and identity dynamics, risks that correspond to three dimensions of protection: the objective and effective protection employed by the 'reasonable man'; the 'relative protection' achieved by various strategies, of which gambling is an example; and the 'absolute protection' achieved by withdrawing from the world of worry. Resus is not reckless, nor a monster, nor a perfectly reasonable being. He is the moving subject of a tension between different ways of subjectively protecting oneself.

The following excerpt from the interview with Marie-Laure and her partner offers another example of this construction of risk within a relationship and the stakes regarding identity. In this example, the meaning of the condom is redefined by being given a meaning at the core of the love relationship.

> I am not the type of man [who goes] for prevention. When you love someone, that person is a normal person. You don't think about the fact that she's picked up that bloody virus. If, when she told me two years ago, 'I have something to tell you. I've got HIV', I had said, 'So long, girl, I'm leaving', would that be a normal reaction for a man? It would only have been a fling. When you love a person, you're not like that.
>
> (Marie-Laure's partner)

Here, not using a condom gives the partner the status of a normal and respectable human being within a structure in which the universe of the normal human relationships of love is contrasted with the world of adventure (Figure 6.2).

Elsewhere in interviews it is clear that the metaphorical aspects of receiving semen (Figure 6.3) and even intimate sexual contact are precisely what is likely to define the other as ideal, whereas the condom, as if a structural mirror, takes on the metaphorical power of the other as 'abnormal', or as having lost his or her exceptional nature. So, Miguel, who is seropositive, explains how important it is for him to receive his seronegative boyfriend's semen:

> Receiving his semen gave me the feeling of having him completely.
>
> (Miguel)

Semen, here, comes to stand for the other through a metaphorical process involving extrapolation and reduction (Ricoeur, 1975; Charbonnel, 1991).

UNIVERSE 1*	UNIVERSE 2
Loving relationship	Fling
When a person loves	(When you're not in love)**
a normal	(Not normal)
person	(Not a person)
You don't think about the fact that she's	(You think about the fact that she's
caught that horrible thing	caught that horrible thing)
(Not leaving)	So long, girl, I'm leaving
Normal reaction	(Abnormal reaction)
of a man or woman (human reaction)	(Non-human reaction)
Not the man for prevention	(The man for prevention)

Figure 6.2   Structure and universes

* A universe is a set of elements that belong together in line with a meaning, intention or plan. This universe is implicitly or explicitly opposed to another manner of seeing the world or another universe of significations.

** What is not stated explicitly but can be deduced logically from the structure of the text's meaning is by convention put between parentheses as a means of separating it clearly from the exact wording.

Not receiving the other's semen thereby carries symbolic dimensions which redefines both the partner and the relationship (Green, 1997; Keogh *et al.*, 1997; Oliviero, 1991).

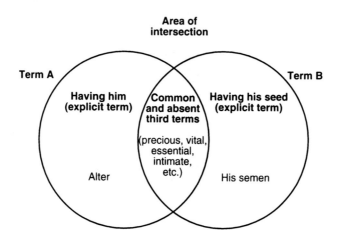

Figure 6.3   The metaphorical translation of semen and partner

HIV risk in occasional relationships

Interviews showed that the condom is seen subjectively by some seropositive individuals as an attribute or mandatory uniform that they fear will reveal their serological status once it is donned. PWHAs feel this most particularly in the context of 'casual' sexual relations. This finding merits more detailed analysis. In the following quotations, it can be seen that the condom was considered by the interviewee before his seropositivity was announced, and compulsory only after the words had been uttered.

> Actually, I think that knowing that condoms were necessary if I didn't want to either catch an additional infection or infect others was a bit difficult, more difficult, in fact, than before, when I had sex before I was infected. It's become a bit more difficult to handle. Giving someone a condom was more difficult to handle, to give, yeah ... because you think, 'If I put on a condom, he's gonna think that I'm infected', and that's why I had that reaction, because at the time I knew full well that I was indeed infected.
>
> (Bernard)

> Although I used condoms then, now it's a problem for me, 'cos it's an obligation. Before it wasn't a problem. On the contrary, it was an additional erotic game that I'd discovered.
>
> (Joseph)

This image of the condom as offering a potential message about serological status is important if we are to understand better the difficulties that PWHAs may feel, notably in occasional relationships. The condom that is worn or imposed by a person with HIV does not have the same subjective meaning as one that is worn or imposed by a seronegative person. Referring to an 'objective' meaning of the condom as a simple means of protection means forgetting that the object takes on an always specific socio-symbolic dimension or meaning, depending on who wears it or who imposes its use.

There is, however, a need to understand better what gives the condom this power of 'denunciation'. The first and underlying rationale seems to be as follows. A seronegative person can wear a condom like an optional piece of clothing or mask, that is to say, without fearing that he or she will be taken for a PWHA, or strong in the knowledge that if he or she is, this can always be denied. A PWHA on the other hand is likely to see the condom as a signalling to others of his serological status while acting as a reminder of this status to the person himself. The logic of these different perceptions is easier to grasp if we take the following imaginary monologue of a police officer going to a costume ball in a distant town:

> If I wear my uniform, someone will surely recognize me and denounce me as a cop, in which case I'll be kicked out. If I say that I am not a police officer I'll be lying, and people will see that I'm lying. In any event, I couldn't lie and enjoy myself at the same time. That is why I won't dress up as a police officer.

However, it is important to understand better why the dominant perception of the condom is that of an indispensable 'accessory' or 'uniform' for and by HIV-positive people themselves. Our hypothesis is that the dominant representation of health linked to the idea of seronegativity or absence of disease serves as the yardstick by which a seropositive person can intuitively be perceived, as a potential 'reservoir of morbidity' both by him- or herself and by others. This image is linked to seeing the condom as an indispensable attribute of seropositive people who, according to society, cannot overlook the presence of the virus, and who consequently bear collective responsibility. Some people would even like to enshrine this responsibility in penal law. Even if seronegative individuals currently force themselves to use condoms, we cannot say that such behaviour is imposed on them by society as is the case for PWHAs. Has the idea of imposing penal sanctions on seronegative persons who do not use condoms systematically ever been brought up? This difference in the way society sees the condom is intimately connected with the way in which each person's perception of the condom differs in line with his or her serological status.

This fear of being recognised as HIV positive is also linked to the experience of rejection when a positive serostatus is revealed. This experience can take various forms:

> When you say it, nine times out of ten it's OK like that. The guy tells you he'd rather not. Or then again, it can be a weirdo who likes that, but I don't agree.
>
> (Eric)

> And it's hard to say. It's very, very hard to say. Because you don't know how the person will react ... They said, 'It was good of you to tell me, but I prefer not to do anything.' And I shut up because they were honest. But you can have refusals where they'll say, 'Hey! That guy's got the virus, he's mad, he comes in here ... '. It can degenerate. Someone who is aware of that possibility just keeps his mouth shut.
>
> (Eric)

Doubts about the condom when facing a true risk

We can deduce from the foregoing that the trust both the seropositive person and the seronegative person who is aware of his or her partner's seropositivity have in the condom's efficacy can be seriously shaken. When, in a one-night stand, an HIV-positive man prefers to 'warn' the other person of his serostatus despite the fact that he is using a condom, he is guided by the thought that if, despite the condom, something happens, he prefers to have been honest. At the same time, after hearing such an announcement, the seronegative person often prefers not to have sex. When the risk is both real and known, trusting an object is problematic when you know from your own experience or hearsay that it is not totally reliable. We can thus understand why, in such circumstances, the seronegative partner may choose not to have sex in order to protect him- or herself. The slightest 'accident' with condoms in the subject's past could trigger serious anxieties about the future, especially if he or she has to deal with a situation of real and known serodiscordance.

Unspeakable fear

Steady relationships and 'casual' sex share at least one feature in common: the influence of fear and the difficulty of speaking about it. The persistence of fear, and its tendency to increase with time, can lead to intense suffering within the relationship, a gradual decline in sexual activity, the break-up of the relationship, or the use of inappropriate precautions leading to HIV transmission – the very opposite of what one set out to achieve.

The difficulties of trusting preventive means are also worth studying, taking account of the various registers to which the 'objects of fear' from which people want to protect themselves belong. In the first register, prevention talk is often of a pragmatic and technical type in which the virus, as the object of fear, and the condom, as the means of protection, are described from the 'reasonable' perspective of de-dramatised risk management. In the second register, the discourse of love offers a more socio-relational way of coping. Certain imaginary perceptions of risk, that is to say, emotions or fears that well up in thought without ever being expressed in speech or discourse, also come to mind. In the third register, death itself or mortality, seen as a risk, and exclusion or flight, seen as a means of protection, can back up each other quite logically. So, through these three registers – which are far from exhaustive – we can distinguish more or less objectivisable, tangible or representable objects of fear from the subjective, emotional or relational objects of fear to the inexpressible or ungraspable objects of fear. The last are what we call 'imaginary objects', to the extent that they escape the control of a symbolic discourse that is supposed to formulate and 'contain' them.

These examples of registers show us that while the objects of fear are always objects of anticipation, such foresight does not always take place in the same plane. Moreover, the tension, necessary hierarchisation and more or less spontaneous and conscious arbitration between these various registers of anticipation and the objects of fear that they contain, may produce inappropriate ways of coping with the virus itself. In the specific case of

AIDS, the virus is a 'pragmatic object' of fear against which condoms or non-penetrative sexual practices are likely to provide adequate protection. The persistence of fear despite the adoption of effective protective means prompts us to posit the existence of another 'object' of fear that is engendered by the virus's actual presence in the interaction. This object may correspond to apprehensiveness about mortality. This hypothesis is supported by both the permanence of, or increase in, the fear, and some of the fascination of being close to HIV that seropositive individuals observe with uneasiness in some of their partners. So, in a sexual interaction with known serodiscordance, two fears may take root (Table 6.1): the fear of the virus itself as a real objectivisable object that can be controlled by specific devices or behaviours, and the fear of one's mortality that comes closer because of the virus – that is to say, a powerfully imaginary element that appears not to be controllable.

We have seen that prevention talk is often pragmatic. Similarly, projects of solidarity with PWHAs are rooted in the promotion of a realistic perception of risk and infection, and in combating what appear to be groundless fears. This promotion, although essential, may make the collective expression or individual confidence concerning residual fears problematic. In the case of serodiscordant couples, a form of taboo may prevent the expression of fears by the couples. Not using preventive means systematically can then be the result of a process of social transaction or complex arbitration through which the couple manages to maintain a certain cohesion and satisfaction for each party. After a while in interview, all of the HIV-positive interviewees began to describe the complexity, difficulty and variability of their behaviour.

Table 6.1   Structured fear in relation to two different objects

	Object of fear	Means of protection
Preventive medicine, 'realistic' or 'pragmatic' axis	Virus	Condom
(Individual and collective) imaginary axis	Death, mortality, contagion with death itself	Flight, heroism, etc.
Tension between the two axes	Ups and downs during which the person either tries to reason or, on the contrary, panics	Variability in words and deeds with regard to the infected partner; inconsistencies between speech and practices, changes of mood, existential tension between the desire to flee and the hero figure

Conclusions

Scientific and preventive actors are usually unable to hear and reassure individuals who are confronted with fears on the imaginary axis, or are the objects of what seem to be unfathomable or inexpressible anxieties. Research and prevention tend together to disqualify these fears by considering them unreasonable and sometimes childish. In so doing, they contribute to inhibiting all talk on this subject and enhance fears, intuitive reactions and discriminatory attitudes. To open up the area of speech to allow the many fears to be expressed, whether in prevention work or inside relationships themselves, is a prerequisite for prevention. Shedding light, together with the people involved, on the complexity of the arbitration with which they must cope, and on the host of processes and registers that are mobilised during such arbitration, thus becomes one of the unavoidable components of a preventive strategy which aims to increase players' abilities to understand themselves and adapt to new situations.

Serodiscordance appears to be illustrative of this type of complex process, to the extent that knowledge of the virus's presence in an interaction triggers uncertainty and a need to readjust. This readjustment takes place at the intersection of several pre-existing registers that are upset by the addition of an actual, known risk and the need for urgent protection. To prevent HIV-related risks lastingly, it is important that PWHAs are understood, respected and given support and guidance in the maelstrom of these processes. Such an attitude requires that the prevention worker gives up the normative or imperative proposition as to 'what must happen' in order to allow for the gradual elucidation of 'what is actually happening'.

In contrast to certain messages or positions that consider it (often naïvely) legitimate and obvious to expect the HIV-positive person always to engage in risk-free behaviour or to protect the other person perfectly by adopting 'safe sex', we should instead focus on how various stakes and thus the various risks belonging to the different registers can influence the ways partners adapt in their relationships. The paradox is as follows. On the one hand, 'reduced risk' (or safer sex) has gradually become the goal of prevention campaigns that have recognised that 'zero risk' is an unrealistic, and therefore counterproductive, objective. On the other hand, the idea that PWHAs might make others run the slightest risk seems intolerable for many people, as a result of which the implicit aim is for a zeroing of risk. By situating risk in the interaction, we shift the emphasis from persons to situations. The risk of AIDS, whether for the self or the other, is part of a hierarchy of concerns, the order of which is not predetermined. The complexity of vulnerability must therefore be understood by means of an analytic framework that allows for this very complexity, yet tries to clarify it for the various agents of prevention. Among these, PWHAs are prime interlocutors.

References

Bastard, B., Cardia-Vonèche, L., Peto, D. and Van Campenhoudt, L. (1997) 'Relationships between sexual partners and ways of adapting to the risk of AIDS: landmarks for a relationship-oriented conceptual framework', in L. Van Campenhoudt, M. Cohen, G. Guizzardi and D. Hausser (eds) *Sexual Interaction and HIV Risk: New Conceptual Perspective in European Research*, London: Taylor and Francis.

Carricaburu, D. and Pierret, J. (1992) *Vie quotidienne et recompositions identitaires autour de la séropositivité, Rapport de recherche*, Paris: CERMES-ANRS.

——(1995) 'From biographical disruption to biographical reinforcement: the case of HIV-positive men', *Sociology of Health and Illness* 17(1): 65–88.

Charbonnel, N. (1991) *L'Important, c'est d'être propre*, Strasbourg: Presses Universitaires de Strasbourg.

Cloninger, C. R., Svrakik, D. M. and Przybeck, T. R. (1993) 'A psychobiological model of temperament and character', *Archives of General Psychiatry* 50: 975–990.

Delor, F. (1997) *Séropositifs. Trajectoires identitaires et rencontres du risque*, Paris: L'Harmattan, Logiques Sociales Collection.

Dubet, F. (1994) *Sociologie de l'expérience*, Paris: Seuil.

Franck, R. (ed.) (1994) *Faut-il chercher aux causes une raison? L'explication causale dans les sciences humaines*, Paris: Institut interdisciplinaire d'études épistémologiques.

Green, G. (1997) 'Positive sex: sexual relationships following an HIV-positive diagnosis', in P. Aggleton, P. Davies and G. Hart (eds) *AIDS, Activism and Alliances*, London: Taylor and Francis.

Ingham, R. and Van Zessen, G. (1997) 'From individual properties to interactional processes', in L. Van Campenhoudt, M. Cohen, G. Guizzardi and D. Hausser (eds) *Sexual Interaction and HIV Risk: New Conceptual Perspective in European Research*, London: Taylor and Francis.

Kennedy, C. A. (1993) 'Psychological distress, drug and alcohol use as correlates of condom use in HIV-serodiscordant heterosexual couples', *AIDS* 7(11): 1493–1499.

Keogh, P., Beardesell, S. and Sigma Research (1997) 'Sexual negotiation strategies of HIV-positive gay men: a qualitative approach', in P. Aggleton, P. Davies and G. Hart (eds) *AIDS, Activism and Alliances*, London: Taylor and Francis.

Lisandre, H. (1995) 'Les homosexuels et le safer sex, une approche psychanalytique', *Sexualité et sida, Recherches en sciences sociales*, Paris: ANRS.

Maasen, T. (1994) 'Challenging the taboo: psychotherapy and sexual risk behaviour among HIV infected homosexual men', in D. Friedrich and W. Heckmann (eds) *Aids in Europe: The Behavioural Aspect, Vol. 2*, Berlin: Sigma.

Niklowitz, M. (1994) 'Sexual risk behaviour in HIV positive individuals', in D. Friedrich and W. Heckmann (eds) *Aids in Europe: The Behavioural Aspect, Vol. 2*, Berlin: Sigma.

Oliviero, P. (1991) 'Le sida et les représentations sociales du sperme', *Le journal du Sida* 30: 40–44.

Remien, R. H., Caraballo-Diéguez, A. and Wagner, G. (1995) 'Intimacy and sexual risk behaviour in serodiscordant male couples', *AIDS Care* 7(4): 429–438.

Ricoeur, P. (1975) *La Métaphore vive*, Paris: Seuil.

Sandfort, T., Clement, U., Knobel, J., Keet, R. and de Vroome, E. (1994) 'Does coping with HIV infection affect safer sexual behaviour?', in D. Friedrich and W. Heckmann (eds) *Aids in Europe: The Behavioural Aspect, Vol. 2*, Berlin: Sigma.
Van Campenhoudt, L. and Cohen, M. (1997) 'Interaction and risk-related behaviour: theoretical and heuristic landmarks', in L. Van Campenhoudt, M. Cohen, G. Guizzardi, and D. Hausser (eds) *Sexual Interaction and HIV Risk: New Conceptual Perspective in European Research*, London: Taylor & Francis.

7 Socio-economic status and HIV prevalence among gay men in Germany[1]

Michael Bochow

There is widespread agreement that, in absolute terms, health standards in the population as a whole have improved throughout Western Europe since the Second World War. Despite such improvements, serious social inequalities in health continue to persist (see e.g. Townsend *et al.*, 1988; Mielck, 1994). At the start of the epidemic, HIV/AIDS offered an exception to the rule (in OECD countries) in that disproportionate numbers of middle-class men were being affected. In most European countries where there is a notable level of HIV prevalence, HIV and AIDS are largely to be found among injecting drug users and gay men. While injecting drug use is a feature of poor and marginalised groups in Europe, gay men on the other hand are often perceived as predominantly belonging to the well-to-do middle classes. That said, the gay population cannot escape the effects of the social inequalities that structure western advanced industrial societies, and it is the goal of this chapter to investigate the class-specific effect of social inequality in two European countries, France and Germany, on the prevalence of HIV among gay men. The comparative study concentrates primarily on France and Germany, but draws nevertheless on recent findings from the UK.[2]

The social context of lower-class gay men

Work carried out in Germany in the early 1970s found that gay men of lower socio-economic origin were on average professionally more mobile (both horizontally and vertically) than their heterosexual counterparts (Dannecker and Reiche, 1974). While this work has not been replicated elsewhere, it is plausible to assume that this process continues in the 1990s. Consequently, it can be hypothesised that the life histories of working-class gay men are more strongly characterised by discontinuity and disruption. For many lower-class gay men, the search for a professional niche in which they are more protected from possible discrimination can lead to their becoming alienated from their families of origin. Often the change in social milieu is connected to a move away from their home town to cities with at least 200,000 residents, with many preferring major conurbations having populations of 500,000 or more.

Middle-class men can seek out supportive social environments without losing their class-related way of life. However, for lower-class men this change in place and job means having to adapt in two ways, both in terms of living their homosexuality and with respect to their class-based behaviour and attitudes. For many of these men, this change means finding a job in the service sector and, when possible, a position of higher social status than their previous employment. Lower-class men, like their middle-class counterparts, often need to leave their home town. But, in addition, they need to leave behind ways of interacting with others that do not fit into the new chosen social environment.

This adaptation process is easier for those men who have managed to develop the typical coping strategy of being able to 'change roles'; that is, of being able to choose when to be open with their homosexuality, and when to give the appearance of being a heterosexual man. This ability to shift from being one's 'gay self' to a heterosexual *façade* is not a given among gay men, but rather a learned coping strategy which is developed over the course of time.

In order to achieve a more or less successful coming out, gay men need to develop the ability to distance themselves from traditional masculine roles, to cope with ambivalent social situations, and to cultivate a greater tolerance of frustration. In this process, gay men develop a specific competence regarding interpersonal communication, including a social flexibility or adeptness comparable with the skills commonly found among the middle class (Bourdieu, 1977). These skills are characterised not only by the cognitive features associated with specific professional qualifications, but also by qualities such as self-confidence, social grace, and being at ease among others. This complex of cognitive, social co-operative and motivational qualifications is encapsulated in Bourdieu's (1979a, 1979b, 1980) concept of *capital culturel*.

The strategies which gay men must elaborate in order to lead a relatively unscathed life as gays endow many of them with specific, highly developed communication skills which are precisely those called for in certain service areas. Although statistics are lacking to back up our claim, we venture to assert that the geographical distribution of gay men in France and Germany is different to that of heterosexual men and the professional distribution of gay men and heterosexual men differs too.

Contrary to the self-representation of many gay public figures, the high proportion of gay men in the service sector does not necessarily mean that gay men figure at the top of wage scales. Particularly in big cities, there is much evidence of an ever-spreading service sector proletariat. Such a group is not composed of traditional blue-collar workers, but is made up of low-grade clerical staff or ancillary personnel. If we are to assume that there is a high proportion of gay men in service industries, then we may further assume that a significant proportion of these men are at the lower end of the pay scales. The jobs they perform as waiters, shop assistants, nurses and cleaners have traditionally been dominated by women 'pink-collar' workers (cf. Connell *et al.*, 1993: 115), and carry with them a great deal of physical and/or mental stress.

The social integration of working-class gay men in the gay community

While many working-class gay men achieve some level of social mobility (not without certain costs), a significant proportion do not for a variety of reasons, including a rejection of middle-class gay 'manners' which may be seen as effeminacy or 'bitchiness' (Dowsett, 1996). The resistance shown by working-class men to middle-class norms and values takes on diverse forms and draws on a variety of motivations. Resistance may spring from an individual's sheer inability to conform to middle-class modes of behaviour. It may be nurtured by indifference or by a lack of ambition to climb the rungs of the social ladder. It may also spring from notions of 'working-class pride'. In Germany, this last form of resistance may be said to be markedly on the decline since the 1950s owing to the disappearance of wide sections of the traditional working class and its assimilation into the ranks of the lower middle class (in France since the 1960s). Furthermore, just as a lack of cultural capital may lead to a dynamic of social exclusion, the lack of skills for dealing with interaction forms in middle-class-dominated gay networks can lead to the social exclusion of gay men of lower social status.

The mechanics for exclusion work differently depending on whether they operate in the bars, backrooms, discos and cafés of the gay scene, or in gay groups, AIDS support networks, or gay sport or cultural groups. But whatever operational differences they display, these processes of social exclusion all veer in the same direction, counteracting the integration of working-class gay men into the networks of the gay community. Recent research by Australian colleagues on the social situation of working-class gay men has arrived at similar conclusions (see Dowsett *et al.*, 1992; Connell *et al.*, 1993; Dowsett, 1996).

Class-specific attitudes towards gay men

A representative survey conducted during 1991 in eastern and western Germany showed that of all the social groups questioned, it was workers and pensioners who were most likely to endorse items portraying gay men either in a strongly disapproving manner, or as trapped in discriminatory stereotypes. In addition, these two groups were least likely to agree with items presenting gay men in a tolerant or egalitarian light (Bochow, 1997a).

The particular attitudes towards homosexuality prevalent in working-class milieux may therefore act as powerful motivators for working-class gay men to leave their home background. If they remain in their original milieu, it is highly probable that they will not be able to live out their homosexuality as openly as middle-class gay men. Hostility to gay men stems only partly from their homosexuality and the fact that they prefer male-to-male sexual contact. More relevant, and scandalous in the working-class context, is their imagined or real lack of manliness. The virulent and often physically violent forms of sanction against homosexuality inflicted by young men from lower working-class backgrounds are extremely threatening to gay men themselves who belong to this stratum (cf. Bourdieu, 1977).

Sampling method and sample composition

In July 1996, and for the fifth time since 1987, a four-page questionnaire was circulated by the most important gay magazines in Germany. Gay men were questioned about their sexual behaviour under the impact of AIDS. All the surveys were commissioned by the Bundeszentrale für gesundheitliche Aufklärung (Federal Centre for Health Education) in Cologne. A total of 3048 men participated (514, or 17 per cent, from eastern Germany including eastern Berlin, and 2534 or 83 per cent from western Germany including western Berlin) (Bochow, 1997b).

Surveys based on a self-administered questionnaire have of their essence 'a built-in middle-class bias'. The surveys in 1991, 1993 and 1996 took the form of a series of 'convenience samples' in which men with lower educational and occupational status and working-class men were clearly underrepresented in relation to the importance of these groups in the overall population (Bochow, 1993, 1994). Even so, the absolute numbers of returned questionnaires were sufficient in themselves to ensure that the responses of underrepresented subgroups of the gay population were available for meaningful statistical analysis.

Three class groups were constituted using data on secondary educational and occupational status: (a) lower-class men with a junior secondary school certificate and unskilled occupation; (b) lower-middle-class men with skilled vocational training and other comparable vocational qualifications; and (c) middle-class men with senior high school and technical college or university qualifications, including students who have not yet finished their studies. Upper-class men, to the small extent that they may have participated in the survey, are included with the middle-class men. Table 7.1 shows the sample composition by class for the surveys of 1993 and 1996 in Germany, and for comparable surveys in 1993 and 1995 in France. The French data also derive from a questionnaire survey conducted via the gay press (Schiltz, 1993, 1998; Schiltz and Adam, 1995).

Class-specific differences in the lifestyles of gay men in Germany

The analysis of class-specific differences in the lifestyles of gay men and in risk behaviour, as well as risk strategies, is based solely on the German data,

Table 7.1   Sample composition by class, in German and French surveys of gay men

Year of survey	Lower class		Lower middle class		Middle class		Total	
	n	%	n	%	n	%	n	%
Western Germany								
1993	175	7	859	36	1359	57	2393	100
1996	259	10	974	38	1301	51	2534	100
Eastern Germany								
1993	26	6	236	50	213	45	475	100
1996	26	5	261	51	227	44	514	100
France								
1993	347	11	969	30	1921	59	3237	100
1995	233	9	760	29	1604	62	2597	100

and a more exhaustive analysis of the class-specific differences concerning working-class gay men in France remains to be carried out.

To analyse the extent to which gays were leading an open gay life, an 'openness' index was constructed based on questions such as whether the mother or father or siblings of the respondent knew about his homosexuality; whether they accepted it; and how far the respondent's friendship circle and colleagues at work were informed. Findings suggested that lower-class gay men in both parts of Germany live substantially more covert lives than their middle-class counterparts. Less than half of German lower-class men live in a relatively open fashion and enjoy acceptance in their social environment. In contrast, two-thirds of German middle-class men live their lives openly as gay men and feel accepted in their social environment. There is almost no difference in the composition of friendship circles between lower- and middle-class men, however, be these composed exclusively of gay men, of heterosexuals, or of an equal mixture of both. Nevertheless, a greater proportion of lower-class gay men – one-tenth – lead socially isolated lives, whereas only about 4 per cent of middle-class gay men stated that they have no close circle of friends.

In 1993 and 1996, a smaller percentage of lower-class gay men in both western and eastern Germany lived in a steady relationship than middle-class respondents (roughly 45 per cent versus 55 per cent). On the other hand, in the twelve-month period before the survey, members of the lower-class group did not have more sexual partners than the middle-class one. Overall, for both eastern and western Germans from the lower and the middle classes, in the past year 16 per cent had one partner, 27 per cent had two to five partners, 16 per cent had six to ten partners, 29 per cent had eleven to fifty partners, and 9 per cent had more than fifty; 3 per cent had no partners. This suggests that 'self-identified' gay men from the lower class do not have substantially more 'anonymous' sex than their middle-class counterparts.

However, when we consider the frequency of sexual contacts, class differences become more apparent. Less than half of German lower-class men have frequent (several times a month or more) male-to-male contact, whereas two-thirds of the middle-class respondents have frequent male-to-male contact. We should note here that explanations for less frequent sexual activity among lower-class gay men should also be understood as being related to class-specific factors. A higher proportion of lower-class gay men live in small towns and cities, and a lower proportion of them live in steady relationships. Both of these factors reduce their chances of sexual contacts.

The western German group of lower-class respondents is large enough to allow for further differentiation with respect to places of residence. In cities of more than 1 million inhabitants, lower-class men report still lower frequencies of sexual contact than their middle-class counterparts. Middle-class men not in a steady relationship report higher rates of sexual contact than their lower-class counterparts. A higher proportion of lower-class men stated that in the twelve months prior to the survey they had no anal–genital contact. This again is related to the fact that at the time of the survey fewer lower-class respondents were living in a steady relationship than middle-class respondents.

Class-specific differences in risk behaviour in Germany

Seventy-six per cent of western German and 72 per cent of eastern German respondents in 1996 (cf. 76 per cent of western Germans and 70 per cent of eastern Germans in 1993) stated that in the twelve months prior to the survey they had no unprotected anal–genital contact with persons whose test status they were unaware of, or who had a discordant test status from themselves.

Analysis of the 1996 western German subsample, however, reveals clear class differences: 69 per cent of lower-class men, 75 per cent of lower-middle-class men and 79 per cent of middle-class men stated that they had not had sexual contact involving risk. For the eastern German subsample the respective figures were 46 per cent, 71 per cent and 77 per cent respectively. These differences are statistically significant at the 0.05 level.[3]

Among men of lower socio-economic status we find not only more subjects who risked HIV infection, but also a higher percentage of men with a high frequency of risk contacts (over fifteen risk contacts in the last twelve months). Table 7.2 shows these class-related difference as reflected in unprotected anal intercourse with partners whose HIV status is not known, regardless of type of partnership.[4] This was possible because information concerning the frequency of the risk contacts for all types of partners (steady, non-steady and anonymous) was collected using the same method.

98   *M. Bochow*

Table 7.2   Socio-economic status and frequency of risk contacts with partners of
unknown serostatus in the last twelve months (western Germans and
western Berliners, figures in per cent, *n* = 2534)

	Number of risk contacts					
Socio-economic status	None	1– 5	6–15	16–35	60–180	n.r.
Lower class (n = 259)	69.5	13.5	7.3	1.9	5.8	1.9
Lower middle class (n = 974)	76.0	12.5	5.6	1.1	3.5	1.2
Middle class (n = 1301)	79.5	11.1	3.9	0.8	3.7	1.0
%	77.1	11.9	4.9	1.1	3.8	1.2

Class-specific differences in HIV prevalence in Germany

In the 1996 survey, there are marked differences between the three socio-
economic groups with respect to the percentage of HIV-positive men.
Among the 73 per cent of western Germans who were tested, 20 per cent of
the lower-class men are HIV positive, as opposed to 13 per cent of the
lower-middle-class men, and 7 per cent of the middle-class men. The
percentage of HIV-positive men among the tested western German respondents in 1993 were as follows: 17 per cent for the lower class; 13 per cent for
the lower middle class, and 8 per cent for the middle class. Thus, the incidence of men with HIV infection or with AIDS is twice as high among
respondents of the lower class than among middle-class men. Figures for the
eastern German subsamples revealed no clear class-specific differences in
both surveys. This may reflect something of the more egalitarian social
structure still found in eastern Germany. In addition, it should be noted that
overall rates of HIV infection are much lower in eastern as compared with
western Germany.

In order to examine the effects of age, the western German samples from
1993 and 1996 were divided into three groups: 16–29 years old; 30–44 years
old; and over 44 years old (most of the subjects in this age group were 45–65
years old). In the 1993 survey, there was no evidence of class-related influences in the over 44 group. Strong class-related differences regarding
infection rate were apparent, however, in the 16–29 and 30–44 age groups. A
chi-square analysis reveals a significant association for both of these age
groups between socio-economic status and being HIV positive ($p < 0.05$)
(see Bochow, 1997a). Within the 1996 data, this association is significant for
all three age groups ($p < 0.05$). Table 7.3 shows the class-related differences
for all age groups of the western German men who had been tested.

Table 7.3   Socio-economic status, age and serostatus (per cent of all tested western Germans)

Socio-economic status	Age and HIV infection				
	16–29	*30–44*	*45+*	*Total 1996*	*Total 1993*
Lower class	11.9	17.3	30.4	19.6	17.1
Lower middle class	9.4	15.3	15.1	13.3	13.1
Middle class	3.1	9.0	7.9	7.0	7.9
N	573	1002	272	1847	1654

Class-specific differences in HIV prevalence in France and England

Results from the 1995 nationwide survey on gay men and HIV/AIDS conducted in France offer a similar picture to that in the German data. The French analysis categorised respondents into class groupings using a method similar to that employed in the German study. The resulting calculations of seroprevalence within the sample also show differences between lower-class, lower-middle-class and middle-class men.

In the French study, 88 per cent of the subjects reported having been tested for HIV at least once (compared with 73 per cent of western Germans in 1996). Of these men 16 per cent were HIV positive (compared with 11 per cent of western Germans). The higher rate of HIV testing and of seroprevalence in France compared with Germany reflects a trend which has been evident since the first Gay Press Survey (1987 in Germany; 1985 in France).

The results of the 1995 French survey also show marked class-related vulnerability for HIV infection. The percentages of those having tested positive among those tested were 25 per cent for lower-class men, 18 per cent for the men of the lower middle class, and 13 per cent for the middle-class

Table 7.4   Socio-economic status, age and serostatus in France 1995 (per cent of all tested French respondents)

Socio-economic status	Age and HIV infection				
	16–29	*30–44*	*45+*	*Total 1995*	*Total 1993*
Lower class	20.5	30.6	26.1	24.9	20.0
Lower middle class	10.8	26.0	6.3	17.8	18.0
Middle class	7.1	19.7	12.4	13.3	16.5
N	1029	1034	176	2239	2619

Source: Marie-Ange Schiltz, CAMS, CNRS Paris

subjects. Table 7.4 shows that these class-related differences hold true for all three age groups.

A chi-square analysis reveals a significant association for all of the age groups between socio-economic status and being HIV positive ($p < 0.05$). Such an association was observed in the 1993 French survey only for the 16–29 age group. The 1993 wave of the French study also shows class-related differences.

However, these differences are not so pronounced as those found in the German data of the same year. Subsequent waves in both countries (France 1995, Germany 1996) show larger class differences compared with the 1993 French data (Bochow, 1997a). Most probably because the HIV epidemic among middle-class French gay men appeared earlier and struck this population more severely compared with their western German counterparts, there was a time lag in the seroprevalence rates among lower-class French men (cf. Pollak, 1988).

A recent survey of gay men in England has shown similar differences between social classes to those found in Germany and France. The British researchers defined social status according to highest attained educational qualification (Table 7.5). Sigma Research recruited 4161 men at gay community festivals in six cities during summer 1997: London, Brighton, Bristol, Birmingham, Manchester and Leeds (Hickson *et al.*, 1998).

Implications for primary prevention

Ulrich Biechele, the author of the sole German study prior to this one on the preventive behaviour of lower-class men, sees experienced gay men as gatekeepers to the gay community. The latter, he claims, do not merely go to the park to pick someone up and satisfy their sexual needs, but are interested both sexually and socio-culturally in the encounter (Biechele, 1996). Biechele recommends that more emphasis be put on the personal communicative

Table 7.5 HIV testing history by highest educational qualification (HEQ)

HEQ	None	O-level	A-level	Diploma	Degree
Never tested (%)	41.7	40.2	42.5	40.1	43.2
HIV negative (%)	47.2	52.7	51.2	54.0	52.5
HIV positive (%)	11.7	7.1	6.3	5.8	4.3
% HIV positive among those tested	19.0	11.9	11.0	9.7	7.6
N	235	860	604	755	1654

Source: Sigma Research, London

Notes:
The proportion never tested did not significantly differ by education.
The prevalence of diagnosed HIV infection decreased, stepwise, with increasing education.

aspects of primary prevention (outreach work) for lower-class homosexual men alongside parallel work in the print media and television.

In the light of Biechele's work and the findings presented above, we can reach some tentative conclusions concerning future prevention efforts for this neglected population. The greater the distance between lower-class gay men and the 'gay scene', the lower is the incidence of gay self-identification (cf. Bochow, 1997a; Dowsett, 1996). This, together with their specific communication and interaction styles, requires a range of specially designed informational and counselling options. Broad appeals through the mass media or the distribution of printed matter can only have a very limited impact on this section of the population. What is called for are special forms of prevention activity based on outreach models. Information, counselling and support agencies need to adapt their work to the needs of specific subgroups. Just what organisational forms and profiles such agencies should seek to promote remains to be seen. However, whatever form they take, it will be vital for them to secure the engagement of activists who either have the same class background as the men they are trying to reach, or have developed a particular social proximity to them.

Notes

1   Translated from the German by Michael Wright, Paul Morland and Brian Hawkins.
2   I would like to thank Marie-Ange Schiltz (CNRS, Paris) and Ford Hickson (Sigma Research, London) for permission to use the necessary data from their relevant surveys. My thanks go to Michael Lange for his help preparing the data from the gay press surveys, to Theo Sandfort for his meticulous reading of the manuscript, and to Stuart Michaels for his help in re-editing this article.
3   These percentages differ slightly from those shown in Table 7.2 because they include unprotected anal contact with partners of unknown and discordant serostatus.
4   One to two risk contacts received the value 1.5; three to four risk contacts, 3.5; five to ten risk contacts, 7.5; risk contact every month, 14; and risk contact every week, 60. It is likely that this method of calculation results in an underestimate of the total risk contacts for men with a high frequency of sexual contacts. This potential problem is, however, not important for the purposes of this study, namely the comparison of the individual subgroups; men without risk contacts; men with few/sporadic risk contacts; men with frequent risk contacts; and men with very frequent risk contacts.

References

Biechele, U. (1996) *Schwule Männer aus der Unterschicht. Sexuelle Identität und HIV-Prävention (Gay Working Class Men. Sexual Identity and HIV Prevention)*, Berlin: AIDS-Forum Deutsche AIDS-Hilfe.

Bochow, M. (1993) *Die Reaktionen homosexueller Männer auf AIDS in Ost- und Westdeutschland (The Reactions of Gay Men to AIDS in eastern and western*

Germany), Report commissioned by the German Federal Centre for Health Education, Berlin: AIDS-Forum Deutsche AIDS-Hilfe.

——(1994) *Schwuler Sex und die Bedrohung durch AIDS – Reaktionen homosexueller Männer in Ost- und Westdeutschland (Gay Sex and the Threat of AIDS – The Reactions of Gay Men in eastern and western Germany)*, Report commissioned by the German Federal Centre for Health Education, Berlin: AIDS-Forum Deutsche AIDS-Hilfe.

——(1997a) *Informationsstand und präventive Vorkehrungen im Hinblick auf AIDS bei homosexuellen Männern der Unterschicht (The Particular Vulnerability of Working Class Gay Men to HIV Infection and AIDS)*, Report commissioned by the Federal Health Ministry, Berlin: AIDS-Forum Deutsche AIDS-Hilfe.

——(1997b) *Schwule Männer und AIDS (Gay Men and AIDS)*, Report commissioned by the German Federal Centre for Health Education, Berlin: AIDS-Forum Deutsche AIDS-Hilfe.

Bourdieu, P. (1977) 'Remarques provisoires sur la perception sociale du corps', *Actes de la recherche en sciences sociales* 14: 51–54.

——(1979a) *La Distinction. Critique sociale du jugement*, Paris: Les Editions de Minuit.

——(1979b) 'Les trois états du capital culturel', *Actes de la recherche en sciences sociales* 30: 3–6.

——(1980) *Le Sens pratique*, Paris: Les Editions de Minuit.

Connell, R. W., Davis, M. D. and Dowsett, G. W. (1993) 'A bastard of a life: homosexual desire and practice among men in working class milieux', *Australian and New Zealand Journal of Sociology* 29(1): 112–135.

Dannecker, M. and Reiche, R. (1974) *Der gewöhnliche Homosexuelle. Eine soziologische Untersuchung über männliche Homosexuelle in der Bundesrepublik*, Frankfurt a.M.: S. Fischer.

Dowsett, G. W. (1996) *Practicing Desire. Homosexual Sex in the Era of AIDS*, Stanford, CA: Stanford University Press.

Dowsett, G. W., Davis, M. D. and Connell, R. W. (1992) 'Working class homosexuality and HIV/AIDS prevention: some recent research from Sydney, Australia', *Psychology and Health* 6: 313–324.

Hickson, F., Reid, D. and Weatherburn, P. (1998) 'Geographic and education variation in HIV testing history among gay men in England', Poster presented at the 12th World AIDS Conference, Geneva.

Mielck, A. (ed.) (1994) *Krankheit und soziale Ungleichheit – Ergebnisse der sozialepidemiologischen Forschung in Deutschland*, Opladen: Leske und Budrich.

Pollak, M. (1988) *Les Homosexuels et le SIDA. Sociologie d'une épidémie*, Paris: Editions A. M. Métailié.

Schiltz, M. A. (1993) *Les Homosexuels masculins face au SIDA: Enquêtes 1991–1992. Rapport de fin de contrat à l'ANRS*, Paris: CAMS, CNRS.

——(1998) *Les Homosexuels face au SIDA: Enquête 1995. Regards sur une décennie d'enquêtes*, Paris: CAMS, CERMES.

Schiltz, M. A. and Adam, P. (1995) *Les Homosexuels face au SIDA: Enquête 1993 sur les modes de vie et la gestion du risque HIV*, Paris: CAMS, CERMES.

Townsend, P., Davidson, N. and Whitehead, M. (1988) *Introduction to Inequalities in Health*, London: Penguin, pp. 1–27.

8 Condom use among 15 to 18 year-olds in France

Changes in behaviour over time

Hugues Lagrange, Brigitte Lhomond and the ACSJ research team[1]

When the AIDS epidemic erupted at the beginning of the 1980s, it raised the practical problem of how best to promote changes in sexual behaviour to a serious and highly diffuse risk. The epidemic did not affect all segments of society at the same time, however. The degree of risk, as measured by the number of new AIDS cases recorded, was and remains variable from one social group to another. At the end of the 1980s, few observers would have ruled out the possibility of the epidemic spreading to a large part of the heterosexual population in Europe, and young people seemed particularly vulnerable. Ten years later, epidemiological evidence shows an increase in the percentage of AIDS cases through heterosexual transmission and concern about AIDS remains high.

Through community action and concerted effort, AIDS came to the forefront of public attention. Information campaigns enabled people to acquire a reasonably good knowledge of the risks involved and the precautions to be taken. But whereas the first studies conducted among the general population (Dab *et al.*, 1988; Aubigny *et al.*, 1990) showed there to be adequate knowledge of how the disease is transmitted, the few studies conducted with teenagers, especially in the USA, revealed little correspondence between the degree of exposure to HIV and the precautions taken. McDonald *et al.* (1990), for example, observed that among US teenagers the number of sexual partners tended to be inversely proportional to the degree of regularity of condom use. Bowie and Ford (1989) and Hingson *et al.* (1990) presented similar findings. According to Binson *et al.* (1993), the systematic use of condoms with 'secondary' (*sic*) partners among middle-class young people aged 18 to 25 decreased as the number of partners increased. Only 14 per cent of persons with four or more partners used condoms systematically. Taking into account the sex of the respondents, Dickson *et al.* (1993) found that for girls condom use declined as the number of partners over the preceding twelve months increased, whereas for boys it remained constant. According to Durbin *et al.* (1993), 50 per cent of the young people not using condoms systematically had more than one partner, but this was the case with only 31 per cent of those using condoms systematically.

In a paper charting changes in sexual behaviour and the risk of exposure to HIV between 1988 and 1993, Robertson (1995) could find no evidence of a systematic reduction in the number of sexual partners. Since the mid 1990s, there is probably even less of an expectation that young people will have fewer partners. After fifteen years of epidemic and ten years of study, some researchers are troubled not to have been able to show a reduction of the number of sexual partners among teenaged young people, many of whom change sexual partners more often than adults over the age of 20. A few researchers have also been amazed that teenagers had not delayed first sexual intercourse[2] or, at least, are not reporting using condoms systematically when having several partners.

By posing the problem in terms of using condoms systematically with 'secondary' partners and/or not distinguishing between multiple simultaneous partners and a succession of partners over time, researchers were – misguidedly, in our view – applying models of sexual behaviour applicable to the adult heterosexual population. The general tone of numerous articles published between 1988 and 1992 reflects the idea that young people, if not ignorant of the health risks they were taking, were at least heedless of them. Why did some teenagers, or certain categories of teenagers, take such serious risks? In order to answer this question it is necessary to acknowledge a certain ambivalence in behaviours linked to the quest for sensations and thrills. Smoking, drinking, using marijuana or ecstasy, and having sex represent not just risks for those who engage in them, but also pleasure, joy, sources of gratification. Teenagers rarely drink and smoke alone (to say nothing of being sexually active), and such practices cannot be understood if we do not take into account notions of exchange and sociability that they involve. Preserving one's health is no doubt important, but we should never forget that health is a condition of existence, not its purpose.

Sexual behaviours are, like precautionary ones, marked by the intersection of a biographical moment – adolescence – and HIV/AIDS. Active sexual life is entered into now in a society that has experienced what Leridon and Toulemon (1987) have called a 'contraceptive revolution', a revolution in which AIDS is now a permanent part.

The aim of this chapter is to describe the use of condoms at first and last intercourse among young people in France. We will analyse these events in a biographical and relational context, taking into account the dynamics of the relationship, the degree of sexual experience of the partners, and the awareness of AIDS.

The study

The population described here is defined by two age limits: 15 is the legal age of sexual consent in France and 18 is the age of majority. The sample consists of 6182 teenagers – 3345 boys and 2837 girls – from regular and technical high schools, and from apprenticeships and other vocational training centres for young people who have left junior high school without a diploma. To reduce organisation and travel costs, data were collected in eighteen *départements* of France chosen in three zones with contrasting rates of AIDS prevalence (high, medium, low). We used a two-level random, stratified sample. The educational establishments to be surveyed were selected from lists of schools and training centres provided by the Ministry of Education, including private institutions as well as public (i.e. non-fee-paying) schools. They were then ranked by number of students and geographical zone of AIDS prevalence in which they were located, so that the strata would be as homogeneous as possible with regard to risk. Within each institution, the individuals to be surveyed were randomly selected from an exhaustive list of students; we did not select entire school classes. The sampling fractions varied according to age and type of educational institution.

Data were collected by face-to-face interviews because this enabled us to adapt questions to the actual experience of the respondents (through the use of filter questions), and offered a more direct means of communication.

The interview schedule explored a wide range of sexual activities including kissing, petting, genital petting, oral–genital relations, and vaginal and anal penetration. Young people who have practised acts involving the genital organs of at least one of the two persons involved were defined as having had sex: 54.6 per cent of our respondents fell into this category. We collected information about the first and last sexual partner and the type of sexual acts practised on three specific occasions: the first sexual intercourse with the first partner, the first sexual intercourse with the last partner for those who had had at least two partners, the last sexual intercourse with the first partner if only one partner, or with the last partner if more than one.

Vaginal or anal penetration had been practised by 44.3 per cent of 15 to 18 year-olds – 47.4 per cent of boys and 41 per cent of girls. Predictably, experience of sexual penetration increased with age: 20.1 per cent of 15 year-olds, 36.3 per cent of 16 year-olds, 52.7 per cent of 17 year-olds, and 66.8 per cent of 18 year-olds reported having had sexual intercourse. The median age of first sexual intercourse was 17 years and 3 months for boys, and 17 years and 6 months for girls. For both sexes, the median age varied with educational status, with those in apprenticeship training centres having intercourse slightly earlier than technical high school students, who in turn started earlier than those in regular high schools.

Among those who had had sex – taken as including any kind of genital contact – 1.4 per cent of boys and 1.3 per cent of girls reported having had a relationship with someone of the same sex. Among those who had practised sexual penetration, 15.4 per cent of the girls and 13.0 per cent of the boys had experienced anal intercourse. Among the boys, 1.2 per cent had experienced receptive anal intercourse.

Finally, for certain comparisons we shall use the results of a study of teenagers' health conducted by the Comité Français d'Education pour la

Santé[3] (CFES). This survey was undertaken in November–December 1997 using a representative, randomly selected sample of 2672 persons – 1370 boys and 1302 girls – aged 15 to 19, living in metropolitan France. Respondents in this survey were interviewed by telephone. In the CFES survey, 50.7 per cent of boys and 46.1 per cent of girls reported having had sexual intercourse.

Condom use

In order to study the types of precautions taken during sexual relations, we focused on those who had practised either vaginal or anal penetration. The following tables only include these people.

In relation to contraception, condoms have become the dominant means of protection used for the self and partner, even for the oldest girls in our sample – this is a new phenomenon (see Table 8.1). The pill comes second and its use increases as young people gain sexual experience. Other methods are used only very rarely. While 'withdrawal' was mentioned by a small minority of respondents in connection with their first sexual intercourse, it disappears entirely thereafter. A small number of sexually active young people did not report using either a means of protection against sexually transmitted diseases or any contraceptive device.

The precautions taken by young people during the second decade of the

Table 8.1   Precautions taken by young people aged 15 to 18 on 1 January 1994 (ACSJ)

	First sexual intercourse		First intercourse with most recent partner		Most recent intercourse regardless of partner, different from first intercourse.	
Percentage using:	*Boys*	*Girls*	*Boys*	*Girls*	*Boys*	*Girls*
Condoms	78.9	74.4	85.0	66.2	72.5	51.1
Birth control pill	22.0	18.6	27.4	28.8	36.2	48.1
Spermicidal creams or suppositories	0.7	0.9	0.7	0.0	0.9	0.8
Attention to timing and calendar	0.5	1.4	0.6	2.0	1.5	1.3
Withdrawal	5.2	5.3	0.0	0.0	1.0	0.9
Nothing*	8.4	12.2	6.6	14.3	6.9	7.8
Base	1842	1314	1033	467	1329**	1180**

* No condoms, pills or any other method, such as withdrawal, timing, etc.
** These bases represent those who had intercourse at least twice with the first or more recent partner.

AIDS epidemic would appear to have evolved remarkably quickly if we take into account the relatively slow transformation of contraceptive habits among adults. More than three-quarters of the boys and girls questioned said they used condoms during their first sexual intercourse, and a still higher proportion of boys said they used a condom during first sexual intercourse with their most recent partner. On the other hand, fewer girls used condoms in that situation than they did the first time. Among people who have had intercourse twice with the same person (be they the first partner or last) the percentage of condom users drops significantly, especially among girls.

Condom use during first sexual relations

Reported condom use is generally higher among boys than girls, and variations in condom use during first sexual intercourse by social milieu are slight and generally not significant. Neither regional cultural differences, nor level of urbanisation, are factors differentiating condom or oral contraceptive use during first sexual relations.

Educational status does make a slight difference here. The use of oral contraceptives is lower among girls studying the sciences and arts than among female apprenticeship trainees. On the other hand, boys' statements suggest that rates of oral contraception among their partners do not vary with educational orientation. During first sexual intercourse, the percentage of condom users is lower among male apprenticeship trainees than among male regular high school students. However, it is difficult to isolate any clear effect due to educational background because the average age and year of first sexual intercourse vary from one type of schooling/training to the next.

We observed an increase in condom use between the 1994 ACSJ study and the 1997 CFES study (Table 8.2). Although these two surveys use different data collection methods, the samples are both representative of the same population. Therefore this global increase is not likely to be due to differences in the samples. Both studies reveal a decrease in the frequency of

Table 8.2 Condom use during first sexual intercourse, by age and sex in the ACSJ and CFES studies

	ACSJ-1994		CFES-1997	
	Boys	*Girls*	*Boys*	*Girls*
15	85.8	92.3	94.6	96.6
16	87.0	78.0	91.9	91.9
17	79.7	72.0	86.8	92.1
18	69.8	67.7	89.0	80.7
19	–	–	87.9	80.6
Base	1842	1314	673	577

condom use between the ages of 15 and 18, but that decrease is sharper in the 1994 study.

The notion of age, in this context, refers to both a moment in the life cycle and the year in which penetrative genital sexuality was first practised. The most remarkable observation is the increase over time in the proportion of young people who used condoms during their first sexual intercourse. This observation encouraged us to consider the date of first penetrative sex as a key variable. The increase is sharper among boys than girls, and occurs first in 1990 and second in 1993 (see Table 8.3, first two columns). After that year, according to the CFES data, there is a slowdown in condom use for first sexual intercourse.

For girls, the dynamic is the same but the increase is not as big. This is due to the fact that their partners belong to more dispersed age categories, primarily 15 to 21. The oldest boys, not in the ACSJ sample, began their active sexual life earlier in time, at a moment when condom use was less frequent; they are much more sexually experienced than the girls, which means, as we will see, that they are less likely to use condoms. For girls, important changes occurred in 1991 and again, as for boys, in 1993. The year at which first intercourse takes place therefore explains why there is an increase in condom use for each age category between the two surveys (shown in Table 8.2).

The observed decrease in condom use with the respondent's age reflects changes between the mid 1980s and the mid 1990s in the protective measures taken in response to the risk of HIV. The oldest respondents in the ACSJ study first had sex at a time when precautions were only beginning to be talked about, whereas the youngest respondents in that study, as well as

Table 8.3   Condom use at first sexual intercourse, by year intercourse occurred and sex, in the ACSJ and CFES studies

Year of first intercourse	ACSJ-1994		CFES-1997
	Boys	Girls	Both sexes*
1989	58.2	55.7	–
1990	73.4	53.4	–
1991	77.8	70.3	–
1992	78.2	72.1	81.3
1993	87.9	82.3	82.0
1994	–	–	81.3
1995	–	–	92.6
1996	–	–	89.6
1997	–	–	85.8
Base	1842	1314	1238**
p***	<0.005	<0.005	–

*	CFES does not provide a tabulation by sexes and *p* value.
**	Twelve respondents did not answer for the year of their first intercourse.
***	The *p* value is associated with the chi-square test.

almost all the respondents in the CFES study, began their active sexual life at a time when condom use was already an established and widespread practice.

The ACSJ data make it clear that we cannot think of early sexual activity as synonymous with risk taking. For a given year, the level of condom use during first intercourse is in fact slightly higher among those starting early. If we look, for example, at the group of individuals who reported having had first intercourse in 1993, we can see that 95.7 per cent of boys aged 15 to 16 used condoms, as against 80.5 per cent of 18-year-old boys. If we keep the year that sexual activity began constant, we can see that boys who began to have sex early used condoms more than boys who began later. For girls, on the other hand, there are no significant variations in condom use with age if we take into account the effect of the year of the first relationship (with the exception of the 1993 group). If we eliminate the cases where the female partner was on the pill and adjust the percentage according to the year of first sexual intercourse (data from logistic regression not presented), we can see that condom use during that experience did not vary with age. Among young people who had their first sexual relationship in one given year, condom use among those who were 18 (91 per cent) and those who were 15–16 (96 per cent) is comparable.

The increase in condom use during first sexual intercourse did not follow a decrease in oral contraceptive use over time. In fact, the use of oral contraception in first intercourse fluctuates around 20 per cent according to the ACSJ report and around 27 per cent according to the CFES study, with no clearly marked tendency to increase or decrease.

Condom use during most recent sexual intercourse

Young people at school in urban areas and in zones where AIDS is relatively prevalent – particularly Paris, Marseilles, Toulouse and Montpellier – do not use condoms any more frequently than those living in rural areas or in zones where AIDS is not prevalent. The geography of the epidemic does not, then, have an effect on young people's precaution-taking behaviour. On the other hand, the effect of age is quite marked in both studies, at least for the most recent sexual intercourse. The youngest teenagers use condoms more frequently than the older ones.

Educational experience also has an influence on precaution taking during most recent sexual intercourse. If age is held constant, apprenticeship trainees differ from regular high school students by using condoms much less: female trainees used them half as often as regular high school students, and the percentage of male trainee users is fifteen points below the students' level. Taking precautions against sexually transmitted diseases and AIDS therefore has a social dimension: in the least prestigious training structures, penetrative genital sexuality begins earlier and is practised with less protection.

The key finding here (see Table 8.4) is that at the beginning of sexual life, when contraceptive habits have not yet been acquired, condoms are massively used in relationships where the male partner is very young – 15 to 16 years old. Between the ages of 16 and 18, contraceptive habits evolve quickly, bringing about changes in the respective use of condoms and the pill. While during the first sexual relationship condom use is practically unaffected by the use of oral contraception, this is not the case for the most recent sexual relation. The frequency of condom use during this last relationship on the part of boys aged 15 to 16 does not greatly depend on whether their partners use oral contraception. Among those aged 17 and 18, however, condom use is less frequent when the partner is on the pill. An analogous phenomenon may be discerned from the girls' statements. During the most recent relationship, the influence of the pill on the level of condom use is decisive, regardless of the respondent's age. The condom loses popularity among boys and even more so among girls as the use of oral contraception becomes more common. It is as if the decrease in condom use were automatically compensated for by an increase in oral contraception.

Total number of partners and age difference

While the majority of 15 to 18 year-olds who have experience of penetrative sex – 65 per cent of boys and 45 per cent of girls – have had several partners since the beginning of their sexual life, in nearly nine out of ten cases these have been successive partners. Very few teenagers report having several partners at the same time (see Levinson, 1997). For most young people, risk lies in the fact that the majority of their partners are new ones. This brings up the question of whether those who have had different partners protect them-

Table 8.4   Condom and birth control pill use during most recent intercourse,* by age and sex (ACSJ)

Age	% using condoms		% on birth control pill	
	Boys	*Girls*	*Boys*	*Girls*
15**	92.8	83.9	21.2	17.2
16	78.4	56.9	35.3	39.2
17	66.4	45.0	38.8	55.7
18	58.8	34.8	54.4	65.8
Base	1419	1208	1419	1208
p	0.01	<0.005	<0.005	<0.005

* Most recent intercourse includes: last intercourse with the first and only partner; and last intercourse with the last partner. For those who have more than one partner, this can be the first intercourse with that partner.
** The sample here is not strictly representative of 15 year-olds: it includes respondents from 15 years 3 months to any age less than 16; not very many persons have intercourse between 15 years and 15 years 3 months old.

selves at last intercourse more than those who have had only one, everything else being equal.

If we do not adjust the percentage calculation to account for the effects of other factors, condom use is practically unrelated to the total number of partners. Those who have had the most partners during their life do not use condoms with any perceptibly greater frequency than those who have had only one sexual partner (Table 8.5). If we adjust for the number of partners during the previous year, however, there is an effect for boys: the more partners they have the more they use condoms (data not presented).

Are there differences in behaviour between boys and girls? Starting at age 17, the percentage of boys using condoms seems to go up with the total number of partners, but the increase is not statistically significant. Among girls, the total number of partners has no effect on condom use. It is as though, because their sexual networks develop over time and they do not have several simultaneous sexual relationships, young people did not really consider the fact of multiple partners to be a significant risk. However, the modest trend that may be observed among certain categories of boys towards an increase in condom use when the number of partners increases should be noted, since it contrasts with the results of several UK and US studies conducted at the end of the 1980s. According to Gottlieb *et al.* (1988) and Bowie and Ford (1989), condom use decreases with the total number of partners. We may here be witnessing, in France at least, a real, if slight, evolution in behaviour.

The combined effect of partners' age on condom use accounts for the contrast between the youngest couples, among whom condom use reaches nearly 80 per cent, and older couples, about 25 per cent of whom use condoms. Furthermore, the most marked decrease in condom use is to be found among the girls who have the oldest partners. This fact singles out a source of risk which has been already underlined for first intercourse: because they are more sexually experienced (they consequently have had more chances to be exposed to HIV) and are psychologically reassuring,

Table 8.5 Condom use during most recent sexual intercourse, by sex, age and the total number of partners in the respondent's lifetime (ACSJ)

No. of partners	Boys			Girls		
	15–16	17	18	15–16	17	18
1	86.4	58.9	43.2	62.6	47.8	38.8
2–4	70.4	69.8	64.9	73.3	40.9	39.6
5 or more	88.0	67.8	66.9	58.2	45.3	32.6
Base	223	310	556	220	402	564
p	>0.1	>0.1	0.08*	>0.1	>0.1	>0.1

* Although with a value slightly higher than 0.05, *p* underlines the behaviour that appears among 18-year-old boys.

older and more experienced boys encourage their younger partners to take fewer precautions, thereby exposing them to a higher risk of infection.

Frequency of sexual intercourse and length of relationships

Length of relationship also affects condom use during most recent intercourse: the longer the relationship, the less likely partners are to use a condom during most recent intercourse. The decrease in the proportion of condom users with length of relationship is not, however, linear: decline in use begins only when relations have lasted three to four months. The decrease is sharper between four and eight months, and then slows down for relationships lasting a year or more (see Figure 8.1).

Condom use also decreases as sexual intercourse becomes more frequent. At the point where intercourse is practised once a week, condom use falls thirty points, and it decreases further when the frequency reaches twice weekly. With greater frequencies, condom use declines slowly and becomes stable at about 15 per cent among those who have sexual relations once every two days or more. Here we must take into account an obvious prac-

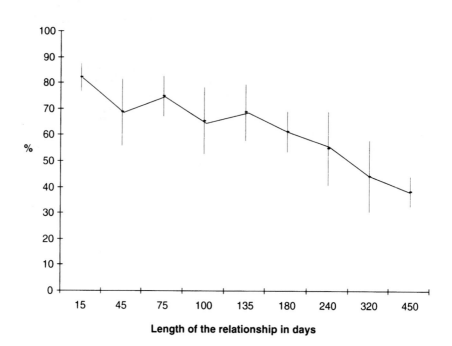

Figure 8.1   Percentage of young people using condoms during most recent intercourse according to length of relationship. Both sexes (ACSJ)

Note: The short thick lines represent average percentages; the light vertical lines indicate the confidence interval for these percentages from the mean to 95 per cent

tical aspect: when sexual intercourse occurs frequently, young people stop using condoms and start using the pill. However, condom use remains close to the maximum level when there is no oral contraception, regardless of the frequency of sexual intercourse. Moreover, there is a relationship between frequency of intercourse and length of the relationship: when oral contraception is not used, the percentage of condom users does not go down with relationship length as long as the frequency of sexual intercourse remains below three times a week. Above that, condom use radically declines. What we have here is the relatively rare case of a long relationship without the use of oral contraceptives, where there is a high risk of unwanted pregnancy.

Co-ordinating condom use and HIV testing

Twelve per cent of boys and 20 per cent of girls have been tested at least once (fairly high percentages). Here we have included only young people who had had penetrative sex with their last partner (who may have been their first), because the partner's getting tested was only envisaged in the context of this last relationship.

Of all the young people who reported having had penetrative sex, some had had a single partner and others had had two or more partners during their life. When they met their most recent partner, the latter were therefore no longer 'virgins' in the usual sense of the term. However many partners they themselves have had, respondents have partners who either had had, or had not had, other sexual partners before meeting them, and this difference affects behaviour.

There is some correlation between the partners' respective levels of experience or inexperience. When the respondent and his or her partner were virgins before meeting, 10.5 per cent got themselves tested for HIV; when neither were virgins, 13 per cent took the test – this is not a significant difference. Two observations may be made about these findings. First, the frequency of condom use is always higher when neither of the partners has had an HIV test following first intercourse – above 80 per cent – and remains high for the most recent intercourse: 60 to 70 per cent. Second, when both partners have had a test, there is a sharp fall in condom use between first and most recent intercourse.

Ceasing to use condoms is associated with getting an HIV test, but is it directly linked? Unfortunately we cannot give a general answer to this question. Testing dates are only known, and then only partially, for respondents themselves and not their partners. When testing takes place between first and most recent sexual intercourse, it is associated with a noticeable decrease in condom use among respondents whose partner was not a virgin, but there is no such decrease when the partner was a virgin. In general, and even though this is not consciously planned, adaptation to the risk of HIV infection combines recourse to the test and condom use. The precautions taken thus *appear* co-ordinated; they consist of using condoms and getting tested for HIV according to relationship characteristics, the year penetrative sex was first practised, and partners' experience.

Perception of risk and precautions taken

Concern about AIDS increased greatly during the first half of the 1990s. In 1991, 50 per cent of respondents who had had their first relationship around that time declared that they were concerned about AIDS; that number went up to 70 per cent in 1993. This increase parallels the increase in condom use, which is the same among girls and boys and is not any more accentuated among young people in vocational or apprenticeship training than among regular high school students. Concern about AIDS is uniformly distributed for all sexually active young people. It is, however, a diffuse phenomenon, not necessarily linked to direct, personal – and therefore variable – experience.

In addition to questions about preoccupation with AIDS, we asked respondents whether they knew anyone who had the 'AIDS virus', regardless of whether that person were close to them or not. Slightly over 20 per cent of 15 to 18 year-olds answered yes. Is this low or high? The answer depends of course on how wide a population of 'people known to you' the respondent had in mind when answering the question. While the percentage of young people who know someone with HIV does not vary according to type of school major or educational orientation, there is a difference according to sex: 27.5 per cent of the girls reported knowing someone with HIV, as against 17.8 per cent of the boys. This result can be partially explained by the age structure of the girls' network of relations, particularly with the opposite sex: the boys that girls know are on average older than the girls and boys that boys know. Furthermore, a much higher proportion of boys (37.1 per cent) and girls (36.5 per cent) who had had homosexual relations knew HIV-infected persons.

On the whole, the HIV-infected persons known to respondents came from circles close to them: nearly 50 per cent are friends or family members. The social spheres involved – family, persons their own age that they see frequently or more distant acquaintances – are the same for boys and girls.

How much do consciousness of risk and perception of a real danger influence precaution-taking behaviour? In order to show the effects associated with pressure from the AIDS epidemic, we have to neutralise the factor that has the most influence on condom use, namely recourse to oral contraception. When this is done, we find that condom use is generally independent of knowing persons infected with HIV. It is true that when oral contraception is used, condom use at last intercourse is higher among respondents who know someone with HIV. How close an HIV-infected person is to the respondent, however, induces consistent variations in condom use: the closer the person known, the more frequently condoms are used.

For both first and most recent sexual intercourse, there is no significant link between frequency of condom use and the personal fear of infection. However, general concern about AIDS is associated with more frequent condom use, except in the relatively rare cases where sex had most recently been had without oral contraception: there the contraceptive intent overwhelmed awareness of risk. In all other situations, concern about AIDS produced significant effects.

Talking about condoms

For sexually active young people today, it is a perfectly ordinary thing to talk about condoms. Ninety per cent of girls and 83 per cent of boys reported talking about them, especially with their friends of the same sex: 73.5 per cent of boys and 61.2 per cent of girls talked about them with friends of the same sex, while 46.1 per cent of girls and 34.6 per cent of boys talked about them with friends of the opposite sex. Is there a connection between talking about condoms and using them? Condom use is not affected by whether young people talk about condoms with friends or not, regardless of the sexual relationship in question. But the role of the peer group in condom use cannot be reduced to the simple fact of talking about condoms, especially since we do not know the content of such discussions. To understand the role of the peer group, we would need to see whether condom use by friends has an influence on the respondent's behaviour, and this would require a different kind of study, in which the whole network of a respondent's friends would be questioned about their preventive behaviours.

Talking about condoms with one's sexual partner does not bring about any variation in condom use as far as boys are concerned. There was, however, a slight tendency to use condoms less during most recent sexual intercourse when a boy had talked about them with his partner (though this variation did not attain the threshold of significance). For girls, the reverse was true. Talking about condoms with their partners went hand in hand with greater condom use, regardless of the sexual relationship in question. When girls talked about condoms with their partners, it was as though talking facilitated use, whereas for boys it was as though that talk enabled some to dispense with condoms during the most recent sexual relation.

Multivariate logistic analysis shows that biographical elements – age, year that active sexual life began – together with relationship characteristics – frequency of sexual relations, length of relationship – play a major role in determining condom use (data not presented). Prevention and contraception choices made 'the first time' affect later practices: boys who used a condom during their first sexual experience continue to do so in greater proportion during later relations, even several years later with a different partner. More surprisingly, the influence of first choice is also manifest among girls: relatively more of those who had their first sexual intercourse with a boy who used a condom also used this kind of protection during their most recent relation. The use of condom at first intercourse has a quasi-initiatory value, and gives condoms more of a biographical than a relational meaning: even with a different partner, the act of using one the first time leaves its mark.

The influence of the first time on precaution-taking behaviours is differential: those whose first time involved practising 'the good habit' retain something of it. But for society as a whole, has the risk of infection decreased? We can assess a possible diminution by means of two comparisons. The first (Table 8.6) involves comparing our results for 18 year-olds – that is, for the year 1994 – with those of the ACSF study for 1992 (Spira *et al.*, 1993). Between 1992 and 1994, there was an appreciable increase in condom use among men and a very slight increase among women. While neither of these differences is significant at the usual threshold, behaviours changed in the right direction.

The second comparison is between the 1994 ACSJ study and the 1997 CFES study. In the former, 64.8 per cent of boys and 44.1 per cent of girls used condoms during their most recent sexual intercourse, whereas in the latter, three years later, 79.9 per cent of the boys and 53.5 per cent of the girls used them. This increase in precaution taking over time, already observed in connection with the first sexual relation, indicates that the new practices are consistently maintained during the first years of active sexual life independently of fluctuations in media coverage of the epidemic.

Young people's adaptive response to the epidemic is not merely a ritualistic gesture performed the first time, it takes the form of a new habit that lasts at least a few months at the beginning of each new relationship and throughout any years in which no single, stable relationship is established. Prevention campaigns have made teenagers feel the necessity of using condoms; that necessity has been understood and the appropriate response put into practice. Today the major question is, do those at risk because they have multiple and/or new partners consistently use protection? The problem is to specify the conditions of safer sex, and this implies a better taking into account of individual situations, biographies, relational contexts – a refining of the map of risk that each person has implicitly drawn in reaching a

Table 8.6   Percentage of 18 year-olds using condoms during most recent sexual* intercourse (ACSF–ACSJ)

	1992 (ACSF)			1994 (ACSJ)		
	%	Standard deviation	Base	%	Standard deviation	Base
Men	50.4	10.7	48	62.4	2.4	755
Women	34.6	11.8	38	36.9	2.3	606

*   Here it is no longer a case of the 'last time' as distinguished from the first, but simply of the most recent sexual intercourse, including cases where this relation is also the first.

compromise between the untenable position of absolute caution and total unawareness or recklessness.

Maintaining a high level of condom use for young people in a long-lasting relationship (eight months to a year or longer) could not be a realistic goal for public policy. This is precisely because establishing a stable sexual relationship, which is associated with the use of oral contraception, seems to be one of the major factors involved in decrease in condom use. Rather than continuing to pronounce general injunctions that will only go unheeded, we might do better to promote systematic condom use at the beginning of each new relationship and for those few young people between 15 and 18 who have several partners at the same time. Furthermore, it would be judicious to promote the idea that the decision to stop using condoms – a fact in 'stable' relationships – should be well thought out; that is, not put into effect until both partners have had an HIV test and know the results. These recommendations are based on observed behaviours and seek to make such behaviours more consistent. They cannot be effective, however, unless they are part of a full, clear and reasoned sex education policy. We cannot promote coherent risk reduction through media campaigns alone. To confront the issue of AIDS today it is necessary, without sacrificing simplicity, to suggest more specific steps, steps that take into account the biographical and relational aspects of young people's sexuality.

Acknowledgements

This chapter was translated by Amy Jacobs.

Notes

1 The present study, entitled 'Analyse du comportement sexuel des jeunes', was financed by the Agence Nationale de Recherche sur le Sida and directed by Hugues Lagrange (CNRS, Paris) and Brigitte Lhomond (CNRS, Lyons). The research team was composed of Marcel Calvez (UHB-CNRS, Rennes), Chantal Darsch (CEFI, Paris), Carinne Favier (MFPF, Montpellier), François Fierro (PRISM, Toulouse), Sharman Levinson (EHESS, Paris), Andrei Mogoutov (ANRS, Paris), Sebastien Roché (CNRS, Grenoble), Josiane Warszawski (INSERM, Paris). Full results of the study have been published in Lagrange and Lhomond (1997).

2 Evidence that the age of first sexual intercourse was increasing would mean that the risk of contracting AIDS had actually reversed the long-term trend of a decrease in the age of first penetrative sexual relations. For a comparative analysis of age at first intercourse in European countries, see Bozon and Kontula (1998).

3 Our thanks to C. Dressen, J. Arènes and M. P. Janvrin, study directors, and P. Guilbert, who were kind enough to communicate their preliminary findings to us (Arènes *et al.*, 1998).

References

Arènes, J., Janvrin, M. P. and Baudier, F. (1998) *Baromètre santé jeunes* 97/98, Paris: Editions du CFES.

Aubigny, G., Berger, P., Bouhet, B., Denni, B., Durif, C., Lagrange, H., Lhomond, B., Roche, S. and Zorman, M. (1990) 'Comportements sexuels et précautions face au sida dans la région Rhône-Alpes en 1989', *Bulletin Epidémiologique Hebdomadaire* 6: 21–22.

Binson, D., Dolcini, M. M., Pollack, L. M. and Catania, J. A. (1993) 'Multiple sexual partners among young adults in high-risk cities', *Family Planning Perspectives* 25: 268–272.

Bowie, C. and Ford, N. (1989) 'Sexual behavior of young people and the risk of HIV infection', *Journal of Epidemiology and Community Health* 43: 61–65.

Bozon, M. and Kontula, O. (1998) 'Sexual initiation and gender in Europe: cross-cultural analysis of trends in the twentieth century', in M. Hubert *et al.* (eds) *Sexual Behavior and HIV/AIDS in Europe. Comparisons of National Surveys*, London: Taylor and Francis.

Dab, W., Moatti, J. P., Abenhaim, L., Bastide, S. and Pollak, M. (1988) 'Le sida et les comportements sexuels de Franciliens', *Bulletin Epidémiologique Hebdomadaire* 40: 193–194.

Dickson, N., Paul, C. and Herbison, P. (1993) 'Adolescents, sexual behaviour and implications for an epidemic of HIV/AIDS among the young', *Genitourinary Medicine* 69: 133–140.

Durbin, M. *et al.* (1993) 'Factors associated with multiple sex partners among junior high school students', *Journal of Adolescent Health* 14: 202–207.

Gottlieb, N. *et al.* (1988) 'Aids-related knowledge, attitudes, behaviors and intentions among Texas college students', *Health Education Research* 3: 67–73.

Hingson, R., Strunin, L. and Berlin, B. (1990) 'Beliefs about AIDS, use of alcohol and drugs, and unprotected sex among Massachusetts adolescents', *American Journal of Public Health* 80(3): 295–299.

Lagrange, H. and Lhomond, B. (eds) (1997) *L'Entrée dans la sexualité. Le comportement des jeunes dans le contexte du sida*, Paris: La Découverte.

Leridon, H. and Toulemon, L. (1987) *La Seconde révolution contraceptive. La régulation des naissances en France de 1950 à 1985*, Travaux et documents, 117, Paris: INED-PUF.

Levinson, S. (1997) 'L'organisation temporelles des premières relations sexuelles', in Lagrange, H. and Lhomond, B. (eds) *L'Entrée dans la sexualité. Le comportement des jeunes dans le contexte du sida*, Paris: La Découverte.

McDonald, N., Wells, G. A., Fisher, W. A., Warren, W. K., King, M. A., Doherty, J. A. and Bowie, W. L. (1990) 'High-risk STD/HIV behaviour among college students', *Journal of the American Medical Association* 263(23): 3155–3169.

Robertson, B. J. (1995) 'Sexual behavior and risk of exposure to HIV among 18–25 year-olds in Scotland: assessing change 1988–1993', *AIDS* 9(3): 285–292.

Spira, A., Bajos, N. and the ACSF (1993) *Les Comportements sexuels en France*, Paris: La Documentation Française.

9 Sexual revolution in Russia and the tasks of sex education

Valeriy Chervyakov and Igor Kon

The so-called sexual revolution of the 1960s in Western Europe and the USA has been thoroughly discussed in the scientific literature (see e.g. Clement, 1990; Haavio-Mannila and Rotkirch, 1997; Reiss, 1990; Schmidt, 1993; Schmidt *et al.*, 1994; Schwartz and Gillmore, 1990). Contrary to media representations and popular belief, this 'revolution' was in fact a multifaceted and contradictory process. Some behavioural and attitudinal changes were substantial whereas others had more of an evolutionary character. Thus, the authors of the US National Health and Social Life Survey (NHSLS) have recently stated that

> social forces – demographic, economic, technological, and social organi-sational – produced the long-term social trends that have culminated in what some have perceived to be the 'revolutionary' transformation of sexuality among young people, while the so-called sexual revolution of the 1960s may have been more of a social construct than a label for concomitant changes in sexual practice.

They conclude that 'these changes may be more appropriately termed evolu-tionary in character' (Laumann *et al.*, 1994: 542).

The term 'sexual revolution' refers to various changes, including those in moral standards, sexual attitudes and practices, number of partners and gender differences. Age at first intercourse is generally considered one of the most significant indicators of changes in sexual behaviour. In all western countries, young people are reported as having become increasingly sexually active over the past 35 years. In particular, the 1960s sexual revolution in the west was characterised by rapid changes in age of sexual debut. Both the tempo and the pattern of these changes do, however, vary between countries (Rademakers, 1997). That is why we focus on this indicator in this chapter.

There exist few reliable data on the sexual behaviour of Russians (for a general overview see Kon, 1995, 1997, 1999). The data that are available, however, show more or less the same general trends as have occurred in the western countries. According to Golod's surveys in Leningrad, in 1965 only 5.3 per cent of sexually experienced university students reported having had first intercourse before the age of 16. In 1972, 8 per cent of the sexually initiated reported having begun their sexual life before the age of 16, and in 1995 this figure had risen to 12 per cent (Golod, 1996: 59). Results from our own 1997 survey among students' parents about the age of their own sexual debut provide evidence to suggest that the observed tendency was valid for other parts of Russia, too. The median age of the first sexual intercourse for the cohort of females born between 1942 and 1951 was 21. In the cohort born between 1952 and 1961 it was 20, while in the cohort born between 1962 and 1966 it was 18. Comparison with twelve European countries for which there is comparable data shows that in cohorts born between 1942 and 1951 and between 1952 and 1961, only Portuguese women reported starting their sexual life later than Russian women, while all the others did so earlier. For those who were born in 1962–1966 the situation has changed. In addition to Portuguese women (whose median sexual debut age was 19.8) women in Greece (median sexual debut age 19.2), Belgium (18.6), Switzerland (18.5) and France (18.2) reported starting later than Russian women (see Bozon and Kontula, 1998: 42–44).

These findings suggest that changes over the last three decades in the sexual behaviour of Russian people show similar trends to those observed in the west. In Russia, however, these changes have had a less definite character and because of political and ideological restrictions have taken place largely 'under cover'.

As might be expected, Gorbachev's *perestroika*, which brought about a general liberalisation of social life, made these changes in sexual attitudes and behaviour both visible and dramatic. As a consequence of increasing freedom of speech and of the press, mountains of erotica and pornography earlier unavailable to the general public appeared on bookstands. Ideological and administrative control lost its strength. Western patterns of behaviour became role models. Modern contraceptives started to be used, while the danger of AIDS, which had long been a reality in the west, remained distant for many Russians.

The aims of this chapter are to discuss the dramatic changes in the age of sexual debut which took place in Russia in the mid 1990s, to analyse the consequences of these changes, and to examine current Russian views on sex education.

Methods

This chapter is based on the results of three social surveys of young people's sexual behaviour and attitudes, conducted by the authors. The first of these took place in 1993 among 1615 secondary school and vocational school students aged 12 to 17 in Moscow and St Petersburg. It was the first-ever survey to examine the sexual behaviour of school students in Russia and its aim was to obtain an overall picture of sexual attitudes and behaviour. A self-administered questionnaire was used. No detailed information on the circumstances of sexual debut, the type of first partner or other sexual activities was gathered.

The second survey, sponsored by The John D. and Catherine T. MacArthur Foundation, was carried out in 1995. A self-administered questionnaire was completed by 2871 respondents aged 16 to 19 in Moscow (large city), Novgorod (medium-sized city), Borisoglebsk and Yeletz (both small towns). Unmarried girls and boys, students of secondary and vocational schools, university students and working adolescents were sampled in equal proportions in each of the four sites. Educational institutions were randomly sampled within each site. The questionnaire contained questions about issues such as the context of sexual debut, the first and the last partner, number of partners, etc. For the first time, a few questions touched on the delicate issues of masturbation and homosexual experience (data not analysed here). In this chapter, and for the sake of comparability, only the findings for secondary and vocational school students are described.

The third survey formed part of the project 'In-school sex education for Russian teenagers' initiated by the Ministry of Education and supported by UNFPA and UNESCO. Data were collected from seventh- to ninth-grade students and their parents and teachers in eight sites throughout Russia (Moscow, Moscow district, St Petersburg, Arkhangelsk, Krasnodar, Krasnoyarsk, Udmurtia and Yaroslavl). The survey was conducted in sixteen schools that had agreed to take part in the project. The aim of the work was to assess students' knowledge and understanding of sexuality, their interest in these matters, sources of information about sexuality, and the dynamics of their sexual behaviour. Since it was planned to evaluate the future educational effects of the family and the school on moral values and students' behavioural patterns, we also assessed parents' views about sex education and collected data regarding parents' own sexual debut and their awareness of sexual problems.

Fieldwork was carried out in the first quarter of 1997. Respondents' participation in the survey was voluntary and self-administered questionnaires were completed anonymously. In total, about 4000 students' questionnaires, 1300 parents' questionnaires and 400 teachers' questionnaires were found to be suitable for data processing.

Changes in age of sexual debut ·

A comparison between the 1993 and 1995 survey data testifies to the fact that a substantial change in the age of sexual debut has taken place. While in 1993 only one of four 16-year-old girls reported having had sexual intercourse at least once, in 1995 a third did so. The proportion of sexually experienced boys of the same age increased from slightly over one-third to a half (see Table 9.1).

Table 9.1   Proportion of sexually active respondents by age and gender

Gender	Survey year	Age							
		12	13	14	15	16	17	18	19
Male	1993	2.3	4.1	11.4	17	38.2	49.3	–	–
	1995	–	–	–	–	50.5	57.1	69.8	77.5
Female	1993	0	1.8	3.7	11.8	25.5	45.8	–	–
	1995	–	–	–	–	33.3	52.4	50.8	54.8

Since young people's sexual behaviour is strongly dependent on social milieu, which is reflected in the type of educational institution attended, we also analysed the data separately by school type (see Table 9.2).

As this table shows, while social differences are important, similar overall changes took place in both types of institutions. This suggests that changes in age of sexual debut cannot be treated as an artefact caused by changes in sample design. We found further evidence of dramatic change in sexual behaviour between 1993 and 1995 when we analysed answers to the question about age at first intercourse independently for different age groups within one and the same sample (survey of 1995). Among 16-year-old women, there were twice as many sexually experienced girls than among the 19-year-old respondents when they were 16 (23 per cent versus 11 per cent). The same difference was found between the 17-year-old women and 19 year-olds who had been sexually experienced at 17 (45 per cent versus 24 per cent respectively). The same tendencies were observed among male students, although the changes were not as large.

Comparing the age of sexual debut across different countries is complicated because of sampling differences and the differences in methods of measurement. For example, differences in social and/or ethnic origins of the respondents cannot always be assigned accurate weightings, and these factors may have a significant effect on studied variables. Moreover, the median, which is often used to describe the average age of sexual debut, varies depending on the age cohorts included in a sample, and does not

Table 9.2   Proportion of sexually experienced secondary and vocational school students, by age and gender, 1993 and 1995 survey samples

Gender	Year	Secondary school		Vocational school	
		16 year-olds	17 year-olds	16 year-olds	17 year-olds
Male	1993	35.7	42.9	41.2	55.9
	1995	44.1	44.1	62.7	71.9
Female	1993	16.4	29.0	39.3	58.5
	1995	23.9	40.3	46.0	60.8

allow correct comparison even using additional mathematical procedures such as survival analysis or life table procedures. The available data, however, do give some idea of how Russian teenagers fare in comparison with those in other countries.

In 1988, in the USA, 33 per cent of white unmarried teenagers reported having had first sexual intercourse by the age of 16, and 53 per cent by the age of 17 (Sonenstein *et al.*, 1991). Among Russian 16-year-old respondents, 39 per cent were already sexually experienced by this age, while among those who were 17, 29 per cent had had such an experience by the age of 16, according to our 1995 survey. In the same survey in the USA, 53 per cent of 17 year-olds and 51 per cent of the 18 year-olds had had sexual experience by the age of 17. If we compare our data with those from this US study, we can conclude that age of sexual debut in the two countries is practically the same. But the US survey had been carried out seven years earlier.

While Russian absolute figures are not in themselves sensational and are in many ways comparable with western survey data (see e.g. Nguyet *et al.*, 1994; Johnson *et al.*, 1994), the pace of change in Russia has been very fast. Moreover, sexual awareness and literacy are poor and adolescent sexuality is strongly influenced by general criminalisation of social life. Because of this, unprotected and early sexual activity may have serious psychological and epidemiological consequences, especially for women.

Circumstances of sexual debut

Our 1995 survey findings shed light on the circumstances in which first sexual intercourse usually occurs. Almost as a rule, girls' sexual debut happens with a partner who is appreciably (two years or more) older than she is herself: 40 per cent of the sexual debuts of 14-year-old girls happen with partners who are 18 or older. One in five boys of this same age is also initiated by a legally adult female. But if girls fairly often have their first sexual experience with men who are more than five years older than they are (as happened with 22 per cent of the female respondents), for boys such an age difference is an exception rather than a rule (less than 5 per cent).

Interestingly, the first sexual partner tends to be someone of the same age when acquaintance before first intercourse exceeded one year. Nearly half (48 per cent) of the girls who had their sexual debuts with boys of the same age did so after knowing him for more than a year. While among teenage girls the majority always comprises those who start their sexual life with partners who are two years older or more, among 15-year-old boys the majority (63 per cent) have their first sexual experience with girls of the same age, and this proportion increases with age.

The portion of sexual debuts in which the partner is quite literally a stranger is surprisingly large: 11 per cent of sexually active girls reported that they did not know their first partners at all, and 9 per cent reported that they had been acquainted with their first partner for about a week. Thus, every fifth girl had her sexual debut with someone she either did not know or had only just become acquainted. Among boys the same thing occurs nearly twice as often: 41 per cent of the boys reported having had their first sexual intercourse with a woman they either did not know previously at all, or with whom they had very little acquaintance. Nearly half of male sexual debuts with much older partners took place at the first meeting. If the boy's first sexual partner happened to be three or more years older than him, the sexual debut happened in nearly two-thirds of the cases no more than a week after acquaintance.

There is a clear trend for the earlier the girl's sexual debut, the shorter the period of previous acquaintance with her first partner. Thus, more than a third of the girls who had had first sexual intercourse by age 13 had done so with a stranger. And, vice versa, the proportion of the same-aged girls who had had their first sex with a partner whom they knew for more than a year was three times lower. Of the girls who had had their first intercourse at 18, 39 per cent had known their partners for more than a year, while those who had had first intercourse with a casual acquaintance comprised only slightly more than 1 per cent of this age group. Such a tendency was not found among boys.

Overall, sexual debut is rarely a conscious, deliberate action prepared for by a long relationship and tender feelings. Only 26 per cent of the males and 31 per cent of the females said that they had foreseen that sex would happen with this particular person. For the rest, the selection of the first partner was more or less by chance; 30 per cent of the girls even said they never felt the desire for sexual intimacy with anyone before it happened for the first time. The same, however, cannot be said about the boys. Only 47 per cent of the girls and 23 per cent of the boys aged 16–17 said that their first sexual partner was their steady boy- or girlfriend. Approximately one-third of the boys had dated their first partner from time to time before first having sex. And nearly every fifth girl and every third boy said that they had had no relationship with their first partner before having sex.

Among the boys who had no acquaintance with their first partner before first intercourse, a third nevertheless felt an attraction towards her or something more (30 per cent of this category said that they liked the girl, and 3 per cent that they were truly in love). However, 58 per cent said that they had no specific feelings about the individual concerned. Among the boys who had a one-week acquaintance with their partner, the proportion of those who experienced feelings of care was twice as large and only one in five had had first intercourse without some feelings of attraction. Yet, in general, only 15 per cent of the boys felt 'true love' for their partner at the time of first intercourse.

Emotional attraction seems to be a more significant factor in motivating sexual intimacy for girls. More than a third of them stated they were 'truly in love' with their first partner. Nearly two times fewer girls than boys experienced first sexual intercourse without any feelings towards their partner.

Table 9.3 Boys' and girls' impressions of first sexual intercourse, by feelings for the partner

Feelings before first intercourse	Sex	Impression				
		Uncondition- ally good	Fairly good	Hard to say, none	Fairly bad	Uncondition- ally bad
No feelings at all	Boys	28.2	37.9	25.2	6.3	2.4
	Girls	4.6	14.9	34.5	19.5	26.4
Liked	Boys	42.0	44.4	9.1	4.2	0.2
	Girls	17.8	33.3	26.3	19.0	3.5
Were truly in love	Boys	47.8	41.3	5.1	5.1	0.7
	Girls	26.2	40.5	17.7	14.8	0.8
Not sure	Boys	30.8	43.6	20.5	3.8	1.3
	Girls	12.8	17.9	28.2	30.8	10.3

Similar gender differences exist in many other countries as well. Yet the respondents' lasting impression of their first sexual intimacy corresponds directly to their feelings towards their partner: the more positively attracted they had felt, the more positively the experience was evaluated (or perhaps remembered) (see Table 9.3).

First sexual intercourse is evaluated differently by boys and girls. The girls who had no positive feelings towards their partners almost never reported unconditionally positive impressions of first intercourse, and every fourth girl in this group gave a definitely negative evaluation. In contrast, more than a quarter of the boys who felt nothing for their first partner gave a positive evaluation of their initiation, while a definitely negative impression was reported by only a few male respondents. In other words, sexual intimacy without emotional involvement can cause negative feelings in some girls (this may even happen in reported cases of 'true love', but the chances are much smaller), while for boys it may only result in less positive emotions.

Although sexual initiation is romanticised in the public imagination, in reality it seems to be a much less romantic experience, especially for girls. One in four girls reported that her first sexual intercourse left no impression on her at all, and only half of all female respondents experienced positive emotions during their first sexual act (see Figure 9.1).

Impressions of first intercourse depend largely on who initiated the sexual contact. Among both boys and girls, positive emotional experiences are most often the result of mutual desire. But the proportion of such debuts is not very large. Only slightly more than half of the boys (56 per cent) and less than a half of the girls (46 per cent) had these kinds of debuts. More often, girls' sexual debuts are initiated by their partners (49 per cent), while they themselves initiate the event very rarely (4.3 per cent). However, women (generally those who are already sexually experienced) take the initiative with sexually inexperienced boys three times more often (13.5 per cent).

According to our 1995 data, 29 per cent of girls' sexual debuts are accompanied by some form of resistance on the part of the girl. Respondents reported that in response to their partner's initiative they either 'first resisted but then agreed' (22 per cent), or 'were against it and fought back till the end' (7 per cent) during first sex. The latter can be characterised as being raped. As a rule, boys in such cases recognised neither the illegality of their actions nor the damage caused by them. One in four boys in fact expressed some agreement with the questionnaire statement that: 'One must not blame a guy if he has sex with a girl whom he has dated for a long time, even if it is against her will.'

artly the consequence of general male lack of understanding of their own, as well as women's, sexuality, and of men's inability to talk about sexual issues. Yet we must also take into account the habit of offering 'token resistance' to sex, which is widespread among Russian women, because of the existence of a strong double standard (Sprecher *et al.*, 1994).

In the 1995 survey, we compared the age at which girls and boys had their

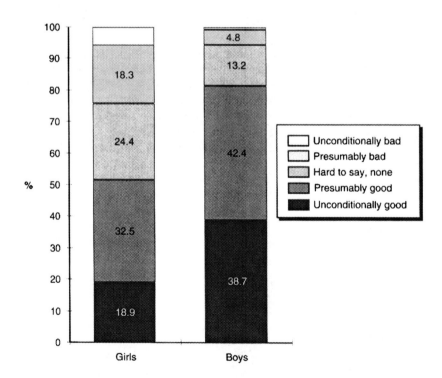

Figure 9.1 Impression of first sexual intercourse

first sexual experience with the age which they considered it best to start. More than half (55 per cent) of the sexually experienced girls were in favour of beginning sexual activity at a later age than they had done themselves. Among boys, the same opinion was expressed by a smaller, but not insignificant, 41 per cent.

All the boys and girls with coital experience were asked how they felt about their sexual initiation with the passage of time. Nearly one-third of the boys answered that they felt they had made the correct decision. Almost the same number did not consider it a major event in their lives. One in four boys experienced mixed feelings, seeing both good and bad in their choice. One in ten felt regret about their sexual debut but only a very few felt it was a serious mistake.

Girls regarded their 'first time' somewhat differently. Only about one in five felt that they had made the correct decision, and the same number felt that they had made a mistake. The most common response was one of mixed feelings, recognising both good and bad sides of the experience. In contrast to boys, far fewer girls regarded the event as being of little importance: only 13 per cent said they considered it an insignificant event in their lives.

Girls' opinion was strongly related to age of sexual initiation. The majority (53 per cent) of those who became sexually active at age 13 or younger expressed regret about the event. As a whole, among those girls who became sexually active before age 16, responses expressing regret outnumbered more positive evaluations.

Consequences of sexual revolution

The changes in age of sexual debut, being part of a world-wide trend, cannot be judged in terms of being 'good' or 'bad'. However, the potential consequences of this rapid change – including increases in teenage pregnancy, STIs including HIV, rape, prostitution and psychological problems linked to early unwanted sex – may be potentially dangerous for society as a whole.

For a variety of reasons, Russian teenagers tend to be poorly prepared for sexual life. For reasons we will return to later, emotionally many may lack adequate preparation for an active sex life. Others may know little about safe sex or the means by which to protect themselves and partners against STIs. Between 1990 and 1996, for example, the incidence of syphilis increase fifty fold in Russia, and seventy-eight fold among young people. In 1996, 265 new cases of syphilis per 100,000 of population were initially diagnosed. The incidence of HIV has also begun to grow almost exponentially (see Figure 9.2). UNAIDS has recently estimated that there may already be more than 40,000 cases of infection in the country.

All these facts suggest that something must be done to limit the potentially negative consequences of the changes that have taken place. The first

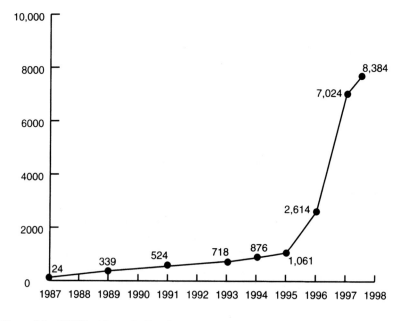

Figure 9.2   HIV incidence in Russia

step may lie in sex education, something which at present does not exist in most Russian schools.

Levels of knowledge about sexuality

According to the 1993 survey findings, only 19 per cent of 16-year-olds reported having received special classes, lectures or seminars on sex education. In 1995, the comparable figure was about 10 per cent, and in 1997 it was 22 per cent. About half of the respondents in each of the samples stated that they had received one or two lectures on problems to do with sexuality (most usually STIs and unwanted pregnancy). Only 2 to 5 per cent of all respondents reported having participated in more than ten lectures or seminars. In the 1997 survey, respondents were asked the question: 'In your opinion, do you have enough or not enough knowledge about sex?' In the seventh grade, 21 per cent of boys and 12 per cent of girls said they knew enough about sex. In the eighth grade, 31 per cent of boys and 17 per cent of girls said so. And in the ninth grade, 34 per cent of male and 27 per cent of female respondents considered that they knew enough about sex. At the same time, only 12 per cent of the teachers consider themselves well prepared to answer students' and parents' questions about sexuality. Only one in three parents gave a clear positive response to the question about whether they thought they have enough knowledge about sex.

The most significant increase in factual knowledge – showing a four-fold increase between seventh and ninth grades – concerns topics directly related to the possible means of sexual gratification (such as the questions about the most sensitive sexual parts of a woman's body, or where the clitoris is located). Of the ninth-grade females 40 per cent answered the first question correctly (compared with 9 per cent of the seventh-grade females), and 40 per cent of ninth-grade females (compared with 5 per cent of the seventh-grade) demonstrated sound knowledge of the clitoris location. However, knowledge about bodily functions and the possible negative consequences of early sexual contact remains grossly inadequate.

Sources of information about sexuality

According to 1997 survey data, young people today have much more information about sexuality at their disposal than did their parents. For members of their parents' generation, the main sources of information about sexuality were conversations with their peers. Today, however, printed materials and electronic media are more important sources of information. However, this often means only the replacement of one source of misinformation with another, more 'virtual' one.

For young people, the main sources of knowledge about sexuality are newspapers, books and magazines. Girls (perhaps because they develop earlier) report starting to read these materials earlier than boys (Table 9.4).

While conversations with friends are not seen as a particular significant source of information among seventh-grade pupils, by the ninth grade girls in particular pay more attention to them than to television programmes. For

Table 9.4 Main sources of knowledge about sexuality, by gender and grade, 1997 survey (%)

Sources of information	Grade 7		Grade 8		Grade 9		Total	
	M	F	M	F	M	F	M	F
Books, magazines, newspapers	52.5	54.1	57.4	63.6	66.5	62.3	60.7	60.8
Conversations with friends	38.8	36.6	54.9	55.8	47.5	56.3	47.7	51.6
Films, TV programmes	39.9	38.7	54.5	50.4	56.1	45.5	52.0	45.4
Parents and other relatives	8.2	32.0	10.2	25.6	12.4	24.3	10.8	26.4
Teachers, lecturers	8.2	7.2	3.3	7.4	9.1	16.5	7.2	11.6
Sisters, brothers	6.6	13.4	9.8	11.6	8.9	6.3	8.6	9.5
Special consultation	4.4	4.6	2.5	4.7	6.1	18.8	4.6	11.3
Medical workers	1.6	9.3	2.0	7.0	3.6	11.0	2.7	9.4
Girl/boyfriend	3.3	2.6	7.0	5.0	4.8	7.5	5.1	5.6
Own experience	7.1	1.5	6.6	4.7	7.9	8.0	7.3	5.5
Other	0.5	2.6	1.2	1.6	0.8	1.8	0.9	1.9

ninth-grade boys, such information from friends is not so significant as that received through television. Given that television deals mostly in erotic imagery of one kind or another – there are no educational programmes about sexuality on Russian TV – it is clear that boys prefer eroticism to factual knowledge about sexuality.

Our analysis of informational sources shows that by speaking to them more about sexuality, the older generation sometimes looks after the needs of girls. Boys, however, receive much less attention. This is true for all institutional forms of information – such as that provided by teachers and medical workers – as well as for parents.

The problem of 'sexual pedagogy'

Generally, Russian public opinion is in favour of sex education. In all national public opinion polls conducted since 1989, the vast majority of adults – between 60 and 90 per cent depending upon age and social background – strongly support the idea of there being systematic sex education in schools. Only 3 to 20 per cent are against it (Kon, 1999). But who should do this work and what exactly should be taught?

Teachers think that parents should provide sex education for their children. According to our 1997 survey, 78 per cent of teachers agreed with this. However, this same survey showed how hard it would be for the family to take on this role. Only about one out of five teenagers considered it acceptable to discuss problems of sexuality with his or her parents. Parents themselves only reluctantly initiate such topics of conversation with their children. More than half of them reported never initiating such talks with their children; another quarter had taken the initiative only once or twice; and only one in five mothers (fathers even more rarely) had initiated such conversations with their children on several occasions. According to parents, the primary restraining factors were psychological and educational unreadiness. This is why more than three-quarters of them were in favour of there being special books explaining what can be said to children about sexuality, and how it can be done best. Approximately two-thirds of parents think it would be useful to have seminars devoted to sex education for parents in the schools their children attend.

At present, schools are not ready to carry out sex education. Three-quarters of teachers were convinced that form teachers (those who are primarily responsible for social and moral education) should discuss issues of gender and sexual relations with their students. However, 65 per cent of teachers report having never done this, and another 15 per cent had done it only once or twice. It is clear why this is the case: only 11.5 per cent of teachers said they were well prepared for such a task; 85 per cent were in favour of special courses on the fundamentals of sexology as part of teacher training.

Attitudes towards sex education

In general, respondents in the 1997 survey were unanimous that sex education courses in schools must be launched. Given other findings, it might be expected that such courses will become one of the favourite curriculum subjects for students: 61 per cent of seventh-grade students and 73 per cent of students in the ninth grade stated that they would eagerly attend such classes. Only 5 per cent of students would prefer to avoid such lessons if they had the chance. To some extent, this distribution of students' responses offers an answer to teachers' worries about the form such education should take – be it a compulsory or voluntary course – when introduced in schools. There are much more serious disagreements among the interested groups, however, in respect to the content of sex education. Teachers would like to offer a detailed treatment of anatomy, physiology and ethics, whereas students have more interest in practical issues (Table 9.5).

Of all the topics proposed in a sex education course for both boys and girls, the greatest preference was for information on STIs and HIV prevention. While other aspects of sexuality are covered in the mass media and in printed materials, these specific medical issues are much less frequently addressed.

Problems of sexual harassment, including rape and unwanted sex, are the second most significant for girls. With age (and consequently with growing interest towards them from the opposite sex) this emphasis increases. Boys do not show as much interest in these issues. They worry much more about how to improve their sexual potency and performance.

Table 9.5 Students' topic preferences in a course on sex education (% of those who called a topic 'very necessary'), 1997 survey

	Grade 7		Grade 8		Grade 9		Total	
	M	*F*	*M*	*F*	*M*	*F*	*M*	*F*
Psychology of gender relationships	54.6	60.8	59.8	69.8	62.2	67.0	59.8	66.4
Conception, prenatal development and childbirth	49.7	64.9	45.5	52.7	39.6	54.3	43.6	56.2
Diversity in sexual orientation, homosexuality, etc.	27.9	26.8	27.0	24.4	18.8	24.3	23.3	24.9
Sexual techniques: how to receive more pleasure from sex	44.3	32.5	55.7	41.5	59.9	43.5	55.2	40.4
Sexual anatomy and physiology	45.4	42.8	43.0	46.5	44.4	45.8	44.2	45.3
Marriage and family life	63.4	79.4	58.2	70.2	56.6	66.5	58.6	70.5
Sexual hygiene (sex organs)	58.5	59.8	53.7	52.3	55.6	50.0	55.7	52.9
Methods of birth control	47.5	63.4	51.6	67.4	62.2	69.3	55.8	67.4
Sexual abuse and avoidance of sexual harassment	50.3	72.2	47.5	74.8	51.0	76.8	49.8	75.1
Prevention of STDs and AIDS	72.1	82.5	76.6	83.3	78.7	84.0	76.6	83.5
Improvement of sexual health	55.7	49.0	56.6	52.7	62.4	52.8	59.2	51.9

More seventh-grade pupils than older students are interested in the problems of marriage and family life. Girls are more interested in family issues than boys, but even among them this interest decreases with age, being perhaps replaced with more 'relevant' problems of gender relationships. The psychology of gender relationships attracts more interest among girls than boys, and this interest grows with age. As they grow older, boys start to pay more attention to feelings, love and interpersonal communication as well.

Girls, much more so than boys, are interested in conception, the development of the human foetus and childbirth. This interest decreases with age equally among boys and girls. Boys have a much higher interest than girls in sexual techniques that enable them to receive more pleasure from sex, and this interest increases with age. Girls also become more interested with age in the 'technical' aspects of sex, though these never become a priority. Apparently such concerns are seen as less relevant in school, an interest in them grows later after the ninth grade, and this lack of knowledge can be easily compensated for using books and other sources of material.

In general, as mentioned earlier, young people give priority to such topics as prevention of STIs and AIDS, methods of birth control, problems of family life and the psychology of cross-gender relationships. Topics such as anatomy and physiology, conception, foetus development and childbirth, and sexual hygiene are regarded as less important along with information about differences in sexual orientation and sexual minorities (perhaps respondents are shy to discuss these matters).

Conclusions

Our data suggest that school students need sex education and are very interested in questions of sexuality. This interest has primarily a pragmatic motivation. Young people's curiosity about sexuality in the absence of an elementary knowledge of human anatomy, physiology and hygiene (to say nothing about psychological differences in the sexual response cycles of boys and girls) makes initial experimentation in sexual relationships potentially dangerous.

At the moment, the pedagogical impact of sex education (so far as there is any) seems limited. In fact, schools hope that sex education will be provided by the family, whereas parents rely upon schools to do this. Meanwhile, the main source of information about sexuality is the printed and electronic media, as well as peers. As a result, young people know little about sexually transmitted diseases, have only an overall idea about contraception, and yet their views and attitudes towards sexual behaviour become more permissive year by year.

At present, neither school teachers nor parents feel that they have enough knowledge about sexuality. Both parents and teachers want there to be preparation for teaching about sex and relationships in both initial and in-service teacher education, as well as at school for parents. At the same time, attention is drawn to the fact that Russia at present lacks appropriate textbooks and methodological materials.

The absolute majority of respondents spoke in favour of introducing sex education into school curricula. Its content, according to the views of students, their parents and teachers, must deal with a wide spectrum of topics, including anatomy and physiology, the psychology of sexual relationships, practical issues of avoiding sexually transmitted diseases and unwanted pregnancy, and the moral aspects of cross-gender relationships.

Our 1997 survey was completed as a part of sociological monitoring for a planned three-year experimental project on in-school sex education sponsored by the Russian Ministry of Education and the United Nations Population Fund (UNFPA) in collaboration with UNESCO. However, before the work had even begun, the project came under heavy attack in the mass media for being a 'Western ideological subversion of Russian children' (see Chervyakov and Kon, 1998). In some small towns, people were asked by journalists on the street: 'Do you want children to be taught in school how to have sex? If not, please sign the petition to ban this devilish project.' Priests and activists alike not infrequently tell their audiences that all bad things in western life are rooted in sex education, that western governments are now trying to ban or eliminate it, and that a corrupt Russian government investigated by the world 'sexological–industrial complex', US secret services and western pharmaceutical companies is acting against the national interests of the country. The Russian Planned Parenthood Association is denounced by the Russian Orthodox Church as being a 'satanic institution' propagating abortion and depopulation. This anti-sexual and anti-western campaign is strongly supported by the communist-dominated state Duma and by the vast majority of Russian newspapers. It has continued for nearly three years. As a result, most attempts to promote sex education for young people in Russia have been stopped, and even those groups that worked on such issues before are finding it increasingly difficult to carry on.

References

Bozon, M. and Kontula, K. (1998) 'Sexual initiation and gender in Europe: a cross-cultural analysis of trends in the twentieth century', in M. Hubert *et al.* (eds) *Sexual Behaviour and HIV/AIDS in Europe. Comparisons of National Suveys*, London: UCL Press.

Chervyakov, V. and Kon, I. (1998) 'Sex education and HIV prevention in the context of Russian politics', in R. Rosenbrock (ed.) *Politics behind AIDS Policies. Case Studies from India, Russia and South Africa*, Berlin: SWZ.

Clement, U. (1990) 'Surveys of heterosexual behaviour', *Annual Review of Sex Research* 1: 45–74.

Golod, S. I. (1996) *XX Vek i Tendencii Seksualnikh Otnosheniy v Rossii*, St Petersburg: Aleteia.

Haavio-Mannila, E. and Rotkirch, A. (1997) 'Generational and gender differences in sexual life in St. Petersburg and urban Finland', *Yearbook of Population Research in Finland* 34: 133–160.

Johnson, A. M., Wadsworth, J., Wellings, K., Field, J., with Bradshaw S. (1994) *Sexual Attitudes and Lifestyles*, London: Blackwell Scientific.

Kon, I. S. (1995) *The Sexual Revolution in Russia From the Age of the Czars to Today*, New York: Free Press.

——(1997) *Seksualnaya Kultura v Rossii*, Moscow: OGI.

——(1999) 'Sexuality and politics in Russia, 1700–2000', in F. H. Eder *et al.* (eds) *Sexual Cultures in Europe. National Histories*, Manchester: Manchester University Press

Laumann, E. O., Gagnon, J. H., Michael, R. T. and Michaels, S. (1994) *The Social Organization of Sexuality. Sexual Practices in the United States*, Chicago: University of Chicago Press.

Nguyet, M. N. T., Mheux, B., Beland, F. and Pica, L. A. (1994) 'Sexual behavior and condom use: a study of suburban male adolescents', *Adolescence* 29: 113.

Rademakers, J. (1997) 'Adolescent sexual development: a cross-cultural perspective', Paper presented at the International Conference on Sexuality Beyond Boundaries, Amsterdam, 29 July–4 August 1997.

Reiss, I. L., with Reiss, H. (1990) *An End to Shame. Shaping Our Next Sexual Revolution*, Buffalo, NY: Prometheus.

Schmidt, G. (ed.) (1993) *Jugendsexualität. Sozialer Wandel, Gruppenunterschiede, Konflikfelder*, Stuttgart: Enke.

Schmidt, G., Klusmann, D., Zeitzschel, U., and Lange, C. (1994) 'Changes in adolescents' sexuality between 1970 and 1990 in West Germany', *Archives of Sexual Behavior* 23(5): 489–513.

Schwartz, P. and Gillmore, M. R. (1990) 'Sociological perspectives on human sexuality', in K. K. Holmes *et al.* (eds) *Sexually Transmitted Diseases*, New York: McGraw-Hill.

Sonenstein, F. L., Pleck, J. H. and Ku, L. C. (1991) 'Levels of sexual activity among adolescent males in the United States', *Family Planning Perspectives* 23: 4.

Sprecher, S., Hatfield, E., Cortese, A., Potapova, E. and Levitskaya, A. (1994) 'Token resistance to sexual intercourse and consent to unwanted sexual intercourse: college students' experiences in three countries', *Journal of Sex Research* 31(2): 125–132.

10 Young people, social relationships and sexuality in Bulgaria

Biliana Vassileva and Milena Komarova

Bulgaria, as a country in transition, faces not only socio-economic problems but also rapid changes in attitudes and behaviour, especially among adolescents. The factors influencing such changes in behaviour, including sexual behaviour, have not been investigated until now and virtually no information exists concerning the impact (if any) of political, social and economic change on young people's behaviour.

There was hardly any tradition of social research in the country before 1988, when the National Centre for Public Opinion Polls was established. Such a sphere of professional activity did not fit easily with the official ideological discourse created by the power holders. Sociology itself was regarded as, and indeed reduced to, the status of courtier to decision makers. As a discipline it was asked and expected to support and legitimise the ideological grounds of the dominant regime, to give it a popular face, and not to question or explain concrete social developments. In 1986, Bulgarian sociology slowly started to change as a result of the changing political climate of *glasnost* and *perestroika*. However, the lack of a long-term tradition of social research remains a disadvantage, especially in relation to issues such as sexual behaviour.

In July 1997, the Joint United Nations Programme on HIV/AIDS (UNAIDS) in Sofia in co-operation with UNICEF agreed to support a research project to identify key elements influencing the sexual behaviour of adolescents in Bulgaria. The focus was on young people's interaction with their immediate social environment. The study was intended to establish a base for future quantitative surveys and to identify priorities for intervention in a pilot peer education project in Bulgaria.

We were especially interested in discovering whether problems in communication increased young people's vulnerability to HIV and AIDS and 'risk behaviour'. There was also another issue we wanted to know more about: while the concept of risk is central to research on the social aspects of AIDS, there has been a tendency to neglect how risk is actually understood by the participants of studies themselves (Rhodes, 1995), and how behaviour is constructed as a socially organised phenomenon. The transition from a totalitarian to a pluralistic society brought with it a complete change in values and reference points. In a short space of time, state ideology lost its validity, and with it a series of unifying values, and norms, disappeared. It was interesting to know, therefore, how the tension between emerging new values, norms, knowledge and independence in young people, alongside the vacuum of values, reference points and norms on the part of the older generations, influenced the behaviour of adolescents.

Although in the course of the work we were able to collect a considerable amount of data on different topics, we focus in this chapter only on those specific areas which are relatively less investigated. We will look in particular at the social environment including parents and friends, and explore the relationships between this and young people's feelings about sex and sexual behaviour.

Approach

We chose to conduct a largely qualitative study. The choice of qualitative methods was influenced by both the study objectives as well as the current state of social research in Bulgaria. Qualitative research was considered especially important because of the lack of previous enquiry that could be used as a reference point. Only a few KAB (Knowledge, Attitudes, Beliefs and Practices) studies had been carried out. While we were able to refer to them, we could not use them constructively for our purposes, because either they were designed to evaluate likely public reactions to the HIV/AIDS epidemic, or they did not include questions about the social environment of young people.

After a literature review on qualitative research methods and techniques we decided on the use of focus groups, not only because they offered a convenient means of data collection, but also because they would allow us to observe participants' communication within groups (Catterall and Maclaran, 1997). Additionally, several narrative research sessions and unstructured key interviews were conducted with young people who were considered 'informal leaders' by their peers. A variety of different pictures of people were shown and participants were asked to pick up one and to develop a story. Objectives were to identify stereotypes of people 'at risk', and the language used to describe relationships and sex.

We stratified the target population on the grounds of sex and age. Since we did not have prior information about when adolescents in Bulgaria begin their sexual lives, we decided to include a broad age range (from 13 to 19 years of age) of participants. In order to capture experience in different socio-economic and cultural settings, we conducted the focus groups in different parts of Bulgaria – in big cities, in small towns, and among ethnic minorities.

The total number of young people participating in the study was 123. Out of these, thirty-five were participants in additional narrative research and key informant interviews of which the results are only briefly mentioned in this chapter. These young people served as a point of reference in our analysis and their responses are used to support some of the arguments in our conclusions. The remainder of the study participants were distributed across the focus groups as follows:

- Boys, one group of eight participants, aged 13 to 14 in a small town; one group of nine participants, aged 15 to 17 in a small town; and one group of seven participants, aged 16 to 19 in the capital city.
- Girls, one group of seven participants, aged 13 to 14 in a small town; one group of six participants, aged 15 to 16 in a small town; and one group of six participants, aged 16 to 17 in a provincial city.

Additionally, one focus group was conducted with eight participants of both sexes from several towns; as well as four focus groups with adolescents from Gypsy and Turkish ethnic minorities[1] comprising twenty-nine participants in total; and one focus group with eight young men currently undergoing military service.

Fieldwork took place between July 1997 and October 1997. For each session, adolescents were invited to a discussion which lasted approximately three hours. Respondents were selected by local NGOs interested in the field of HIV/AIDS prevention with whom a working relationship existed. Focus group discussions took place in local halls or at summer camps in locally available facilities and were led by a moderator who followed a discussion guide that had been developed beforehand. Participants were asked to take part in a general discussion concerning everyday-life issues such as communication, love, sex and interaction with their immediate environment. The questions in our discussion guide were grouped in three parts:

Part 1: Cultural context This part aimed at collecting information about the adolescents' perceptions of their immediate environment (family, friends), men and women, love, norms and authorities, punishment and sanctions.

Part 2: Images of sex In this section, participants were asked to verbalise in association games, and to visualise, by making collages and drawing pictures, their images of sex.

Part 3: Sexual behaviour The block of questions about sexual behaviour asked about specific sexual attitudes and practices, as well as risk perceptions.

All the focus groups were tape-recorded and discussions were fully transcribed for the purpose of analysis. What we attempted afterwards was a comparative analysis of the discussion dynamics within each focus group and of the issues discussed within each of the groups. The main issues explored were what seemed to be the most common across-groups denominators, with respect to both repeated patterns of group dynamics and theme content.

Immediate social environment

This part of the discussion guide aimed to collect information about if and how adolescents' perception of their immediate social environment triggered particular reactions, responses and modes of communication both with the environment and among themselves. We left it to respondents to identify and name the people in their immediate social environment. The question asked was 'Let us talk about the others in your immediate environment – the people that you deal with, communicate with, and get in contact with. Who are these people in your life?' Answers varied in content and order of appearance, but in all the groups two types of people were invariably mentioned – parents and friends.

Parents

When preparing the discussion guide, we included a block of questions about the *family* in general in which probing for parents was included. Though in opening up this part of the discussion the word in use was *family*, it was systematically understood and substituted by the respondents with *parents*.

Following the cut-and-paste approach of deriving common themes from the data content, we tried to divide young people's responses into descriptive and functional perceptions. We were impressed by the lack of functional definitions of parents. Descriptive phrases about parents included, for example, 'the people that gave birth to us and then brought us up', and 'the people that we live with'. The only more or less functional perception was formulated as 'the people who look after us and take care of our upbringing and education', a definition in which respondents seemingly identified themselves not as subjects but as an object of the relationship. Most of the respondents across the groups said they rarely talked with their parents. Exceptions in this respect were the groups of younger respondents – boys and girls of between 13 and 15 years of age. To the question 'Why is that?', the following types of answers were given:

They set limits to our communication in thinking they know everything.

They think it is them who have to say what is to be done.

They want to know what's up – how is life going but they always make annoying comparisons between them and us.

They should know how it feels to want to do something but not to be allowed to do it.

They are a different generation, their way of thinking is completely different.

They stress things which are not of great importance for us.

When asked what they 'shared' with their family, young people responded in a variety of ways. These varied from the positive and the inclusive to those that were seemingly lacking in involvement:

I often talk with my father about the outside world, he tells me how I should react to it, what my attitude towards people should be.

I keep them informed, in order not to worry, but I never go into details.

Almost nothing, because they don't understand me.

When asked why they feel misunderstood, respondents described negative reactions (interdictions) by their parents to their interests (computers, access to information, gaining their own experiences), lifestyles (sports, friends, clothes), freedom of choice (travel, business, studies), and entertainment (discos, cinema).
   When asked 'Do you look for advice from your parents? When do you turn to them and about what?', responses included:

If a friend has lied on me the first people I will turn to are my parents.

If I have to make up my mind about general things in life – education or future profession.

When asked 'Is there anything about which you would turn only to your family?', young people replied:

The little nothings in life – it is about them, that we feel very uncertain. The bigger problems are easy to solve – the options are limited – the question is just to choose the better one.

Problems in school. Health problems.

Not untypical responses to the question 'Is there anything about which you will not turn to them?' included:

Personal matters, because they always tell us what is right and wrong.

I never share with my parents things which I know that they will not approve.

I can't share intimate matters with my father because I know what he is going to tell me.

When asked about how they knew their parents would react negatively to things they wanted to talk about with them, such as love, sex and intimate matters, the answers given either were from 'personal experience', or took the form of extrapolations from cases of talking to parents on other topics. An additional source of information was observed patterns of communication in the families of friends.

With regard to discussion dynamics, what to us seemed crucially important were the negative initial reactions of respondents when talking about their parents. At the start of the discussions, we always and invariably observed a strong reaction of rejection towards parents. Only later did positive opinions appear as though to soften this initial impression. Another seemingly important point was that respondents would commonly state that they were ashamed to talk about sex with their parents. They were, however, unable to explain clearly where this shame came from and what exactly feeling shameful meant. With respect to parents, shameful was explained as not knowing when and how to start a conversation.

Discussion

Overall, parents were seen as prescriptive, oppressive and belonging to a different generation. Their ability to 'understand' was questioned to a great extent. It became obvious that understanding was measured by adolescents comparing their interests, lifestyle, freedom of choice, etc., with the values and norms of their parents.

Child–parent relationships were often based on inequality, which makes adolescents feel undervalued. Communication with parents was often perceived as a violation of the young person's own personality, because most of the time parents' knowledge (including their norms and values) served as a base for judgements and comparisons. The consequence was a self-limited form of communication, because adolescents felt they 'knew' what would be the reaction of their parents.

Didactic ways of transferring knowledge from parents to children were seen as preventing young people gaining their own experience. As regards help, parents are kept on 'standby' in case problems arose that could not be solved either by the young people themselves, or by friends. Even where there was a smooth and understanding relationship, parents were perceived as too biased to share ideas and feelings with, because they were seen as being emotionally involved.

Discussing sexual issues with parents was perceived as shameful, and if such discussions took place within the family they were usually in the form of a monologue on the side of the parents.

Adolescents' perception of friends

To purloin respondents' own phrasing, a friend is: 'somebody of the same age sharing the same ideas', 'somebody with whom one has common interests', 'somebody from the same generation, because each generation is characterised by its own ideas', and 'somebody who is like you, who means a lot to you'.

Functionally, a friend is 'somebody who can help, who can understand you', 'someone you trust', 'somebody one can go to for advice and help', 'a person with whom one shares things that one can't share with parents', 'somebody to whom you can reveal the essence of your inner feelings', 'somebody you can go to if you have a problem', 'somebody who can support you', 'somebody with whom you can exchange information', 'somebody who will ask you for help', and 'somebody who you turn to in sadness and happiness'.

With their friends, respondents reported talking about problems that they had. These were commonly described as general issues ('things to do with life'), intimate issues ('about sex', 'about relationships'), and depressing things ('unwanted pregnancies', 'problems with parents').

Young people talked about sex spontaneously with their friends in almost all of the groups, with the exception of the youngest group of girls. When asked, respondents said that they talked about sex a lot. It was clear from the dynamics of discussions that sex as a topic held a special meaning in respondents' conversations with their friends, as it seemed an illegitimate subject to talk about either with their parents or at school. On the whole, talking about 'intimate' and 'personal' issues such as relationships and feelings about the opposite sex seemed to be exclusively confined to the circle of friends. This particular impression was also supported by data from the analysis of narrative games. In these, respondents were asked to explain what sex is, either in an imaginary conversation between parents and children, or to an extra-terrestrial. They demonstrated a complete inability to do so, not because they did not know what sex is, but because they had difficulties talking about it without having to use euphemisms.

Nevertheless, respondents reported a fear of revealing too much about themselves. When asked 'Are there limits to friendship?', there was a consensus that no friendship lasts for ever, and that therefore there were certain things that should not be shared:

> I share with friends only after I have made an assessment of the consequences.

> If you share too much, rumours will start to spread and you will not be able to stop them.

> With friends one has to be on the alert.

> If I drop a brick, if I make a mistake, I will never share it, because they will laugh at me. This is so because people experience fear – inner fear – of failure as regards all aspects of their lives.

There was a certain ambiguity in responses to questions about friends. Some participants had a positive approach, others highlighted more negatively the limitations in friendship. Although these were often followed by more positive descriptions of friendship, later more fears and anxieties would appear, often ending with phrases such as 'actually you cannot trust anyone'.

Discussion

Overall, friends were perceived as being members of a group/community that respondents see as belonging to their 'generation'. The most common variables by which this group/community was characterised were age, shared views and ideas, and a common lifestyle. Understanding, help and support are important functional determinants of friendship. There seems to be a reflected and felt necessity of help and support which adolescents feel they do not receive from people other than their friends. More than this, the fact that respondents spontaneously and pointedly talked about friends as being the only people capable of understanding and support seems to a certain extent to be a compensatory effect of their inability to communicate with parents.

That said, young people's perceptions of friends are organised around a contradiction. Because of similarities (being of the same generation) friends perceive each other as able to understand and help. On the other hand, they also see each other as a threat since sharing too much may impact negatively on future life. Communication with friends is therefore limited by trying to avoid the largely imaginary negative consequences of sharing.

Sex is seemingly a very important topic of discussion among friends. The term covers relationships, gossip and rumours. Its importance in communication with friends to some extent compensates for respondents' inability (real or assumed) to talk about sex outside their circle of peers.

Sexual behaviour

> Years ago there existed a lot of dogmatic principles in Bulgaria. But now we can find out what is happening around the world as we have more information, and it turns out to be that sex is normal.

As a child I believed that in socialist countries women take special pills in order to have children and only in the capitalist countries did people have sex.

Before discussing findings from the sexual behaviour block of questions, it should be mentioned that the focus group guide also included questions about respondents' ideas and stereotypes about sex. Young people also made collages (by drawing and gluing together pictures from magazines) and played association games with the word sex. In general and very abstract terms, 'sex' appeared to be perceived rather romantically by all the groups. Their pictures showed attractive couples, weddings, babies, sunsets and beaches; word associations frequently mentioned feelings, closeness, happiness and love.

The block of questions about sexual behaviour asked about specific sexual attitudes and practices, both of their peers and themselves. On the whole, early sexual relations and sex before marriage were perceived as normal and widespread practices (see also Stoilova and Popova, 1994). Nevertheless, sex and age differences existed in young people's responses. While boys, and especially the older ones, were more inclined to think of sex as a necessary practice that 'helps one acquire experience and emotional stability', girls on the whole were more hesitant in defining sex as 'necessary'. Also among boys, lack of early sexual relationships was thought to endanger the proper development of masculine abilities and eventual family stability.

The reported sexual behaviour of respondents seemed to a large extent to be influenced by existing group norms. Sex and girls were said to be topics often discussed with friends, especially among the older boys, and participating in this kind of communication was described as one of the factors influencing sexual début. If friends are sexually active, one has to follow in order not to lose their respect:

they do it because the environment puts pressure on them

many of my friends do not experience pleasure, they do it without feelings

if you don't have sex you will be accused of being blocked

In descriptions of sexual behaviour and experience we were confronted in several groups with the phrase 'it [sex] was quick and shameful'. Again, the word 'shame' could not be defined by participants, but referred to something which was considered as 'not quite right'. This links to the peer pressure described above: one has sex (quickly and without feelings) because of existing group norms; on the other hand it is 'shameful' because one is not expected to have sex.

Parties, discos and places of entertainment were said to be the locations and occasions where and when contacts with other young people more often end with sex. Especially for younger age groups, parties are the place. In this respect we came across two findings of particular interest.

First, as a result of talking with friends, boys usually know which girls are already sexually active. The latter are considered 'easy to get' and 'date-rape' seemingly occurs quite frequently at parties, as was mentioned by several participants. Second, alcohol commonly plays an important role in approaches to the opposite sex. Although young people talk a lot about sex with their peers, talking about sex with a member of the opposite sex is close to a taboo. Alcohol is used to overcome existing limitations on social inter-action and sex often occurs without any discussion.

There were also indications to suggest the existence of group pressures (which were more clearly articulated in the male groups) encouraging adolescents to have sex. There was evidence too that girls more often than boys self-consciously succumb to the pressure of group norms when starting a sexual life. However, they claim to feel pressured to have sex not so much by their female friends as indirectly by the male friends of their boyfriends, and by boyfriends themselves.

Risk perceptions

When they were asked to nominate words that come to mind regarding sex, respondents did not tend to associate sex with risk or with danger. When specifically asked about the risks connected to sex, answers included: unwanted pregnancies,[2] punishment by parents, negative reactions by society (being cited as a 'bad example' by adults, teachers, the parents of classmates, etc.), and sexually transmitted infections.

Group dynamics showed a rather heterogeneous pattern. Initially, when specifically asked about 'risks', rational answers like sexually transmitted diseases and unwanted pregnancies were given. These were replaced at a later stage with phrases describing fears:

That my parents, friends know about.

That my parents (mother) will force me to undergo an abortion.

That I will be worn out ... if my parents know, they will send me to a doctor.

A changing society

There are clear indications of generational conflict between adolescents and their parents in Bulgaria. This is, however, neither country specific, nor a particularly startling conclusion to reach. What is perhaps more original is the way in which this generational conflict has been aggravated by the post-totalitarian loss of reference points, norms and values that indirectly seem to affect the sexual behaviour of adolescents.

Until 1989, the so-called 'iron curtain' prevented the free exchange of ideas in Bulgaria and between Bulgaria and the outside world. All information coming into the country, and the dissemination of information within the country, was controlled. People could only access a limited range of information and technology. This shaped the generations living under the socialist system, and influenced the range of knowledge individuals had access to. The state system tried to replace individual beliefs and values with 'proper' ideological ones, and indeed succeeded to a great extent. Party discourse was one of uniformity (for the sake of transparency and control) in each and every niche of society. Not only that, people were not expected to question this discourse, and it was dangerous if they attempted to do so.

After 1989 when the totalitarian system fell into disorder, unification ceased to be the underlying principle that had for so long penetrated all different levels of society. The country entered a stage of serious and multi-dimensional transitions. With the transition from a totalitarian to a pluralistic society, old values, norms and reference points were no longer valid and/or widely promoted.

The generation of parents of contemporary Bulgarian adolescents was shaped and influenced by a political system which neither expected nor allowed them to make their 'own choices' and take their 'own decisions'. Before 1989, travel was restricted, literature was censored, cinemas showed only movies produced in Bulgaria or other communist bloc countries, and individual behaviour was controlled by party and social committees. This system no longer exists but has left its legacy. In contrast, the environment in which young people now live is one of more open access to information and technology. Young people have a broad range of choices, and articulate a clear wish to learn in ways whereby they can define and make their own experiences. To be understood is an important factor for adolescents, if they are to accept help, advice and guidance from others.

Our findings show that many young people feel misunderstood and there-fore not supported by their parents, not only because of generational conflict (the need to be emancipated and to live their own lives), but because of gaps in knowledge (things 'normal' for them were not known about by their parents) and the application of outdated norms and rules, which are the result of the former political system. The last seems to have blocked their parents from developing adequate communication skills. They were substi-tuted for by politically correct notions, ideas and ways of transmitting them.

Thus, adolescents' perception of being misunderstood leads to restricted communication with their parents and a rejection of even valuable advice. This triggers self-fulfilling responses on the part of young people and increases their vulnerability. It is more important to reject parents' opinion than to increase possible behavioural options through communication.

There is a clear tension between emerging new values, (group) norms, knowledge and independence on the part of young people, and the vacuum of values, reference points and norms on the part of older generations. This is partly managed in the context of 'old' norms and rules. Inexplicable feelings of 'shame' still influence the behaviour of adolescents, and a rejection of their parents' values increases vulnerability.

In young people's eyes, sexually transmitted infections, including HIV/AIDS, are not a major concern. The decision to engage in sex is mainly influenced by group norms that are quite different from those of the older generation and are shaped by a feeling of liberation from outdated values and norms. At the same time, however, these norms are linked to fears that the system to which this behaviour is a reaction may sanction them. We believe these phenomena play an important role in the socio-epidemiology of HIV/AIDS in Bulgaria. A challenge for future research lies in deepening our understanding of socio-cultural changes in countries undergoing transition from former totalitarian regimes, and the impact of these changes on behaviour.

Notes

1   Together, these two ethnic minorities comprise close to 15 per cent of Bulgaria's population. Recent socio-economic change in the country, among other things, has enlarged the number of mobile populations in the country. Many people travel to and from Turkey as well as around the country. It is popularly believed that gypsy girls comprise a considerable number of those involved in prostitution.
2   We cannot fully explain the perceived risk of unwanted pregnancies as abortions are still accepted in Bulgaria. In 1997, abortions cost less than one month's supply of an oral contraceptive and outnumbered deliveries by four to one.

References

Catterall, M. and Maclaran, P. (1997) 'Focus group data and qualitative analysis programs: coding the moving picture as well as the snapshots', *Sociological Research Online* 2: 1.

Rhodes, T. (1995) 'Theorizing and researching "risk": notes on the social relations of risk in heroin users lifestyles', in P. Aggleton *et al.* (eds) *AIDS: Safety, Sexuality and Risk*, London: Taylor & Francis.

Stoilova, M. and Popova, V. (1994) *The Value System of the Contemporary Bulgarians*, Sofia: Microcosmos.

Part III

Drug use
User and policy perspectives

11 Risk behaviour and HIV infection in European prisons

Michel Rotily and Caren Weilandt[1]

Identifying the prevalence of diseases and related risk behaviour is necessary for the implementation of appropriate prevention programmes. Although the routes of HIV transmission have been clearly identified, social, economic and psychosocial risk factors associated with HIV transmission are not well understood and change over time. Imprisonment has often been identified as a risk factor for HIV infection (Bird *et al.*, 1995; Gore *et al.*, 1997; Rotily *et al.*, 1994; Malliori *et al.*, 1998).

In European countries, the size of the prison population has increased dramatically over the last two decades. Social and psychological factors including poverty, migration, violence, education and living conditions have contributed to this trend. Other reasons include changes in incarceration policies (Raynal, 1998), and the widespread repressive legislation against drug usage in the context of an increasing drug consumption. Although reliable estimates are not available in Europe, several studies suggest that a comparatively high proportion of people entering prison have a history of drug use before imprisonment (10–65 per cent). Studies have also highlighted the interaction between injecting drug use and viral infections (such as those of HIV and viral hepatitis). Among non-imprisoned French patients infected with HIV through drug use and followed up by medical units, half had already been incarcerated (Cavailler *et al.*, 1997). Furthermore, as we will see, HIV seroprevalence has always been found to be higher in prison than in the general population (Gore *et al.*, 1997; Bird *et al.*, 1997, Rotily *et al.*, 1994). Thus, there are strong interactions between incarceration and diseases that are sexually transmitted or blood-borne.

Given the paucity of knowledge about the epidemiology of HIV and hepatitis in prisons and existing prevention measures, as well as the small number of researchers in this field, it was decided in 1995 to create the European Network for HIV/Hepatitis Prevention in Prisons. The work of this network has identified a series of directions for socio-behavioural and epidemiological research, and for future interventions.

Approach

In 1998, the national co-ordinators of the Network prepared reports on the current situation of HIV/hepatitis in prisons from national and local published reports. They also distributed standardised questionnaires to national prison and health systems, as well to prison directors and chief medical officers. The objectives of these surveys were to describe existing HIV/hepatitis prevention policy and to provide an overview of the current situation. Because situations vary within countries, it was sometimes difficult for respondents to provide answers relevant to the whole country. Published papers identified via the Medline database provided supplementary information, especially on risky behaviours in European prisons.

Socio-demographic data

Around 350,000 people are in prison in the fifteen European Union (EU) states, a rate of 94 per 100,000 inhabitants (compared with 645 per 100,000 in the USA). The ratio of prisoners per inhabitant varies significantly between European countries, being higher in Portugal, Spain and the UK, and lower in Sweden, Finland and Ireland. The percentage of women in the prison population varies between 2.5 and 5.5 per cent, except in Spain and Portugal, where the female prison population is 8.6 and 9.9 per cent respectively. The proportion of prisoners of foreign nationality or of minority ethnic origin (as far as figures are available) is high in most countries, reaching 46 per cent and 60 per cent in Italy and The Netherlands, respectively.

HIV screening/testing

HIV tests are generally available in prisons. In some countries, tests are offered on a voluntary basis to all prisoners on entering prison.[2] In others, the test is only carried out on prisoners identified by the medical officers as being at risk. In The Netherlands and Scotland, they are carried out on individual request only. While we do not have reliable estimates of the proportions of HIV-tested prisoners, the range is likely to be wide. In Germany, it varies between 15 and 95 per cent depending on how official testing policy is implemented in practice. In France, where HIV testing is offered systematically to prison entrants, two-thirds accept it (Rotily *et al.*, 1996). Prisoners' compliance with HIV testing when offered is quite good, especially among injecting drug users. However, agreement is most likely related to the prison's capacity not to segregate HIV-positive prisoners, and to protect confidentiality.

Answers to questions concerning pre- and post-test counselling reveal that HIV counselling is not carried out in an appropriate way in all prisons. Some prisons do not offer pre-test counselling, and in others post-test counselling is carried out only in the case of a positive result. In most prisons, HIV test results are not communicated to the prison administration and are strictly confidential. However, in some European prisons HIV-positive results are communicated to prison directors. As the majority of medical officers are employed by the prison service, breaches in confidentiality are possible.

In a few countries, a positive HIV test has certain consequences for the prisoner. In parts of Germany (e.g. in North Rhine Westphalia), Belgium and Greece, HIV-infected prisoners can be placed in single cells, and if they prefer to share a cell with other persons, the cell-mates have to be informed about their serostatus. In some countries, HIV-positive as well as Hepatitis-B- and C-positive inmates are excluded from kitchen and/or barber work. Here again, the situation is difficult to evaluate because prison directors have discretionary powers that allow them to designate the jobs and locations to which prisoners will be assigned.

No systematic HIV surveillance system has yet been implemented in European prisons. In Scotland, cross-sectional surveillance studies have, however, been carried out in many establishments (Gore and Bird, 1995). In England, similar studies have been implemented in some prisons (Bellis *et al.*, 1997). Elsewhere, a few one-off studies allow an estimation of HIV sero-prevalence (Rotily *et al.*, 1994, 1997a; Malliori *et al.*, 1998; Pont *et al.*, 1992). In France, a routine survey is carried out annually on a given day using anonymous reports of HIV-infected cases from medical officers (Bourdillon *et al.*, 1995). All these studies tend to show that HIV seroprevalence is much higher – about ten times higher – in prison than in the general population. However, owing to the paucity of data and the absence of a proper surveillance system in prisons, we know little about time trends in HIV seroprevalence. Data on the incidence of HIV/AIDS in prison are scarce (Brewer *et al.*, 1988), and no European data are available at the present time.

Risk behaviour in prison

Several studies have examined past patterns of risk behaviour among people entering prisons (e.g. Bird *et al.*, 1992, 1997; Rotily *et al.*, 1994), especially women (Rotily *et al.*, 1995) and injecting drug users (Rotily *et al.*, 1996). A study carried out in a large prison in south-eastern France in 1992 showed that HIV seroprevalence was six times higher among prisoners who had already been incarcerated than among prisoners incarcerated for the first time (Rotily *et al.*, 1994). Two hypotheses, which are not exclusive, are suggested by these results. First, it may be that prisoners who have been incarcerated several times have more risky behaviour, evidenced in higher drug consumption, more sharing and less cleaning of injection equipment, and in more risky sexual behaviours. A second hypothesis is that some prisoners may have been infected during previous incarceration because of needle sharing and/or risky sexual behaviours, such as unprotected intercourse and rape.

Methodological issues

The Network has collected published European data on risk behaviour during incarceration. The variety of methodologies and surveyed populations calls for caution in the interpretation of the results. Some surveys have been carried out among ex-inmates, others on current inmates, often with different conditions of anonymity. Surveys that do not guarantee anonymity, or that are performed by an investigator linked to the prison administration, are likely to provide unreliable data. Surveys performed outside prison offer a better guarantee of independence, since ex-prisoners are unlikely to fear reprisals from the prison administration. However, such studies may suffer from selection and recall biases. Even if the quality of data from a face-to-face interview is usually better than that from a self-completed questionnaire, a face-to-face interview may not be the best way of exploring intimate issues such as sexual behaviour or drug injection practices in prison. Even under conditions of anonymity it is likely that inmates interviewed in prisons tend to underreport prohibited and stigmatised behaviour.

Sexual behaviour in prisons

Data concerning the incidence of sexual behaviour within European countries are scarce and not easily interpretable owing to the variety of duration and conditions of imprisonment. Most of the time, surveys have dealt with homosexual intercourse (Table 11.1). Two studies have reported no homosexual intercourse within prisons (Power *et al.*, 1992; Bird *et al.*, 1992), but it is important to recognise that Power *et al.*'s study used a face-to-face questionnaire. Anal penetration has been reported in several Scottish and English surveys (Carvell and Hart, 1990; Gore *et al.*, 1997; Taylor *et al.*, 1993), and also in other European studies (e.g. Rotily *et al.*, 1997b).

No survey has yet investigated heterosexual intercourse, particularly in visiting rooms. The only available results come from the feasibility study carried out in six European prisons (Rotily *et al.*, 1997b), in which 85 out of 537 respondents (16 per cent) reported having had heterosexual sex in prison, most usually in the private visiting rooms of German and Swedish prisons. Interviews with prisoners, staff and physicians suggest that heterosexual intercourse can frequently occur in visiting rooms (Welzer-Lang *et al.*, 1996). As with the general population, prison prevention policy must not neglect this potential form of HIV transmission.

Drug injection in prison

Published data on injecting drug use in prison are more numerous (see Table 11.2). Surveys have been carried out in French, Greek, Scottish and English prisons (Carvell and Hart, 1990; Turnbull *et al.*, 1992; Dye and Isaacs, 1991;

Table 11.1 Published data on homosexual behaviour in European Union state prisons

Country	Year	Authors	Sample size	Questionnaire	Have ever had anal sex in prison
England	1989	Carvell and Hart (1990)	42[1]	Self -administered	6%
Scotland	1991	Bird *et al.* (1992)	378	Self -administered	0%
Scotland	?	Power *et al.* (1992)	559[2]	Face-to-face	NA[3]
Scotland	1993	Taylor *et al.* (1995)	227	Self-administered	0.5%
Scotland	1995	Gore *et al.* (1997)	282	Self-administered	1%
France, Germany, Italy, The Netherlands, Scotland, Sweden	1996	Rotily *et al.* (1997b)	720[4]	Self-administered	1%

Notes:
[1] Ex-inmates injecting drug users.
[2] The survey was carried out in nine prisons.
[3] The question did not specify anal sex.
[4] The survey was carried out in six sites, one in each country.

Bird *et al.*, 1992, 1995, 1997; Gore *et al.*, 1997; Power *et al.*, 1992; Bath *et al.*, 1993; Rotily *et al.*, 1998; Taylor *et al.*, 1993; Malliori *et al.*, 1998). One European survey has been conducted in six prisons in France, Germany, Italy, The Netherlands, Sweden and Scotland (Rotily *et al.*, 1997b). All surveys reported injecting drug use (13–85 per cent) and needle sharing (50–100 per cent) during incarceration. Results are consistent across methodologies (face-to-face or self-completed questionnaire), and the surveyed population (remand or sentenced prisoners, ex- or current inmates).

Although the proportion of injecting drug users in a prison population varies within and between countries, there is evidence that it is higher among women and remand compared with convicted prisoners (Rotily *et al.*, 1995). The figures in Table 11.3 have been provided by the country co-ordinators of the Network, and are based on estimates from prison services and/or results from recent prison surveys. Estimates of injecting drug use range between 15 and 65 per cent of the total prison population. In France, the proportion of injecting drug users (IDU) who have ever been incarcerated has been estimated at between 40 and 45 per cent (Facy, 1993), and 60 per cent of IDUs incarcerated at a given time have been imprisoned before (Rotily *et al.*, 1994). On average, Berliner IDUs have been in prison 2.7 times since they

Table 11.2   Published data on injecting drug use in European Union state prisons

Country (year)	Authors	Sample size	Population	Questionnaire
Germany (1993)	Muller et al. (1995)	418	Ex-inmates	Face-to-face
England (1989)	Carvell and Hart (1990)	50	Ex-inmates	Self-administered
England (1990)	Turnbull et al. (1992)	164	Ex-inmates	Face-to-face
Scotland (1991)	Dye and Isaacs (1991)	43[1]	Inmates	Face-to-face
England (1997)	Bellis et al. (1997)	260[2]	Remand prisoners	Self-administered
Scotland (1991)	Bird et al. (1992)	66	Inmates	Self-administered
Scotland (1992)	Power et al. (1992)	154[2]	Inmates	Face-to-face
Scotland (1992)	Bath et al. (1993)	67	Ex-inmates	Self-administered
Scotland (1994)	Bird et al. (1995)	327	Inmates	Self-administered
Scotland (1994)	Gore et al. (1995)	75	Inmates	Self-administered
Scotland (1996)	Bird et al. (1997)	116[2]	Inmates	Self-administered
		53	Inmates	Self-administered
Scotland (1995)	Gore et al. (1997)	82[2]	Inmates	Self-administered
		58 (women)	Inmates	Self-administered
France (1996)	Rotily et al. (1998)	68	Remand prisoners	Self-administered
France, Germany, Sweden, The Netherlands, Scotland (1996)	Rotily et al. (1997a)	210[2]	Inmates	Self-administered
Greece (1996)	Malliori et al. (1998)	544[2]	Inmates	Face-to-face

Notes:
[1] Sample unrepresentative of the prison.
[2] Multisite survey.

No. of sites	Injected	Shared	Comments
One	48%	75%	50% of IDUs who injected prison did so more than 50 times
One	66%	78%	Many injected products were reported
One	27%	75%	Mean no. of injections in prison: 18.7 (1990)
One	67%	76%	Reports of drug injection higher in short-term and remand prisoners (1991)
One	16%	56%	
One	47%	–	
Nine	28%	74%	Inmates declared lower risks than outside
One	21%	50%	
One	50%	–	
One	59%	–	
Two	57%	–	
	74%	–	
Two	85%	–	
	57%	–	
Two	13%	44% (4/9)	Prisoners were interviewed about the first 3 months of incarceration
Five	49%	–	
Two	69%	69%	

started to inject (Kleiber and Pant, 1996). A European multicentre study showed similar high multiple incarceration rates among IDUs (Rotily *et al.*, 1997b). The period immediately after discharge is one of high risk for IDU prisoners (Dye and Isaacs, 1991). Recently, it has also been shown that mortality rates after discharge, mainly due to overdoses, were very high among IDUs in Scotland (Seaman *et al.*, 1998).

Other evidence of the risk of HIV/hepatitis transmission in prisons comes from non-European incidence studies. Brewer *et al.* (1988) reported an HIV-1 incidence rate of 0.4 per cent per person-years in the Maryland state prison system. In Australia, Crofts *et al.* (1995) reported an hepatitis C incidence rate of 41 per cent per person-years among IDUs reincarcerated within the year, but no HIV infection. However, in the latter study, it was difficult to disentangle infections related to incarceration from those related to risk behaviour outside, especially at discharge.

Strong evidence for the risk of HIV/hepatitis transmission in prison derives from the HIV outbreak which occurred in a Scottish prison (Taylor *et al.* 1995) where eight cases of HIV transmission occurred within the first half of 1993. More generally, outbreaks of HIV infection or viral hepatitis

Table 11.3   Proportion of injecting drug users (IDUs) in prisons of the European Union states

Country	Proportion of IDUs in the prison population
Austria	14% in remand prisons and 17.5% in penal institutions (estimated by prison medical doctors, high numbers of unreported cases suspected)
Belgium	Approx. 15%
Denmark	Approx. 35%; 25% of them are IDUs
England and Wales	15–29% IDU use prior to incarceration
Finland	Figures not known, estimated to be high
France	Exact figures not known, estimated at 22% for IDUs (min. 0%, max. 33%) in west and south-east France
Germany	Approx. 30% of male and over 50% of female prison population
Greece	31% in the Athens prison
Ireland	Approx. 35% are drug users; proportion of IDUs not known
Italy	Approx. 25%
Luxembourg	Approx. 30%
The Netherlands	Approx. 30% used hard drugs like heroin and cocaine; no information about injection behaviour; IDU supposed to be low
Portugal	Estimated at 65% by the Ministry of Justice
Scotland	About 33% of adult prisoners are drug users (one-third IDUs)
Spain	54% drug users; 40% of total prison population had consumed heroin or cocaine within a day of their arrest
Sweden	25–65% (varies dramatically between prisons)

Note: The statistics have been provided by the country co-ordinators of the European Network for HIV/Hepatitis Prevention in Prisons. They are based on prison administration estimates or are derived from prison survey results.

are rarely documented as national surveillance centres do not routinely collect data on recent incarceration and its location (Gore and Bird, 1998).

Drug testing is performed in almost all countries but with varied frequency, mainly as a disciplinary measure or as a component of therapeutic settings like drug-free units. The UK is the only EU member state with a systematic policy of mandatory drug testing for inmates in all prisons. This policy has been criticised for different reasons (e.g. for encouraging drug users to switch from drugs with long urinary half-lives such as cannabis to those with shorter half-lives such as heroin (Gore *et al.*, 1996)), and may be revised soon.

Drug treatment and harm reduction programmes

Procedures regarding drug treatment/drug substitution programmes vary considerably between EU member states (Table 11.4). In Sweden, methadone maintenance is not provided in prison. In Italy and Greece, treatment is only available to those individuals who were enrolled on a methadone programme before imprisonment. Some countries offer only short-term detoxification therapy and no methadone maintenance treatment, or do so only for HIV-positive individuals on combination therapy. In Denmark, France, Scotland, Spain and The Netherlands, detoxification as well as methadone maintenance are available for most prisoners. The effectiveness of these approaches has yet to be evaluated, and it has not been possible to ensure their widespread implementation. The concept of drug-free units established in several European prisons (Portugal, Scotland, The Netherlands) seems well accepted by medical and prison staff, and by the prison administrations. However, these projects too need proper evaluation.

Needle exchange programmes (NEPs) have rarely been implemented in European prisons. Because many prisoners are imprisoned for drug or drug-related offences, and drug use is prohibited in most countries, prison administrations tend to consider such programmes inappropriate. To facilitate their more widespread use, NEPs must be evaluated and show clear efficacy. This is methodologically difficult, especially in a context where there is much resistance. However, since the first pilot NEPs in Switzerland were established and were shown to be feasible as well as effective (Nelles and Harding, 1995), other pilot projects, several currently under evaluation, have been implemented in Germany and Spain.

Bleach and sterilising tablets have been distributed in all Scottish prisons since 1993, together with an information leaflet and video tapes containing practical instructions about how to clean syringes. In most EU member states, bleach is either not available or used for general cleaning purposes, without information on how to use it to sterilise injecting equipment. Resistance to bleach availability in prison can be explained by the fact that, like NEPs, it means acknowledging drug injection in prison. Additionally, some health workers and prison staff believe that bleach availability could

Table 11.4 HIV testing and harm reduction programmes in prisons of the European

Country	HIV testing on admission	Counselling pre-/post-test	Segregation	Drug substitution programme
Austria	Offered on admission in most prisons/voluntary	Most cases	Exclusion from kitchen work	Yes
Belgium	Offered to at-risk prisoners	No/only when positive	Single cell, no kitchen work	Only in 4 prisons, for detox. if treatment initiated
Denmark	On request of prisoner	Yes/yes	No	Yes (methadone maintenance and detox.)
England and Wales	On request of prisoner	Yes/yes	No	Only for detox. and remand prisoners already receiving treatment
Finland	Offered on admission/voluntary or on request of prisoner	Yes/yes	No	Yes
France	Offered on admission in most prisons/voluntary	Most of the time	Sometimes exclusion from kitchen work	Yes
Germany	Offered on admission/voluntary	Most of the time/only when positive	Single cells, no kitchen or barber work	Detox. and maintenance in some prisons
Greece	Offered voluntarily	Yes/yes	Single cells/no kitchen work	No (except for prisoners who were enrolled in a methadone programmer before incarceration)
Ireland	Offered on admission/voluntary	Yes/yes	No	Only for detox., maintenance just for HIV-pos. prisoners on tri-therapy
Italy	Offered on admission/voluntary	Yes/yes	No	Only for prisoners enrolled on a methadone programme before incarceration
Luxembourg	Offered on admission but done after 2 months	No systematic counselling, only on request	No	Yes (only for detox.)
Netherlands	Only on request	Yes/yes	No	Most prisons
Portugal	Offered/voluntary	Most cases	No	Only in 3 prisons
Scotland	Only on request	Yes/yes	No	Yes
Spain	Offered/voluntary	Yes/yes	No	Yes (detox. and maintenance)
Sweden	Offered/voluntary	Yes/sometimes	No kitchen work	No

*   NA: not available.

Union states

Needle exchange	Condoms/lubricants available	Bleach in prison	Conjugal visits
No	Yes/only in a few prisons	No	No
No	Yes/NA*	Some prisons for cleaning/no data on how to clean syringes	No
No	Yes/no	Yes (+ brochures)	Yes
No	On prescription if prison doctor believes there is a risk of STD transmission	No	No
No	Yes/no	Yes	Yes
No	Officially available in the medical service in all prisons	Yes (since 1/98), not yet practised in all prisons, without brochures	Only in 2 prisons (pilot projects)
4 pilot programmes in different prisons	Most prisons/in some prisons	Some prisons for cleaning purposes/no information on how to clean syringes	Some prisons
No	No/no	Yes (+ brochures)	No
No	No (sexual relations are prohibited)	No	No
No	No/no (sexual intercourse is prohibited)	Some prisons	No
No, but a pilot project is being considered	Yes/yes	No	No
No	Yes/ NA*	Available, but not distributed officially	Yes, in remand prisons
No	Yes (in the medical service)/no	Yes (in most prisons)	Only in 1 prison
No	No (condoms only for home leaves and as part of release pack)	Sterilisation tablets in all prisons (since 1993)	No
1 pilot	In all prisons/no	Yes	Yes, in all prisons
No	Yes/NA*	No	Yes, in all prisons

thwart drug treatment efforts within prison, and harm reduction programmes on the outside. Furthermore, it is not clear whether the use of bleach for cleaning purposes offers an effective approach to preventing hepatitis C transmission.

Prevention of HIV sexual transmission

In Scotland, Italy and Ireland, sexual relations are openly prohibited in prison, and consequently condoms as well as lubricants are not available to prisoners. They are sometimes distributed to home leavers and/or as part of the release pack. In England and Wales, prisoners can get condoms on prescription if the prison doctor believes that there is a risk of STD transmission. In all other countries, condoms are (as a rule) available for prisoners, but the modes of distribution/availability vary considerably and have not been appropriately evaluated.

In the majority of European member states, conjugal visits are not allowed. In some countries (e.g. Germany, France, Greece and Portugal), some pilot projects have been implemented. Private visiting rooms, where prisoners can visit with partners and also have sexual intercourse in privacy, exist for all prisons in only three European countries (Sweden, Denmark and Spain). Evaluations of such strategies are not available, but apparently both prison staff and prisoners find them acceptable.

Conclusions

Our analysis shows that European health and prison administrations are concerned with the issue of HIV/AIDS in prison, and improvements in prevention policy have already been achieved. However, all published data highlight the frequency of risk behaviour among prisoners, before, during and after incarceration, and the inadequacies of current prevention policy. Access to harm reduction measures in European prisons still falls short of the World Health Organisation's 1993 *Guidelines on HIV Infection and AIDS in Prisons*. This situation presents public health and penitentiary administrations with a tremendous challenge to provide much-needed educational, prevention and treatment services. A number of research and intervention priorities suggest themselves.

First, reliable HIV and hepatitis surveillance systems should be implemented in European prisons, and multicentre studies carried out to provide trend estimates not only of the prevalence of HIV and hepatitis antibodies, but also of risk behaviour in prison. The need to include the information on imprisonment in HIV/hepatitis notification by monitoring centres should be discussed, taking into account issues of confidentiality. Incidence studies should also be conducted to highlight the need to strengthen harm reduction policy (Gore and Bird, 1998).

Second, an analysis of the impact of harm reduction measures introduced in some prisons, such as free and anonymous access to condoms, bleach, sterile injection equipment and methadone maintenance treatment, suggests that few obstacles are encountered. Prisoners and prison staff and administration tend to be supportive (Nelles and Harding, 1995). It is difficult, however, for both health and administrative staff to acknowledge the reality of prohibited behaviour and the need for a harm reduction policy. All actors in the field should recognise that the major objective of incarceration is social rehabilitation, which implies an improvement in mental and physical status. Therefore the provision of health education, including ready access to condoms and lubricants, safe and humane conditions for sexual intercourse (i.e. family visit units), and an efficient harm reduction policy aimed at IDUs should be included. Research should be undertaken to analyse reluctance to strengthen harm reduction policy in prison. In particular, we need to identify the level and the nature of resistance to harm reduction strategies among health workers and prison staff.

Third, there is an urgent need to enhance current harm reduction policy, and to disseminate findings from pilot projects already tried in some European prisons, especially drug maintenance programmes (i.e. methadone), NEPs, drug-free units and private visiting rooms. In each country, these projects should be implemented in pilot sites, with close collaboration between health, social and administrative staff, and alongside rigorous evaluation.

Although it has been shown that prevention strategies aimed only at eliminating drug use are inadequate among IDUs living in the community, there is still a tendency in European prisons to adhere to this old belief. Debates about harm reduction in prison are not broad enough, and are less advanced than those held by people in general. Such debate is crucial. Prisoners are part of the community, and they come from and return to the community. They deserve the same level of information, protection and care received by people outside prison. Communicable diseases in prisons should be considered as a general public health issue and not one restricted to this subgroup of the population.

Acknowledgements

The Network is funded by the European Commission. Neither the Commission nor any person acting on behalf of the Commission is responsible for the use that might be made of the information contained in this chapter.

We would like to thank Sheila Gore, Kerstin Käll, Emma Iandolo, Marteen van Doorninck, Flip Maas, Peer Brehm Christensen, Fabienne Hariga, Leena Arpo, Meni Malliori, Andrew Weild, Carlo Reuland, Maria Manuela dos Santos Pardal and Julia Munarriz for their previous contributions within the Network.

Notes

1   This chapter was written on behalf of the European Network for HIV/Hepatitis Prevention in Prisons.
2   Our surveys among physicians and prison administrations have shown that there is no mandatory HIV testing policy in European prisons. When a test is offered to prisoners, it is on a voluntary basis. However, in the context of incarceration, especially when the physicians are employed by the prison administration, some prisoners can feel that the offer is mandatory and that testing is carried out without their consent.

References

Bath, G. E., Davies, A. G., Dominy, N. J., Peters, A., Raab, G. and Richardson, A. M. (1993) 'Imprisonment and HIV prevalence', *The Lancet* 342: 1368.

Bellis, M., Weild, A., Beeching, N., Mutton, K. J. and Syed, Q. (1997) 'Prevalence of HIV and injecting drug use in men entering Liverpool Prison', *British Medical Journal* 315(7099): 30–31.

Bird, A. G., Gore, S. M., Jolliffe, D. W. and Burns, S. M. (1992) 'Anonymous HIV surveillance in Saughton Prison, Edinburgh', *AIDS* 6: 725–733.

Bird, A. G., Gore, S. M., Cameron, S., Ross, A. J. and Goldberg, D. J. (1995) 'Anonymous HIV surveillance with risk factor elicitation at Scotland's largest prison, Barlinnie', *AIDS* 9(7): 801–808.

Bird, A. G., Gore, S. M., Hutchinson, S. J., Lewis, S. C., Cameron, S. and Burns, S. (1997) 'Harm reduction measures and injecting inside prison versus mandatory drugs testing: results of a cross sectional anonymous questionnaire survey', *British Medical Journal* 315(7099): 21–24.

Bourdillon, F., Bonnevie, M. C. and Martinez, R. (1995) 'Enquête un jour donné, en milieu pénitentiaire, sur l'infection par le VIH. Principaux résultats', *Ministère des Affaires Sociales, de la Santé et de la Ville, Direction des Hôpitaux – Mission Sida, Ministère de la Justice – Direction de l'Administration Pénitentiaire*.

Brewer, T. F., Vlahov, D., Taylor, E., Hall, D., Munoz, A. and Polk, B. F. (1988) 'Transmission of HIV-1 within a statewide prison system', *AIDS* 2: 263–367.

Carvell, A. L. M. and Hart, G. J. (1990) 'Risk behaviours for HIV infection among drug users in prison', *British Medical Journal* 300: 1383–1384.

Cavailler, P., Obadia, Y., Rotily, M. and Moatti, J. P. (1997) 'Pratiques à risque chez les usagers de drogues intraveineuses séropositifs', Presentation at the conference on Epidémiologie et Evaluation en Toxicomanie, Lausanne, Switzerland.

Crofts, N., Stewart, T., Hearn, P., Yi Ping, X., Breschkin, A. M. and Locarnini, S. A. (1995) 'Spread of bloodborne viruses among Australian prison entrants', *British Medical Journal* 310: 285–288.

Dye, S. and Isaacs, C. (1991) 'Intravenous drug misuse among prison inmates: implications for spread of HIV', *British Medical Journal* 302: 1506–1508.

Facy, F. (1993) 'Toxicomanes consultant dans les institutions spécialisées en 1991–1992', *INSERM U 302*.

Gore, S. M. and Bird, A. G. (1995) 'Cross-sectional willing anonymous HIV salivary (WASH) surveillance studies and self-completion risk factor questionnaire in establishments of the Scottish Prison Service', *AIDS New Supplement to the*

Weekly Report of the Scottish Centre for Infection and Environmental Health, AM-15 WR 95/39:1–4.

——(1998) 'Study size and documentation to detect injection-related hepatitis C in prison', *Quarterly Journal of Medicine* 91: 353–357.

Gore, S. M., Bird, A. G., Burns, S. M., Goldberg, D. J., Ross, A. J. and MacGregor, J. (1995) 'Drug injection and HIV prevalence in inmates of Glenochil Prison', *British Medical Journal* 310: 293–296.

Gore, S. M., Bird, A. G. and Ross, A. J. (1996) 'Cost implications of random mandatory drugs tests in prisons', *The Lancet* 348(9035): 1124–1127.

Gore, S. M., Bird, A. G., Burns, S., Ross, A. J. and Goldberg, D. (1997) 'Anonymous HIV surveillance with risk-factor elicitation: at Perth (for men) and Cornton Vale (for women) Prisons in Scotland', *International Journal of STD and AIDS* 8(3): 166–175.

Kleiber, D. and Pant, A. (1996) 'HIV-needle sharing-sex', Paper presented at Nomos, Baden-Baden.

Malliori, M., Sypsa, V., Psicogiou, M., Touloumi, G., Skoutelis, A., Tassopoulos, N., Hatzakis, A. and Stefanis, C. (1998) 'A survey of bloodborne viruses and associated risk behaviours in Greek prisons', *Addiction* 93(2): 243–251.

Muller, R., Stark, K., Guggenmoss-Holzmann, I., Wirth, D. and Bienzle, U. (1995) 'Imprisonment: a risk factor for HIV infection counteracting education and prevention programmes for intravenous drug users', *AIDS* 9: 183–190.

Nelles, J. and Harding, T. W. (1995) 'Preventing HIV transmission in prison: a tale of medical disobedience and Swiss pragmatism', *The Lancet* 346: 1507–1508.

Pont, J., Kahl, W. and Salzner, G. (1992) 'HIV epidemiologie und Risikoverhalten für HIV Transmission in Haft in Österreich. Sonderanstalt Favoriten', *Bundesministerium für Justiz des Republik Österreich*.

Power, K. G., Markova, I., Rowlands, A., McKee, K. J., Anslow, P. J. and Kilfedder, C. (1992) 'Intravenous drug use and HIV transmission amongst inmates in Scottish prisons', *British Journal of Addiction* 87: 35–45.

Raynal, F. (1998) 'Une seule punition, l'enfermement?', *Le Monde Diplomatique* Juillet: 22–23.

Rotily, M., Galinier-Pujol, A., Obadia, Y., Moatti, J. P., Toubiana, P., Vernay-Vaisse, C. and Gastaut, J. A. (1994) 'HIV testing, HIV infection and associated risk factors among inmates in south-eastern French prisons', *AIDS* 8(9): 1341–1344.

Rotily, M., Galinier-Pujol, A. and Vernay-Vaisse, C. (1995) 'Risk behaviours of inmates in south-eastern France', *AIDS Care* 7 (Suppl. 1): 91–95.

Rotily, M., Vernay-Vaisse, C. and Messiah, A. (1996) 'HIV testing prevalence and risk behaviours among prisoners incarcerated in south-eastern France, TuC2632', Paper presented at the XIth International Conference on AIDS, Vancouver, July.

Rotily, M., Vernay-Vaisse, C., Bourlière, M., Galinier-Pujol, A., Rousseau, S. and Obadia, Y. (1997a) 'HBV and HIV screening, and hepatitis B immunization programme in the prison of Marseille, France', *International Journal of STD and AIDS* 8: 753–759.

Rotily, M., Weilandt, C., Gore, S. M., Käll, K., Jandolo, E., De Jong, W., Van Haastrecht, H. and Rousseau, S. (1997b) 'Prévalence des pratiques à risque de transmission du VIH et des Virus des Hépatites chez les usagers de drogues intraveineuses en Milieu Carcéral: Une enquête multicentrique européenne', Paper presented at the conference on Epidémiologie et Evaluation en Toxicomanie, Lausanne, Switzerland, September.

Rotily, M., Galinier-Pujol, A., Escaffre, N., Delorme, C. and Obadia, Y. (1998) 'Survey of French prison found that injecting drug use and tatooing occurred', *British Medical Journal* 316(7133): 777.

Seaman, S. R., Brettle, R. P. and Gore, S. M. (1998) 'Mortality from overdose among injecting drug users recently released from prison: database linkage study', *British Medical Journal* 316(7129): 426–428.

Taylor, A., Goldberg, D., Frischer, M., Emslie, J., Green, S. A. and McKeganey, N. (1993) 'Evidence of risk', *British Medical Journal* 307: 623.

Taylor, A. *et al.* (1995) 'Outbreak of HIV infection in a Scottish prison', *British Medical Journal* 310: 289–292.

Turnbull, P. J., Dolan, K. A. and Stimson, G. V. (1992) 'Prison decreases the prevalence of behaviours but increases the risks', Internal Document, Centre for Research on Drugs and Health Behaviour, London.

Welzer-Lang, D., Mathieu, L. and Faure, M. (1996) 'Sexualités et violences en prison', *Observatoire International des Prisons, Editions Aleas*, Lyons.

12 Drug users' views and service evaluation[1]

Joanne Neale

In the UK, evaluations of drug service provision have tended to examine the views of service providers rather than service users (e.g. Greenwood, 1992; Carroll, 1993; Bond and Matheson, 1997). With a few notable exceptions (e.g. Jones *et al.*, 1994; Sheridan and Barber, 1996), drug users' views are seldom encountered within the literature. The objective of this chapter is to help to redress this imbalance by examining the role of drug users' views in evaluating two key HIV prevention strategies: substitute methadone prescribing and the provision of sterile injecting equipment.

Injecting drug use, HIV infection and service provision

Injecting drug users are at risk of infection with HIV and other blood-borne pathogens both through the sharing of injecting equipment and through unsafe sexual behaviours. Because drug injectors are often affected in the early stages of HIV epidemics, it is essential to control HIV infection amongst injecting populations in order to control HIV epidemics in the wider society (Stimson *et al.*, 1998).

In the UK, concerns about HIV infection have prompted a number of changes in drugs policy and service provision for drug users. Although abstinence remains the ideal treatment outcome, it is now widely accepted that there are a range of important 'harm reduction' measures which people with drug problems might take in order to curb the spread of HIV and lessen some of the other dangers of drug injection. These harm reduction measures include less sharing of injection equipment, a cessation of sharing injection equipment, a move from injectable to oral drug use, a stabilisation of drug use, and a lowered level of drug use.

Recent studies have shown that harm reduction initiatives (such as methadone prescribing and the provision of sterile injecting equipment) have had beneficial effects on the behaviour of drug users. Methadone programmes have been associated with reduced rates of illicit drug use; injecting; criminal behaviour; other HIV risk-related behaviours (such as needle sharing, number of sexual partners, and exchange of sex for money or drugs); overdose; and death (Gronbladh *et al.*, 1990; Bertschy, 1995;

Deglon, 1995). Needle exchanges, meanwhile, appear to have prevented a substantial proportion of HIV infections (Gruer *et al.*, 1993; Durante *et al.*, 1995) and led to a significant reduction in syringe sharing (Peters *et al.*, 1994; Stimson, 1995).

Despite these valuable achievements, high-risk drug-related activities have not been eradicated. The injection of oral methadone syrup is widespread in some areas (Darke *et al.*, 1996), methadone leaked from prescriptions may be contributing to drug deaths (Bentley and Busuttil, 1996), and injecting equipment continues to be shared (Barnard, 1993; Dear, 1995). Additionally, drug users often fail to recognise that 'frontloading' and 'backloading' (drug-sharing techniques which utilise a communal syringe to measure and distribute 'fair shares' of the drug or drugs to the syringes of other injectors) and the sharing of other injecting paraphernalia (such as filters, spoons and water) are also high-risk behaviours (Power *et al.*, 1994). In order to reduce these dangers, both new intervention initiatives and the regular monitoring and evaluation of existing drug services are required.

In England, the Task Force to Review Services for Drug Misusers (Polkinghorne, 1996) has recommended that performance indicators be used to evaluate drug service provision. These performance indicators include the number of clients entering methadone programmes, the percentage becoming drug free within set time periods, the cost of the service per client, the number of exchange packs given out per month, the number of needles/syringes sold to drug users per month, and the return rates of used equipment. Although evaluations of this kind provide important informa-tion about existing drug service provision, they do not offer a complete picture of service effectiveness. This is because they investigate only a narrow range of easily measured aspects of service delivery and do not consider provision from the perspective of drug users themselves. Consequently, they provide a business-like cost–benefit analysis and not a more humanitarian overview of service quality.

The process of evaluating drug services, such as methadone treatment and needle and syringe provision, is complex and requires a detailed examination of various aspects of service delivery. In the language of public service evalua-tion, these aspects are commonly referred to as 'inputs', 'processes', 'outputs' and 'outcomes' (Klein and Carter, 1988; Smith, 1996). 'Inputs' are the resources required to provide the service, 'processes' describe the way the service is delivered, 'outputs' measure quantifiable rates of change in the behaviour of drug-using individuals, and 'outcomes' consider the impact of provision on individuals receiving the service. Outcomes provide a valuable qualitative indicator of performance but are difficult to measure and tend not to be well researched. This is because they focus on relatively intangible aspects of service delivery, such as how drug users feel that methadone and the provision of injecting equipment have effected their quality of life. In order to evaluate the outcomes of methadone prescribing and needle and syringe provision, it is necessary to ask drug users how they feel about such services.

Interviewing drug users

During 1996, semi-structured qualitative interviews were conducted with 124 illicit drug users in rural, urban and inner city areas of Scotland. The recruitment sites included twenty-two pharmacies and eight drug agencies. The pharmacies were identified from a national pharmacy survey (Bond and Matheson, 1997) as having varying degrees of involvement with illicit drug users. The eight drug agencies included five specialist drug agencies offering a prescribing service and/or needle exchange; a drop-in centre; a project offering supported accommodation for people experiencing difficulties related to drug dependency; and a self-help organisation providing support to recovering addicts.

Letters explaining the research were distributed to drug users who were then asked whether they would be willing to participate in the study. Although most individuals were happy to be interviewed, it is possible that drug users who refused and drug users not in contact with drug agencies had views of services that were more negative, lifestyles that were more chaotic, and behaviour that was more risk orientated than those who were interviewed. The findings of the study may consequently underestimate the true extent of negative opinions and high-risk drug-related behaviour occurring among the drug-using population as a whole.

In view of the above, some interviewees were asked to introduce the researchers to friends who were non-service users (snowball sampling). Interviews with these individuals provided a useful check on how the opinions of those not in contact with agencies differed from those who were. Although the number of non-service users included was too small to allow for any detailed independent analysis, the opinions of the non-service users were considered in conjunction with the views of service users not receiving prescribed methadone in order to obtain a broader overview of substitute prescribing. Similarly, some comparisons between the opinions of the interviewees who were current injectors, interviewees who had ceased injecting, and interviewees who had never injected regarding the provision of sterile injecting equipment were made.

The interviews were conducted in local cafés, pubs and parks, interviewees' homes, private rooms in drug agencies and pharmacies, and the researchers' cars. Confidentiality was assured and the researchers emphasised that they were undertaking independent research and had no connections with any service providers. This, it was hoped, would reduce the risk of the interviewees identifying the researchers with the recruitment sites and thus being reluctant to criticise provision, or misunderstanding that their comments might have consequences for them as service users.

During the interviews, in-depth information was collected about a range of topics. These included the provision and administration of substitute drugs, the availability of injecting equipment, and the roles of different service providers. The semi-structured interview format enabled a similar range of topics to be covered in each interview, whilst also offering respondents maximum opportunity to express their views and experiences in their own words. All interviews were tape-recorded with full transcription, and analysis of the transcribed material was then carried out using *Winmax*, a software package suitable for the computer-assisted interpretation of qualitative data.

The interviewees

Of the 124 individuals interviewed, seventy-seven (62 per cent) were male and forty-seven (38 per cent) were female. This reflected the existing gender imbalance in this drug-using population (*Drug Misuse Statistics Scotland*, 1995). Most interviewees were aged between 21 and 40 years (age range 16 to 56 years) and ninety-one individuals (73 per cent) had injected drugs. Of the ninety-one individuals who had injected drugs, sixty-two (68 per cent) were male and twenty-nine (32 per cent) were female, while the thirty-three others had never injected drugs.

At the time of the study, eighty of the 124 respondents were receiving prescribed methadone and sixteen were receiving other substitute drugs, such as diazepam and dihydrocodeine. Of the eighty individuals receiving methadone, forty-one were receiving methadone only and thirty-nine were receiving methadone and at least one other substitute drug. The duration of methadone prescriptions ranged from one day to eight years, and daily dosages ranged from 8 mg to 230 mg (mean 54 mg). Of the forty-four interviewees not currently receiving prescribed methadone, eleven had previously had a methadone prescription and thirty-three had never had a methadone prescription. Only thirteen individuals had never had a prescription for any type of substitute drug.

Drug users' views of prescribed methadone

In this section, the interviewees' views of prescribed methadone are discussed. The benefits and disadvantages identified were not categories introduced by the researchers. Rather, they emerged inductively from the interviewees' responses to questions such as 'How has methadone helped you?' and 'What problems have you experienced?'

On the whole, drug users felt that methadone was a valuable substitute drug and dispensing through pharmacies an important service. It would, however, be inaccurate to claim that the respondents were either 'for' or 'against' the prescribing of methadone. Most drug users believed that methadone was a complex substitute drug which had many advantages but also caused many problems for drug users. Furthermore, respondents reported that the impact of prescribed methadone on any given individual depended on a number of factors. These included the individuals' determination to stop taking drugs, their personal support systems and interests, the length of time they had been on methadone, and any conditions (such as supervised consumption) involved in the prescribing process (Neale, 1998a).

Interviewees who were not currently receiving prescribed methadone were the most critical of its use as a substitute drug. These individuals were most likely to argue that there should be stricter conditions and controls attached to the prescribing process. Likewise, they most frequently stressed that methadone did not work or that it would only work for a short period of time or for some individuals or under certain circumstances.

Box 12.1

Most frequently discussed benefits of prescribed methadone (listed in descending order of priority):

1   Reduced illicit drug use
2   Positive health effects
3   Crime prevention
4   Harm reduction
5   Increased physical and emotional resources
6   Financial benefits
7   Improved personal relationships

A very large number of respondents, regardless of whether they person-ally had a methadone prescription, stressed that methadone was valuable in preventing illicit drug use (see Box 12.1). First, methadone lessened the craving for other drugs and, second, it reduced the painful withdrawals asso-ciated with heroin use and thus made abstinence easier. Many respondents (again both those receiving and those not receiving methadone at the time of the study) stated that prescribed methadone improved drug users' emotional and physical health. That is, it made them feel 'normal', reduced painful heroin withdrawals, increased weight, and facilitated sleep.

A large number of interviewees (but especially those not currently receiving a methadone prescription) also reported that prescribed methadone was beneficial because it prevented crime. That is, drug users no longer had to commit crime because they no longer needed large amounts of money to access illegal drugs. Furthermore, they no longer ended up in jail or in trouble with the police as a result. Additionally, many respondents (both those currently with and those without prescriptions) argued that methadone reduced the various harms caused by illicit drugs. For example, methadone stopped drug users from injecting and was cleaner and safer than street drugs.

Some respondents (mostly individuals currently receiving methadone) reported that legal prescriptions increased drug users' physical and emotional resources. This was because drug users receiving a prescription no longer needed to spend the entire day running around looking for drugs. Consequently, they could think about other things, but also had the time and energy to do other things, for example to be more involved with their children or to seek paid employment. A methadone prescription also benefited drug users financially because it reduced their need to work as a prostitute, sell personal belongings, borrow off others, or accumulate debts. Finally, a small number of individuals (all currently prescribed) felt that methadone improved their personal relationships because it made them more stable and less argumentative.

Box 12.2

Most frequently discussed disadvantages of prescribed methadone (listed in descending order of priority):

1   Negative health effects
2   Similar problems to, or worse problems than, heroin
3   Abuse of the system
4   Problems with the prescribing process
5   Constraint on personal resources

In spite of these benefits, many respondents (both with and without current prescriptions) complained that substitute methadone caused significant detrimental effects to drug users' health (see Box 12.2). The main health problem discussed was damage to teeth, but other common difficulties included weight changes (both weight loss and weight gain); stiffness and soreness; hallucinations; constipation; sweating; sleeping problems; and tiredness. Additionally, some individuals believed that prescribed methadone made drug users violent and aggressive, while others felt that individuals being prescribed sometimes became depressed with their situation and committed suicide.

Frequently, drug users complained that prescribed methadone was responsible for causing similar problems to, and sometimes worse problems than, heroin and other street drugs. These problems included severe addiction and unpleasant withdrawal symptoms. This criticism was made by many individuals who had been prescribed methadone, but was particularly common amongst individuals who had never been prescribed. Abuse of the prescribing system was a further common concern, particularly amongst respondents who had never personally had a prescription. This abuse included prescriptions being sold, given away and swapped, but also the 'topping up' of medication with illicit drugs.

Some drug users (especially those currently prescribed) also discussed problems relating to the prescribing process (e.g. being given insufficient dosages of medication or the prescribing agency being too strict about reducing them). Additionally, several respondents felt that drug users receiving a methadone prescription suffered unnecessarily in prisons because medication was terminated too abruptly by the prison authorities. Finally, some respondents (both those with and without a prescription) argued that the collection of methadone was a very time-consuming process which restricted their freedom and impinged upon the quality of their lives. This was particularly a problem when collection prevented people going away on holiday or made it difficult for them to sustain a job.

The respondents' evaluations of methadone prescribing were largely consistent with the benefits and problems often discussed by policy makers, providers and researchers. That is, drug users appreciated methadone's capacity to reduce illicit drug use, decrease drug-related harms, minimise HIV risk behaviours, and prevent crime. Simultaneously, they were concerned about abuse of the prescribing system, methadone's addictive nature, and its potential to cause similar problems to, or worse problems than, heroin. Additionally, however, drug users (and particularly those currently receiving prescribed methadone) emphasised a much broader range of less immediately obvious effects. These included the positive and negative impact of methadone on health, increased physical and emotional resources (particularly time and energy), financial benefits, improved personal relationships, flaws in the prescribing process, and problems associated with collection.

From the interviewees' comments, it was evident that drug users' concerns extended beyond the limited range of performance indicators recommended by Polkinghorne (1996) and included a broader range of less tangible aspects of service delivery, such as the impact of methadone on the quality of service users' lives. A further finding, meanwhile, was the contradictory nature of many of the benefits and problems discussed by the respondents. Thus, some individuals emphasised positive health effects; some opposite negative health effects; and others a mixture of the two. Such contrasting opinions can be explained in a number of ways.

Methadone, like all opioids, has many potential side effects. Some of these (e.g. excessive sweating and insomnia) can disappear with prolonged use; others (such as tooth decay and constipation) can be minimised or treated; and others (such as respiratory depression and death) will only occur in non-tolerant individuals or in cases of overconsumption. Many of the potential problems caused by methadone may also be exacerbated by individual lifestyle factors: poor diet, lack of exercise and insufficient dental hygiene. For example, methadone promotes the growth of plaque, attacks tooth enamel, and decreases the production of saliva, all of which contribute to tooth decay. Nevertheless, these hazards can be reduced by changing to sugar-free methadone, rinsing the mouth with water, cleaning the teeth, and chewing sugar-free gum.

Further to the above, the side effects of methadone can become confused with general symptoms of opioid withdrawal (such as aching joints) and with a general restabilisation of the body as an individual reduces drug consumption and adopts a less chaotic lifestyle. So, weight changes may occur because individuals are beginning to eat more regularly. Similarly, depression might resurface in individuals who have ceased using heroin to repress negative emotions. In summary, respondents' contradictory comments about the benefits and disadvantages of methadone probably reflect the fact that drug users are individuals whose views and experiences depend on their particular circumstances and behaviour at any given moment in time.

Drug users' views of accessing and disposing of injecting equipment

As discussed in Neale (1998b), most interviewees knew of local agencies (mostly pharmacies or needle exchanges) from which sterile injecting equipment could be obtained. Current injectors were, however, the most informed about outlets offering injection-related services whilst those who had never injected and those who no longer injected often distanced themselves from the need to know such information. Most respondents recognised that access to sterile injecting equipment had increased over recent years and described this as an important improvement. Nevertheless, twenty (22 per cent) of the ninety-one individuals who had ever injected, and two (6 per cent) of the thirty-three interviewees who had never injected, still believed that the current level of availability was insufficient and more provision was required. Additionally, where sterile equipment was not on hand, injectors (both current and ex-injectors) believed that drug users often shared.

Only three individuals (one individual who had never injected and two individuals who had ceased injecting) argued that providing easier access to sterile equipment was harmful because it encouraged people to inject. More individuals (mostly current injectors) stressed that there should be at least one local source of clean equipment in each area of town and outlets should be open for longer hours, especially in the evenings and at weekends. Others felt that there should be more publicity regarding which pharmacies were providing needles and at what times. For drug users visiting unfamiliar areas, a lack of such information was considered especially problematic.

The ninety-one respondents who had ever injected reported that they obtained sterile equipment from a wide range of sources: pharmacies; needle exchanges; other specialist drug agencies; friends or partners; medical supplies; mobile buses; health centres; doctors; and hospitals. Some injectors explained that they always acquired their equipment from the same source, but most maintained that they used different outlets depending on which was convenient at the time. Although many of the ninety-one interviewees who had ever injected said that they had shared or used discarded needles, many stressed that they had not engaged in such high-risk behaviour since sterile equipment had become more accessible and since they had become more aware of the dangers. When respondents did share, this was often related to situational factors, such as the pharmacy or needle exchange being shut or respondents being too far away from these facilities. Additional reasons for sharing included feeling invulnerable, lack of self-control, not caring, being in prison, and not feeling at risk from other individuals involved.

Although some interviewees felt that it was not difficult to enter a pharmacy and ask for needles, others found it extremely awkward or degrading. Some individuals felt able to obtain needles from the pharmacy where they obtained their prescription for substitute drugs; others felt that this was not possible because the pharmacist would not allow it or because they were personally too embarrassed. Some injectors stressed that they preferred to use a pharmacy where they were known and did not have to explain what they wanted. Others simply asked friends to collect or dispose of equipment on their behalf. Men were more likely to report that it was easy to use a public place for accessing injecting equipment; women were more likely to ask friends to deal with equipment on their behalf. There was also some evidence that older injectors collected for younger injectors and that sterile equipment was sometimes transferred from urban pharmacies to drug users in rural areas where injecting equipment was less accessible.

The ninety-one injecting respondents also reported using various strategies for disposing of their used needles. In Scotland, many agencies encourage drug users to place their used equipment in specially designed plastic disposal containers or 'cin bins' and then return them for incineration. Some injecting respondents reported that they complied with these arrangements; others confessed that they had carelessly discarded used cin bins into rubbish bins, or abandoned needles and syringes in blocks of flats, streets and parks. Alternative disposal techniques described by the respondents included needles being thrown down drains, wrapped in black binliners, squashed in soft-drink tins, buried in gardens, burned on fires, flushed down toilets, and stored in bedroom drawers.

In spite of the dubious nature of some of these strategies, almost all ninety-one injectors stressed that they personally disposed of their equipment safely. Whilst it was likely that unsafe disposal occurred more frequently than reported because respondents were unwilling to discuss their own dangerous practices, it also seemed that many respondents genuinely misunderstood what actually constituted 'safe'. Nevertheless, both injectors and non-injectors recognised that abandoned needles posed a serious public health hazard in many areas and, when questioned about this, reported that this occurred because 'some' users were thoughtless or too intoxicated to care.

When respondents discussed whether they preferred to use a pharmacy or a centralised needle exchange to access and dispose of injecting equipment, a complex picture emerged. In general, drug users felt that pharmacies were the most accessible sources of clean needles and syringes, although they tended only to provide limited kinds of assistance. Centralised needle exchanges were less convenient in terms of location and opening hours, but offered a more comprehensive range of assistance (such as sterile swabs, cin bins, general health care, advice and information). Accessibility, friendliness and discretion emerged as the most important characteristics of needle and syringe provision.

Finally, the data indicated that the use of issue and return rates as performance indicators for evaluating exchange services is problematic. This is because the number of drug users actually using the services of a pharmacy or an exchange is not necessarily reflected in the number of individuals physically presenting themselves at the agency doors. Many drug users donate sterile equipment to others. Additionally, used equipment is not always returned to the same outlet from which it is acquired. Consequently, some providers have artificially high and others artificially low return rates. Moreover, some used equipment is disposed of safely, even though it is not returned to an official agency.

The way ahead

The study has shown that the opinions of drug users are similar to those often expressed by policy makers, providers and researchers. Nevertheless, it has also been evident that drug users have additional concerns about service provision. Moreover, the opinions of service users vary depending on the individual concerned and the particular circumstances of that individual at any given moment in time. Drug users' views are, in other words, diverse but also susceptible to change over time. Furthermore, individuals with drug problems often demonstrate a high level of insight into their personal circumstances and seem well placed to make a contribution to decisions about their own treatment and service requirements. Inevitably, some drug users will require services which they dislike (such as prison) or their views will differ from those of other professionals or from research evidence. For example, some individuals may be offered very low levels of substitute medication and others forced to comply with conditions (such as urinalysis, supervised consumption or compulsory counselling) in order to receive their prescriptions. Such potential sites of conflict require further consideration.

First, it is not always possible to predict which services particular individuals will like and which they will dislike. In this study, some interviewees described prison as a welcome break from drug use and an opportunity to 'straighten out' and to recover physically and mentally from life on the outside. Similarly, many interviewees were very happy with the conditions they had to fulfil to receive their medication because they felt that these conditions helped them to stick to the programme and prevented abuse of the system. Drug users will not, in other words, always disagree with what appear to be infringements of their personal liberty.

Second, when disagreement between involved parties does occur (e.g. in the case of an unwelcome prison sentence), it may still be possible to offer services (such as substitute medication, accommodation in a drug-free wing or counselling) which the user may actively desire. In less extreme circumstances than imprisonment, meanwhile, there will be scope for at least some discussion, compromise and conflict resolution. Open discussion, without conflict resolution, will in any case provide all participants with a greater understanding of the issues and the opportunity to incorporate this knowledge into future decisions.

Finally, it should be remembered that services imposed upon individuals against their will are unlikely to succeed. Moreover, it is in everybody's interests to understand why some services will not work, or are not beneficial, for some individuals under certain conditions. Although drug users cannot provide the definitive statement about the value of service provision, their views are important and deserve careful attention from policy, practice and research.

At an individual provider level, professionals (such as general practitioners, counsellors and drug workers) can ascertain drug users' views through regular consultation with their drug-using clients. Additionally, they can canvas their clients' opinions through feedback forms or small-scale surveys. At an interagency level, user participation in service evaluation is perhaps best achieved through independent research. This could include interviews, surveys and focus groups with drug users in and out of treatment. Unfortunately, resources for such independent research are not always available and so it may be necessary also to seek cheaper, second-best alternatives. For example, if the consent of drug users is obtained, details of their consultations with practitioners could be recorded formally and fed back into policy evaluations.

More radically, drug users may self-organise and form drug users' organisations for the purpose of advocating on behalf of drug users or even for implementing and monitoring their own services. Additionally, drug users can participate in service evaluation by working as outreach workers or peer educators, reducing HIV risk behaviour and HIV infection rates by demonstrating the value of prevention strategies through their own behaviour and by attracting more injectors into effective forms of treatment where HIV prevention efforts may be implemented. Ultimately, such advances in user involvement can only flourish in a supportive political, legal and cultural environment where injecting drug users and individuals with HIV infection are not marginalised, but are recognised as individuals entitled to the same basic rights as all others. Where this is not yet the case, community education (see also Ball, 1998) is an important first step in ensuring that drug users will one day be able to participate positively in all forms of service evaluation.

Acknowledgements

The author would like to thank the Scottish Executive for funding this study; Catriona Matheson (Department of General Practice and Primary Care, University of Aberdeen) for conducting some of the interviews; and Annick Prieur for helpful comments on an earlier draft of the chapter.

Note

1   The Centre for Drug Misuse Research is funded by the Chief Scientist Office of the Scottish Executive Health Department. The views reported in this chapter do not necessarily reflect those of the Executive Health Department.

References

Ball, A. L. (1998) 'Overview: policies and interventions to stem HIV-1 epidemics associated with injecting drug use', in G. V. Stimson *et al.* (eds) *Drug Injecting and HIV Infection: Global Dimensions and Local Responses*, London: UCL Press.

Barnard, M. (1993) 'Needle sharing in context: patterns of sharing among men and women injectors and HIV risks', *Addiction* 88: 805–812.

Bentley, A. J. and Busuttil, A. (1996) 'Deaths among drug abusers in south-east Scotland (1989–1994)', *Medicine, Science and the Law* 36: 231–236.

Bertschy, G. (1995) 'Methadone-maintenance treatment – an update', *European Archives of Psychiatry and Clinical Neuroscience* 245: 114–124.

Bond, C. and Matheson, C. (1997) *Community Pharmacists' Involvement with Drug Misusers: a Scottish National Survey of Attitudes and Practice*, University of Aberdeen, Department of General Practice and Primary Care.

Carroll, J. (1993) 'Attitudes of professionals to drug abusers', *British Journal of Nursing* 2: 705–711.

Darke, S., Ross, J. and Hall, W. (1996) 'Prevalence and correlates of the injection of methadone syrup in Sydney, Australia', *Drug and Alcohol Dependence* 43: 191–198.

Dear, L. (1995) 'Negotiated safety – what you don't know won't hurt you, or will it?', *Drug and Alcohol Review* 14: 323–329.

Deglon, J. J. (1995) 'Methadone treatment – a necessary and efficient therapy for chronic addicts', *Therapie* 50: 537–542.

Drug Misuse Statistics Scotland (1995), Edinburgh: ISD.

Durante, A. J., Hart, G. J., Brady, A. R., Madden, P. B. and Noone, A. (1995) 'The health of the nation target on syringe sharing: a role for routine surveillance in assessing progress and targeting interventions', *Addiction* 90: 1389–1396.

Greenwood, J. (1992) 'Unpopular patients – GPs' attitudes to drug users', *Druglink* July/August: 8–10.

Gronbladh, L., Ohlund, L. S. and Gunne, L. M. (1990) 'Mortality in heroin addiction: impact of methadone treatment', *Acta Psychiatrica Scandinavica* 82: 223–227.

Gruer, L., Cameron, J. and Elliott, L. (1993) 'Building a city wide service for exchanging needles and syringes', *British Medical Journal* 306: 1394–1397.

Jones, S., Power, R. and Dale, A. (1994) 'The Patients' Charter: drug users' views on the "ideal" methadone programme', *Addiction Research* 1: 323–334.

Klein, R. and Carter, N. (1988) 'Performance measurement: a review of concepts and issues', in D. Beeton (ed.) *Performance Measurement: Getting the Concepts Right*, London: Public Finance Foundation.

Neale, J. (1998a) 'Drug users' views of prescribed methadone', *Drugs: Education, Prevention and Policy* 1: 33–45.

——(1998b) 'Reducing risks: drug users' views of accessing and disposing of injecting equipment', *Addiction Research* 6: 147–163.

Peters, A. D., Reid, M. M. and Griffin, S. G. (1994) 'Edinburgh drug-users – are they injecting and sharing less?', *AIDS* 8: 521–528.

Polkinghorne, J. (1996) *The Task Force to Review Services for Drug Misusers. Report of an Independent Review of Drug Treatment Services in England, Department of Health*, London: HMSO.

Power, R., Hunter, G. M., Jones, S. G. and Donoghoe, M. C. (1994) 'Correspondence: the sharing of injecting paraphernalia among illicit drug users', *AIDS* 8: 1509–1511.

Sheridan, J. and Barber, N. (1996) 'Drug misusers' experiences and opinions of community pharmacists and community pharmacy services', *Pharmaceutical Journal* 257: 325–327.

Smith, P. (ed.) (1996) *Measuring Outcome in the Public Sector*, London: Taylor & Francis.

Stimson, G. V. (1995) 'AIDS and injecting drug-use in the United Kingdom, 1987–1993. The policy response and the prevention of the epidemic', *Social Science and Medicine* 41: 699–716.

Stimson, G. V., Des Jarlais, D. C. and Ball, A. L. (eds) (1998) *Drug Injecting and HIV Infection: Global Dimensions and Local Responses*, London: UCL Press.

13 Between public health and public order

Harm reduction facilities and neighbourhood problems

Dominique Malatesta, Daniel Kübler,
Dominique Joye and Dominique Hausser

Swiss and European studies have shown that the provision of harm reduction facilities to the users of illegal drugs has largely positive effects. Harm reduction facilities are central to HIV prevention among injecting drug users and make a significant contribution to the improvement of their state of health as well as their social situation (Hausser *et al.*, 1991; Dubois-Arber *et al.*, 1994; Cattaneo *et al.*, 1993; Ackermann-Liebrich and Coda, 1996; Gervasoni *et al.*, 1998).

Switzerland is characterised by the rapidity with which it recognised that the HIV epidemic required a new preventive approach when it came to marginalised groups within the population, such as homosexual men and injecting drug users (Malatesta, 1993/1994). Measures aimed at reducing the risk of infection for people who injected drugs, mainly by distributing sterile syringes, were quickly adopted. These measures were based on the principle that drug injectors, like anyone else, have a right of access to AIDS prevention programmes. Over the past two decades, the Swiss Confederation and local authorities have therefore promoted the development of drug policies that include harm reduction facilities for drug users (Malatesta, *et al.*, 1992; Kübler *et al.*, 1997; Kübler, 1998, 1999).

The implementation of harm reduction programmes has, however, given rise to serious difficulties. Since these facilities are accessible to a part of the population that continues to live in conditions of illegality and whose behaviours are considered 'taboo', their presence not infrequently triggers hostile reactions from neighbourhood groups. Quite often, these reactions appear in the form of NIMBY (Not In My BackYard) syndromes, where it is not so much the principle of setting up a facility as its location that is questioned (Allison, 1986; Burnett and Moon, 1983; Mair, 1986; Laws, 1992; Dear and Gleeson, 1991; Dear, 1992). In many cities, action from neighbourhood groups has led to the closing down of harm reduction facilities, and made the setting up of new ones extremely difficult (Malatesta *et al.*, 1993).

The study on which this chapter is based (Kübler *et al.*, 1997) was conducted to understand better the problems involved in the implementation of such programmes. In particular, it asked why and how neighbourhood reactions appear, develop, are debated, and usually change when the harm reduction professionals intervene co-operatively.

Background

Introducing a harm reduction facility in an urban neighbourhood creates various types of interaction between actors of differing motivations and interests, namely authorities, neighbours, drug users and professionals. Harm reduction facilities are thus to be considered as 'urban' services, in the sense that they constitute an interface between drug users and the urban social environment (Amphoux and Jaccoud, 1992). The above actors and their interests influence the place and reception of the harm reduction facility in the neighbourhood. The attitudes of various actors towards the drug problem, towards drug policy and towards the integration of drug users in the city play a central role in the implementation process.

Local authorities often define the goals and measures to be adopted in the policy fields of public health and public order. Local political authorities are also involved in political debate about drug policy. These debates may involve large sections of the population, or may be restricted to certain closed groups of experts, authorities and professionals working in the drug field.

Neighbourhoods are fully fledged actors in the implementation process and the advent of harm reduction programmes involves them in a new type of interaction. To them, harm reduction facilities may be perceived as a threat to safety and public order, as well as to standards of environmental hygiene. In general, harm reduction facilities are viewed as a new element that defines the quality of life in a neighbourhood. The issue of democratic participation in policy making is of particular significance to neighbourhoods, enabling them to exert influence on local authorities. In this context, associative structures at neighbourhood level play an important role.

In the past, drug users could only become partners in a dialogue once they were committed to detoxification. Those who refused to do so were taken into the custody of the police and courts. Today, it is accepted in Switzerland that drug users have the right of access to harm reduction facilities and to social integration. They have thus been granted the opportunity to become full 'users of the city' – in other words, they have been given a form of freedom through equal access to resources promoting health.

The role of the professionals involved in disease prevention and in the treatment of drug users has changed in parallel with the evolution of the theories concerning care and prevention, so as to include the concept of harm reduction. From the moment when the concept of harm reduction and free access to services was formalised, they have also become actors in the *urban* implementation of prevention policies.

These are the different actors involved in the implementation of harm reduction programmes. Their motivations and interests shape the problems that emerge once harm reduction policies are put into practice and facilities established. Indeed, the opening of such facilities in urban contexts compels cities and their population to take part in the realisation of a harm reduction policy (Malatesta *et al.*, 1993). Authorities and harm reduction professionals need to be supported in managing these new forms of interaction.

Approach

In order to identify the factors that explain neighbourhood conflict over harm reduction, we conducted a comparative analysis of a number of such facilities in Switzerland (Kübler *et al.*, 1997). Twenty-seven facilities, located in twelve different cities, were investigated. The selected cities belonged to three linguistic areas, and included the five main Swiss urban centres as well as a couple of smaller cities. They differed from one another in terms of political representation and institutional structure.

To be eligible for inclusion in our research, harm reduction facilities had to fulfil three criteria: (a) offer medical or social services to users of illegal drugs; (b) provide services on an outpatient basis; and (c) be entirely or partially financed by public authorities. These three criteria ensure that the facility can be considered as directed towards the management of the *drug problem* (users of illegal drugs), as having an *urban impact* (since the drug users become users of the neighbourhood outpatient facilities), and as part of a *public policy* (involving public authorities).

Two different enquiries were carried out. The first was largely qualitative, based on case studies of neighbourhood conflict with respect to harm reduction facilities. Over 100 semi-directive in-depth interviews were conducted with the actors involved, directly or indirectly, in the implementation of the harm reduction facilities in the twelve cities. These semi-directive interviews followed a general format, covering the relations between the main actors involved in the neighbourhood conflicts, the way in which the facility was implemented and the response generated.

The second enquiry was quantitative in nature, and focused on the attitudes of neighbours towards harm reduction facilities. In four cities, Bienne, Geneva, Basle and Zurich, a sample of 900 people living within a 200 metre radius of a harm reduction facility was selected (250 in each city). They were interviewed by telephone using a standardised questionnaire focusing mainly on how they perceived their environment and how they assessed changes brought about by the introduction of harm reduction facilities.

Through the comparative analysis of neighbourhood conflicts in various local contexts, two main factors influencing the implementation process of harm reduction facilities were identified: the problems brought by the service to the neighbourhood; and the strategies adopted by harm reduction professionals and public authorities.

The problems brought by the services to the neighbourhood

The problems mentioned by the neighbourhoods were connected to perceived intrusions and/or nuisances affecting the public order that a neighbourhood implicitly takes for granted. Social/environmental nuisances were mentioned, both concrete ones and those that people thought likely to be produced by harm reduction facilities. Criminality was referred to, as well as filth (vomit, garbage, etc.), and in particular discarded syringes. In general, it appeared that the presence of a high number of drug users contributed to the perception of an insecure urban environment.

What is the extent of these problems both from a temporal and spatial perspective? In relation to time, qualitative analysis showed that the implementation of harm reduction policies encountered particular difficulties initially, that is in the late 1980s. However, even if such problems seem less urgent today, comparisons between cities shows that fears and hostile reactions towards the setting up of harm reduction facilities appear with some regularity.

Nevertheless, the survey carried out among local inhabitants shows a high rate of acceptance of the harm reduction facilities in general. According to the majority of inhabitants interviewed, drug users have had fewer negative effects on the neighbourhoods than, for example, motorised traffic (noise and pollution): 38 per cent of the respondents considered traffic to be a significant problem, whereas only 17 per cent regarded drug use to be a real problem in their neighbourhood. Moreover, about half of the respondents believed that the opening of harm reduction facilities did not cause any real inconvenience in the locality. Only a minority felt inconvenienced (see Figure 13.1). About two-thirds said they would agree to the opening of a new facility. These figures show that a large majority of the population supports the work done by the services, which confirms the findings of other national studies (Gervasoni *et al.*, 1998).

Generally speaking, the nuisance problem arises when different groups, with diverging interests, have to share the same space. Our case studies show that contracts and agreements between harm reduction facilities and their drug-using clients can reduce these levels of conflict. These contracts and agreements may include principles concerning the behaviour that will be accepted in and around the facility (no dealing, no drug use, etc.), as well as rules formulated by the neighbourhood or by the police to make cohabitation as easy as possible.

The management of the harm reduction facilities

What are the political conditions that influence the success or failure of implementing a harm reduction facility in its neighbourhood? Our case

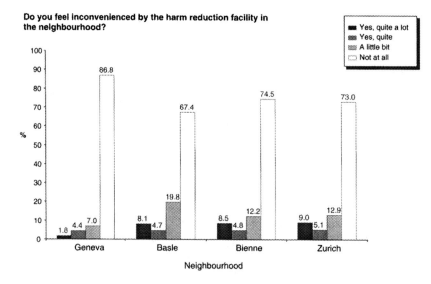

Do you feel inconvenienced by the harm reduction facility in the neighbourhood?

Figure 13.1   Nuisances of harm reduction facilities

studies show that failures are due mainly to three main factors: the political constellation; the resources invested by the actors; and the contact strategies adopted by harm reduction professionals and public authorities.

In terms of political constellation, a compromise is hardly possible when the problems connected to the implementation of the service are influenced by ideological or party conflict. This is also true when political organisations, in pursuit of electoral goals, capitalise on the situation and amplify neighbourhood reactions. This was the case in Zurich, for example, where a right-wing party used the drug problem to argue against the general policy of the leftist city government. On the other hand, some political contexts enable harm reduction professionals to work at implementing a prevention policy on the basis of an objective and non-emotional approach, as has been the case in Geneva.

Second, in terms of resources of action, whenever the involved actors occupy strong positions in the decision-making process, they can influence whether a project is a success or a failure. In other words, implementation always takes place in the context of networks including a number of dominant actors. In this context, it is worth noting that local authorities are increasingly tending to take up a role of deliberate leadership.

Third, in terms of contact strategies, a strategy that tries to downplay existing problems and outpower neighbourhood actors will not make for successful implementation. This is particularly true in cities where there are strong neighbourhood associations. Through these associations, neighbourhoods demand to be kept informed and want to be able to participate actively in the management of the facility. This participation will thus need to be formalised and institutionalised, since these neighbourhoods are to be considered significant actors at the global level of local policies.

Towards urban compatibility

In general terms, conflicts between neighbourhoods and harm reduction facilities result from the tension between two connecting logics of action: the logic of *public health* (the need to provide health and social services for drug users) and the logic of *public order* (the need to maintain the security of the population). Neighbourhood conflicts are thus implementation conflicts and do not always involve general and ideological tensions between different approaches to the drug policy field (e.g. repression versus harm reduction policy).

Our study has shown that in the context of harm reduction facility implementation, important experiences of cohabitation take place at all levels: between organisations, between the police and harm reduction professionals, or – on a more daily basis – between users of the same neighbourhood. Urban compatibility is achieved on the basis of processes linked to the progressive amelioration of the mental and physical health of the facility's clients; behaviour and self-presentation (including style of dress); and the creation of communication channels between all involved actors, especially between harm reduction professionals and local people.

It is worth noting that much effort is invested, sometimes unconsciously, in creating structures of mediation that will favour exchanges between the facilities, their clients and their neighbourhoods. These concrete exchanges can eliminate social distance and misunderstanding. In neighbourhoods where a positive form of cohabitation is still to be found, these exchanges can help foster the acceptability of harm reduction facilities. Local people need to know that facility staff are willing to listen to possible complaints and to take appropriate action to keep disturbances in the neighbourhoods to a minimum. Quite often local people themselves make proposals, thus attempting to eliminate the distance between themselves and the staff, but also to have better control over a new type of social interaction.

Mediation and legitimacy

In general, the legitimacy of public policy depends on both the trust put in policy makers and the degree to which this policy corresponds to what citizens want. This last requirement necessitates a dynamic and dialectic relationship; either the policy will be adapted or the interests expressed by the citizens will evolve, thus creating a new 'fit'. It is at this level that mediation mechanisms may be useful: the integration of different interests within a harm reduction facility may help create a specific system of support. Mediation will also influence the development of trust between citizens and policy makers. In so far as it creates interaction between them, it may potentially serve as a means to renew political trust.

Mediation practices mainly involve harm reduction professionals and their clients, on the one hand, and the neighbourhood actors on the other. Yet it would be wrong to believe that the tension between *public health* and *public order* only exists between these two actors. Those who 'defend' one or the other attitude – the police, politicians and journalists – are also involved. For instance, it is impossible to try to solve the tension between public health and public order without the participation of the police. In so far as the police are part of the administrative structure, it is relatively easy to ask them to collaborate in attempts at internal integration.

Mediation and neighbourhood

It is important to distinguish between two main forms of mediation at the neighbourhood level. The first type takes place during the period preceding the implementation of a service, and the second occurs while the service is actually functioning.

Mediation before the implementation of a service

Our case studies demonstrate that, very often, as soon as a neighbourhood has been informed that facilities for drug users are to be installed in its locality, its inhabitants will react violently and with evident hostility. The manner in which this information is provided may, however, greatly influence the extent to which the service is accepted. Indeed, in order to cultivate a relationship based on trust it is essential that professionals remain open-minded and understand that the implementation of the service may provoke certain fears or objections in the neighbourhood. In this sense, the time and styling of a facility's presentation is crucial to the whole process of implementation. This event is often the first opportunity for contact between professionals and local people. The image that the actors in the neighbourhood will hold of those who are responsible for the facility will be greatly influenced by the manner in which its opening is announced. At this level, trust in the policy makers depends on how sensitive the latter have been to fears expressed by local inhabitants.

The initial announcement of the opening of the facility constitutes a useful opportunity for all actors to familiarise themselves with their respective objectives and interests in relation to the facility. This must be a first step towards integrating the varying viewpoints. Before different viewpoints can be integrated, however, the actors concerned must know what their respective positions and opinions are, and it is easier to become aware of these in neighbourhoods where inhabitants have formed well-established associations. Quite often, it is through these associations that the neighbourhood's position is initially clarified and defined. It is also with their help that demands may be properly channelled.

The forms that mediation can take during this period may be extremely varied. In some cases, meetings were organised, during which members of the neighbourhood were able to ask questions about the objectives and the management of the planned facility. In other cases, harm reduction professionals directly contacted each of the inhabitants in the neighbourhood.

Mediation once the service is functioning

Contacts between harm reduction professionals and the neighbourhood that take place *after* the opening are mainly aimed at checking that agreements are being respected. These contacts also offer neighbours an opportunity to express their opinion concerning the problems and social nuisances induced by the facility. The staff can receive complaints and, in return, provide information about the measures taken (or planned) to improve the situation. During these contacts, each side assesses the situation according to its own viewpoint and communicates this assessment to the other side. Each side is thus continually aware of the other's judgement and may react when this seems useful. This regular contact helps to create a relationship of mutual trust.

As far as harm reduction professionals are concerned, regular exchanges with the neighbourhood are a way of 'taking the temperature' and reacting to possible problems as soon as they become manifest. For the inhabitants of the neighbourhood, these exchanges offer a guarantee that their viewpoint will be taken into account, even after the facility has been opened. In this sense, regular contact between neighbourhood and facility may become a genuine form of monitoring.

In some cities, this contact takes place informally via telephone calls when problems appear, or in chance meetings between neighbours and professionals, and so on. In other cities, it has become more formalised: regular public meetings are organised during which the inhabitants of the neighbourhood may share their feelings, or 'support groups' have been created, including delegates from all the groups concerned by the activities and by the management of the harm reduction facility (professionals, neighbours, police, etc.).

Conclusions

Our conclusions draw on the basic finding that there are harm reduction facilities for drug users that are widely and well accepted by their city neighbourhoods. Based on this, we have formulated recommendations concerning the processes that allow this objective to be achieved. A first step in the learning process is to understand the local political context. This means assessing the degree of political support for the harm reduction policy. If the creation of a facility is the result of a clear political statement in favour of harm reduction, its meaning and objectives are unlikely to be discussed. However, if the harm reduction approach is not (yet) politically stabilised, the facility will soon find itself in the turmoil of a general political debate about drug policy. This initial diagnosis will help define the strategy used in informing the neighbourhood before the opening of the facility, and make it possible to reach a compromise.

Second, the opening of the facility requires particular attention, even if contacts with the neighbourhood have already been made. It is at this very point that the experience of cohabitation starts. The contracts binding facility and clients play an important role in this since they define the manner in which the clients have agreed to integrate into the neighbourhood. Daily experience of cohabitation between facility and clients, and between clients and neighbourhood, may bring proof that this type of drug policy can be successful. The stakes are therefore high. During this phase, it is important that contact with the neighbourhood becomes more personal. Professionals need to show and introduce themselves, playing the role of go-betweens between neighbourhood and drug users. Open days may be suggested, or more personalised contacts may be made with people who are thought to be representatives of the neighbourhood. These people may be school principals, presidents of parent–teachers associations, work in day-care centres for children, or publicans.

Third, the setting up of a communication system between neighbours and facility staff constitutes an important step towards the integration of a facility into its neighbourhood. Communication systems should be *visible* from the beginning. Neighbours must know that contact between them and the facility staff will continue as long as the facility is operating in the neighbourhood. In order to build a spirit of co-operation, it may be necessary, at least initially, for harm reduction professionals to take the first step and go out and meet the neighbours. Later, and once contact has been established, neighbours may also be invited to contact professionals inside the harm reduction facility.

The integration of a harm reduction facility in city neighbourhoods and the sustainability of this integration are dependent on the processes of adaptation and change. If facilities are integrated on a flexible and negotiable basis, the neighbourhood may come to understand that its requests and needs will be taken into account. Gradually, the representations that the various groups have of the others (neighbours–professionals, professionals–drug users, drug users–neighbours) will start to change. It is possible to influence this evolution consciously by paying attention to the modalities of the social experience that the opening of the service represents. Here we see similarities with the work of community development projects in which the aim has been to bring together actors who do not necessarily want to cohabit.

References

Ackermann-Liebrich, U. and Coda, P. (eds) (1996) *Evaluation niederschwelliger Hilfsangebote im Drogenbereich. Supplementum zu Sozial- und Präventivmedizin*, Basle: Birkhäuser.

Allison, L. (1986) 'On dirty public things', *Political Geography Quarterly* 5: 241–251.

Amphoux, P. and Jaccoud, C. (1992) *Des services pour habiter: orientations de recherches et expérimentations*, Lausanne: IREC-DA/EPFL.

Burnett, A. and Moon, G. (1983) 'Community opposition to hostels for single homeless men', *Area* 15: 161–166.

Cattaneo, M., Dubois-Arber, F., Leuthold, A. and Paccaud, F. (1993) *Evaluation of the Federal measures to reduce the problems related to drug use, Phase I. Initial report*, Lausanne: Institut Universitaire de Médecine Sociale et Préventive.

Dear, M. (1992) 'Understanding and overcoming the Nimby-syndrome', *Journal of the American Planning Association* 58: 288–300.

Dear, M. and Gleeson, B. (1991) 'Community attitudes towards the homeless', *Urban Geography* 12: 155–176.

Dubois-Arber, F., Jeannin, A., Meystre-Augustoni, G., Gruet, F. and Paccaud, F. (1994) *Evaluation of the Aids prevention strategy on Switzerland mandated by the Federal Office of Public Health. Fourth assessment report 1991–1992*, Lausanne: Institut Universitaire de Médecine Sociale et Préventive.

Gervasoni, J.-P., Dubois-Arber, F., Benninghoff, F., Spencer, B., Devos, T. and Paccaud, F. (1998) *Evaluation des mesures de la Confédération destinées à réduire les problèmes liés à la toxicomanie. Deuxième rapport de synthèse 1990–1996*, Lausanne: Institut Universitaire de Médecine Sociale et Préventive.

Hausser, D., Zimmermann, E., Dubois-Arber, F. and Paccaud, F. (1991) *Evaluation of the Swiss Aids Prevention Policy. Third assessment report 1989–1990*, Lausanne: Institut Universitaire de Médecine Sociale et Préventive.

Kübler, D. (1998) 'Politique de la drogue dans les villes Suisses entre ordre et santé. Analyse des conflits de mise en oeuvre', PhD thesis, University of Lausanne.

——(1999) 'Beyond nimbyism: urban conflict resolution in Swiss drug policies', in U. Khan (ed.) *Participation Beyond the Ballot Box. European Case Studies in State-citizen Dialogue*, London: UCL Press, pp. 43–64.

Kübler, D., Malatesta, D., Joye, D. and Hausser, D. (1997) *Entre santé publique et ordre public. L'impact urbain des services pour consommateurs de drogues en Suisse*, Lausanne: IREC-DA/EPFL.

Laws, G. (1992) 'Emergency shelter networks in an urban area: serving the homeless in metropolitan Toronto', *Urban Geography* 13: 99–126.

Mair, A. (1986) 'The homeless and the post-industrial city', *Political Geography Quarterly* 5: 351–368.

Malatesta, D. (1993/1994) 'Le sida et les consommateurs de drogue: la prévention à l'épreuve de la ville', *Ethnologica Helvetica* 17/18: 201–218.

Malatesta, D., Joye, D. and Spreyermann, C. (1992) *Villes et toxicomanie. Des stratégies urbaines de prévention du sida en Suisse*, Lausanne: IREC-DA/EPFL.

Malatesta, D., Kübler, D. and Joye, D. (1993) *Zone et quartier. Rapport sur une étude de faisabilité présenté à l'Office fédéral de la santé publique*, Lausanne: IREC-DA/EPFL.

14 Drug use, AIDS and social exclusion in France

France Lert

Throughout Europe, the AIDS epidemic has brought about major changes in public policy on drug abuse. While harm reduction policies were firmly established in the UK and the Netherlands by the early 1980s (Berridge, 1994), such was not the case in countries such as France. Here, the response differed both from the UK and The Netherlands and from the zero-tolerance option in the USA where, for example, needle provision remains unsubsidised by public funds (Des Jarlais, 1995).

In countries which introduced harm reduction strategies early on a fairly broad scale, access to sterile injection significantly reduced, but did not eradicate, HIV risk-related injection practices (Stimson, 1996; Stimson *et al.*, 1996; Booth and Watters, 1994; Hurley *et al.*, 1997; Benninghoff *et al.*, 1998; Drucker *et al.*, 1998). Mortality studies on European cohorts of drug users point to an increase in mortality associated with AIDS, overdoses and violent deaths (Goedert *et al.*, 1995; Orti *et al.*, 1996; Van Haastrecht *et al.*, 1996).

France offers an unfortunate illustration of how delays in the implementation of harm reduction policies provoked a health catastrophe among injecting drug users (IDUs). Epidemiological surveys carried out in the 1980s in prison or drug treatment settings showed that by then over 50 per cent of tested IDUs were HIV positive. This rapid spread of the epidemic among members of this population can be directly linked to the stringent legal restrictions on the sale and availability of syringes which were initial characteristics of drug policy in France. AIDS activists and their allies in the health profession subsequently reacted strongly to alert public opinion and politicians, and to modify health care professionals' attitudes towards addiction and drug treatment (Coppel, 1996). They succeeded in convincing public authorities to pass a decree in 1987 which abolished the necessity of a medical prescription for the sale of syringes in pharmacies.

Until 1993–1994, however, this legal change remained the only official public health measure to prevent HIV transmission among IDUs. Despite enduring opposition from many pharmacists to the sale of syringes (some continued to refuse to sell syringes to drug users, some charged excessive prices, others required the purchase of a full box of thirty syringes when they were asked for one), this single measure had an important effect on the course of the epidemic (Lert and Lert, 1998). It is only in the mid 1990s that more drastic changes in French drug policy occurred with the introduction of programmes offering direct support to drug users and drug maintenance treatment. Interestingly, these innovations were all developed outside the framework of already-established drug treatment settings.

It is conventional to account for these changes in drug policy in terms of increasing medical attention to the physical problems experienced by IDUs, and growing concern about preventive measures such as drug maintenance treatment, vaccination against hepatitis B, etc. The purpose of this chapter, however, is to offer a broader alternative interpretation which suggests that changes in French drug policy were part of a broader global renewal of social policy for health.

Our hypothesis is that the evolution of the French drug policy is related to a major shift in the basic principles of social policy. The social and health conditions of IDUs were no longer to be seen as an individual phenomenon, but were viewed as a consequence of *social exclusion*. This process, which will be described in detail below, is an effect of the functioning of health and social institutions themselves. Social exclusion as a phenomenon is not specific to drug users, but common to a wide variety of marginalised population groups. The new paradigm of 'social exclusion' challenged traditional welfarist approaches which treated poverty and marginalisation as individual problems due to catastrophic individual life events (e.g. the occurrence of a major disease or accident) or individual maladaptation.

In the traditional European conceptualisation of the 'welfare state' which emerged after the Second World War, income as well as social rights were seen as linked to participation in the workforce, and social policies were designed mainly to provide financial support to people temporarily excluded from the labour market. Harm reduction strategies for IDUs informed by notions of social exclusion work from a different balance between public order and public health, by putting the emphasis on interventions based on proximity, social and material support, and on user participation. Similar changes can be observed in other fields of French social policy such as with respect to homelessness, illegal immigration, unemployment, urban poverty and prostitution.

The French paradox

For non-French readers, it may come as something of a surprise to learn that drug-related interventions in France have historically been the prerogative of psychiatrists, particularly those with an interest in psychoanalysis (Lert, 1998). According to the psychoanalytic paradigm, addictive behaviour is to be viewed as an individual proneness to use psychotropic drugs in response to a disturbed self. Drug use is seen as a symptom of a disturbed personal and family history. The 'addict' uses drugs as a protection against anxiety and other dysphoric states, and as a means of dealing with a frightening outside world. Psychoanalytic-oriented therapies are not directed towards substance use itself but towards the mental and psychological functioning of the individual. According to classic psychoanalytic therapy, detoxification is considered first proof of the subject's willingness to enter the therapeutic process, and social interventions are viewed as providing a support for it. One can easily imagine how such a psychoanalytic approach might have difficulties in accommodating more pragmatic measures such as syringe and needle exchange.

French authors (e.g. Coppel, 1996) attribute the belated change in drug policy to resistance from poorly informed politicians and public opinion, supported by drug treatment health care professionals sticking rigidly to psychoanalytic theories of addiction. Interestingly, sociological studies undertaken in the 1980s show that the psychoanalytic paradigm was already facing difficulties in the more general aftermath of AIDS, although no clear alternative had emerged.

The paradox of the French situation is that the dominance of psychoanalysis within the drug treatment community was in many ways a departure from the medical mainstream and from more traditional coercive psychiatric approaches. While in other countries, similar values and motivations had led to a critical appraisal of conventional drug treatment and to a shift towards harm reduction policies, in France the effect was exactly the reverse. Guerrieri and Pinell (1984), in their account of the Marmottan Hospital, one of the most famous French centres for drug treatment, show how this system of treatment developed in the 1970s, being built on innovative approaches to psychiatric work, including anti-psychiatry. At that time, outpatient clinics and later in-patient treatment functioned in ways diametrically opposed to the established models in the psychiatric sector. The staff structure was not hierarchical, few restrictions were imposed on patients, and role distinctions were blurred.

Research in the sociology of organisations (Bergeron, 1996) shows how the psychoanalytic paradigm failed to meet the needs of many drug users. Drawing on fieldwork conducted in 1990 and 1993 in two areas in the Paris region, Bergeron points out that while in theory the psychologist/psychiatrist was in charge of drug treatment institutions, with psychotherapy being the major treatment modality, in reality the staff of specialised centres were mainly composed of educators and social workers. These were the individuals who had to deal with the social, and sometimes medical, emergencies that keep drug users from entering fully into the therapeutic process. Commencing psychotherapy after detoxification was considered the ultimate goal of the social worker's intervention. In fact, most drug users dropped out after the first stages and only a few were included in the full cycle of treatment. Hence, a significant number of first visits or first contacts in drug treatment settings had no follow-up (Curtet and Davidson, 1979; Moutin and Briole, 1984). In Bergeron's words:

The very notion of a social emergency is giving rise on the practical level to a growing confrontation between political reasonings and psychotherapeutic thinking … It is thus the very role of psychologists in such a context which is being questioned. Can they remain in a system where social pressure and the politicized issue of drug addiction lead them to give up their professional methods and in the long run to change careers?

(Bergeron, 1996: 125)

This situation is similar to that described by Mino and Arsever (1996) in Switzerland. As head of a drug treatment programme in Geneva, Mino reports that in 1990 she replaced a psychologist and an educator by a doctor and a nurse, thereby seizing the chance to

change an approach which she had disapproved of for a few years already, and which implied that the psyche dominated the body.

(Mino and Arsever, 1996: 142)

The stigmatisation and marginalisation of IDUs

There has been much debate about the stigmatisation and marginalisation of IDUs in France. Questions of marginalisation have been central at most of the conferences on drug use and AIDS. In January 1993, for example, the French Ministry of Health organised an international conference entitled 'AIDS, Drug Addiction and Marginalisation'. In February 1994, during a meeting on AIDS prevention among IDUs, Lowenstein, one of the leaders in medical care for drug users, focused his address on the issues of limited access to care, prevention and drug maintenance treatment. In October 1994, a meeting organised by UNESCO was entitled 'Drug Addiction – AIDS, Human Rights and Deviancy' (*Actes…*, 1994). The Henrion Commission, an expert committee mandated by government to develop an advisory report on drug policy, concluded in early 1995 that there needed to be changes in policy aimed at 'abolishing the marginalisation of drug addicts' (*Rapport…*, 1995).

A range of perspectives on the social marginalisation of IDUs have been offered. Some referred to addiction as a process which itself leads to the marginalisation of the dependent individual. Tonnelet (1994), head of the French drug professionals' association, declared that 'drug addicts try to escape into an experience which becomes totalitarian' and described 'a dropping-out process [which deprives them] of any sense of belonging to a social world for which they might choose to feel responsible'. Charles-Nicolas, one of the first physicians involved in AIDS care for IDUs, said 'another virus may be more dangerous still [than the HIV], which some would wish to spread, namely marginalisation' and exhorted people 'not to buy social order at the price of marginalisation' (1989). Several key actors in the field have looked upon marginalisation as a process generated by the 'dogmatic and sectarian' project of drug treatment services (Tremblay, 1994), and/or by legal interdictions which deprive drug users of their basic rights (Caballero, 1992). They have advocated together for harm reduction and the legalisation of drug use (Drucker, 1993), claiming at the most extreme that 'drugs are not prohibited because they are dangerous, but that they are dangerous because they are prohibited' (Stevenson, quoted by Marks, 1994).

With the spread of HIV among French IDUs, it became clearer that legal and practical barriers to the access of clean needles and syringes, and drug treatment professionals' denial of the physical consequences of drug use, were the main factors fuelling the epidemic. It also became clear that the psychoanalytic paradigm, by considering that the drug user unconsciously seeks to risk his or her life through the consumption of drugs and that needle sharing is a necessary component of the drug users' community subculture (Maxence, 1991), was to some extent responsible for this situation. Some drug treatment professionals themselves became aware of the counterproductive public health effects of their usual terms of reference. As Mino and Arsever put it:

> The real scandal ... consists in having made speeches about a needle-sharing culture, when sharing was in fact the direct outcome of the scarcity which we brought about by prohibiting their sale or making them more difficult to get; it consists in having asserted that drug addiction was a suicidal choice when it was our policy which condemned drug addicts to risk death at each injection.
>
> (Mino and Arsever, 1996: 244)

In the late 1980s, hospitals were faced with a growing number of IDUs suffering from AIDS. Some hospital staff supported these patients in their fight against discrimination and advocated for more research and solidarity (e.g. Hirsch, 1991). Simultaneously, however, they often forced drug-dependent patients to stop using illegal drugs, at least during hospital stays, without providing them with any treatment to prevent the symptoms and pain associated with withdrawal. Drug-using patients therefore often chose to leave hospital as soon as the medical emergency was over, or ended up being excluded for their 'antisocial' behaviour. Many IDUs, who were thought unable to comply to therapeutic drugs regimens and to medical follow-up, were denied AZT treatment and were excluded from clinical trials (Lert and Marne, 1992), a situation which appears to have persisted since (Carrieri *et al.*, 1999).

Health care workers sometimes used drug users' deviant, manipulative or suicidal behaviour to justify their own negative attitudes and behaviours. Because these attitudes violate medical ethics and principles of equal access to care, guilt and frustration soon appear among some of those in charge of AIDS patient care. Closer links have been forged with drug treatment settings in order to provide better quality care. Drug treatment professionals, after a period of anger and denial similar to that described by Des Jarlais (1990) in the USA, felt unable to offer help to HIV-infected clients, many of whom were becoming severely ill and/or dying. Both groups tried to reach some kind of compromise.

While discrimination against drug-using patients was common among general practitioners (GPs) (Morin *et al.*, 1997; Boullenger, 1994), a minority of GPs started to prescribe benzodiazepines, buprenorphine (Temgesic®), morphine sulphate and dextromoramide (Palfium®) to relieve withdrawal symptoms. This practice put the physicians at risk of disciplinary proceedings or prosecution. Interestingly, this 'spontaneous' response among some doctors appeared little grounded in scientific evaluations of methadone maintenance, almost as if French GPs were themselves 'reinventing' opiate maintenance therapy (Carpentier, 1994).

IDUs also had difficulty accessing housing services, shelters for the homeless, training centres, and even some drug treatment centres which denied access to those who were still injecting heroin. Since 1988, this has led to the creation of some limited housing facilities specifically for HIV-positive drug users.

In spite of the universal coverage guaranteed by the French Social Security Sickness Fund, various subgroups (to which HIV-infected drug users often belong) face multiple barriers when it comes to accessing care. These include economic barriers. In 1996, for example, 16 per cent of a representative sample of the French general population reported having delayed or given up medical care in the last twelve months because of financial constraints (Dumesnil *et al.*, 1998). Homeless people and sometimes the elderly seeking care in hospital emergency departments are often denied in-patient treatment by hospitals which prefer to concentrate their activity on high-technology interventions (Camus and Dodier, 1994; Legrain, 1995; HCSP, 1998). Other groups such as prostitutes do not seek medical care because of stigmatising and rejecting attitudes on the part of many health professionals (Coppel *et al.*, 1990).

With the notable exception of the authorisation of legal pharmacy syringe sales without prescription in 1989, no major innovation took place in French drug policy until the early 1990s when a dramatic shift towards the introduction of harm reduction policies took place. Inadequate access to health care in prisons had long been denounced by non-governmental organisations fighting for prisoners' rights, and AIDS made the seriousness of the situation more obvious when it was found that most HIV-positive inmates were drug users. Allowing hospital specialists in HIV medicine access to prison populations was one of the first steps to integrating prison health services with the general medical care system. Since 1994, prison medical services have been part of the local general hospital system and are no longer dependent on the prison administration.

From 1992 onwards, needle exchange programmes were piloted in the major French cities, and were legally authorised in 1995. During 1995, experiments with syringe vending machines (which exchanged used syringes for sterile ones) were started in some cities (Obadia *et al.*, 1999). The most spectacular shift, however, concerned the introduction of drug maintenance treatment whose adoption and diffusion in France had been blocked for decades.

Until 1995, methadone maintenance treatment had been restricted to experimental settings (involving fewer than 300 patients nationally), and while the prescription of morphine sulphate to IDUs was tolerated, prescribing physicians risked legal penalties. Initial approval of methadone maintenance treatment was given in March 1995 and the number of patients included in such programmes reached 3000 one year later. The initial prescription of methadone remains, however, restricted to a limited number of services (mainly hospitals or specialised units), family physicians being authorised to renew these prescriptions only after the patient has stabilised his or her use of illegal substances. The use of buprenorphine for mainte- nance treatment was authorised in July 1995 and three dosages of buprenorphine (0.4, 2 and 8 mg, under the brand of Subutex®) have been available in French pharmacies since February 1996, allowing any physician, including GPs, to prescribe such treatment. Each prescription can legally cover a maximum of twenty-eight days' treatment. No registration is neces- sary. After the prescription of morphine sulphate for maintenance drug abuse treatment was forbidden in December 1996, buprenorphine became the treatment of choice in French general practice. Current Ministry of Health estimates (December 1998) suggest that about 55,000 IDUs are on buprenorphine substitution and 7000 are in methadone maintenance programmes (Emmanuelli *et al.*, 1999).

The emergence of the 'social exclusion' paradigm

A key factor influencing this switch in policy was the growing popularity of social exclusion as a framework by which to understand drug-related vulner- ability to HIV. The 'social exclusion' paradigm goes beyond concepts of discrimination and marginalisation that may be more familiar for North American and other European readers. The concept of social exclusion not only relates to the marginalisation of stigmatised groups such as drug users to structural inequities of income and access to economic as well as 'cultural' capital, but also emphasises how institutional and social mecha- nisms, including public policies supposedly aimed at increasing social support for marginalised groups, may consciously or unwittingly contribute to this process of exclusion.

In time of economic growth, poverty and precariousness were perceived as a legacy of the past which affected only those individuals unable to adjust to the modernisation of the economy and society because of family, cultural, physical or educational deficiencies. Massive unemployment, which appeared in European market economies in the 1980s, totally changed the picture. Unemployment sharpened competition on the labour market and threatened the living conditions of increasingly large portions of the population, including groups which were previously protected from social deprivation. Systems of social security based on participation in the workforce no longer protected a growing sector of the population from the loss of housing, access to medical care or social and political rights. The growing number and the diversity of cases of exclusion made some sectors of public opinion aware that social cohesion might be endangered. Social exclusion is not compatible with the egalitarian ideals of a democratic society and therefore represents a danger to the social order. The integrating mechanisms of the welfare state could no longer meet the basic needs of a large number of citizens (Paugam, 1996). Thus, new policies were called for.

For example, until the 1980s France had never acknowledged the value of a systematic welfare allocation for the poor. Instead, it was felt that income should be obtained from the labour market in the form of salary or unemployment benefits for those who had lost their job. A welfare allocation (an RMI or Minimum Income for Social Reinsertion) was instituted in 1988, long after similar mechanisms had been introduced in Northern European countries. The fight against social exclusion was, however, not only a matter of income redistribution. It sought to rebuild social ties and affiliations. Humanitarian and other non-governmental organisations played a major role here.

Concurrent with the development of new approaches to understanding social marginalisation came a range of new social interventions. During the late 1980s, Restaurants du Cœur (soup kitchens) were set up in France. Since 1986, the French domestic branch of Médecins du Monde has provided medical care to patients excluded by hospitals and ignored by primary care practitioners (Aeberhard, 1993). And since 1993, there have been more institutionalised interventions (including the already-mentioned RMI) and programmes for outreach work for homeless people (SAMU Social). New activist organisations have given a voice to the unemployed, the homeless and illegal immigrants, indeed to all the 'socially useless' groups (*inutiles au monde*) described by Castel (1995). Many of these organisations have challenged public opinion by organising public demonstrations involving famous artists and personalities as well as strong media coverage. The emergence of harm reduction policies in the field of drug use can only be understood in this context of new social movements and public interventions against various forms of social exclusion; and they share features in common with other new interventions in favour of excluded populations.

The common denominators of new interventions

Innovative interventions against social exclusion share three main features in common: (a) a concern for citizenship, the defence of human and civil rights and active political participation; (b) a commitment to collaboration with humanitarian and activist movements; (c) a concern for strengthening social bonds through community interventions, material assistance and peer participation.

Citizenship

Political action against the exclusion of IDUs from health services and struggles to achieve recognition of their basic human rights are dependent on more general claims for 'citizenship'. Until AIDS, no self-help organisations had existed among IDUs in most European countries (Friedman *et al.*, 1990), with the exception of the Dutch *junkiebonds* in the early 1980s. In France, IDUs' interests were only represented through the mediation of those drug treatment professionals who refused to comply with the 1970 Act relating to the prosecution and care of drug users. In 1986, when the Minister of Justice first attempted to institute compulsory treatment, he faced such a strong opposition from treatment professionals that the project had to be abandoned. This commitment to the rights of drug users in the political arena was, however, not exempt from some elements of paternalism.

In France, IDUs remained without any means of expressing their needs until they began to organise their own self-help groups within AIDS-related NGOs. The first leaflet about safe injection practices was published by AIDES, the most important NGO working with people living with HIV/AIDS, in 1986. AIDES activists were the first to offer assistance to drug users and to make them part of the organisation. In 1992, the first autonomous self-help group, ASUD, was created within APPARTS (an NGO providing access to accommodation for HIV-infected drug users) and subsequently relocated to AIDES. In 1993, the main NGOs working in the field of HIV and AIDS co-ordinated their efforts under the banner 'Limit the Catastrophe' to urge the government to change its drug policy and to implement harm reduction strategies on a larger scale. AIDES again supported the organisation of this group through both funds and management. Act Up, the most radical NGO, has already protested against the prohibition of drug use and in favour of a greater access to drug maintenance treatment. Act Up even supported the implementation of injectable heroin trials as a means of drug maintenance treatment. Self-help and peer education remain a limited part of these organisations, however, which instead acted as interest groups through their journals and their communication activities involving the media.

Humanitarian organisations in social interventions

Humanitarian organisations, previously known best for their emergency interventions in developing countries, entered the French domestic scene in the mid 1980s using the media to publicise their actions. The buses of Médecins du Monde and the clinics run by Médecins sans Frontières, both NGOs already well known for their work in the Third World, offered free medical care to patients excluded from the health care system. Their work was seen by many as being at the forefront of the fight against social exclusion. Médecins du Monde also played a pioneering role when it opened a facility for anonymous free HIV testing in 1987, and the first French needle exchange programme in 1989. The same organisation also initiated the first methadone programmes in France in 1994 and, in January 1998, the first mobile methadone bus.

At first, humanitarian organisations saw these actions both as a form of lobbying and as ways of piloting new social interventions. They progressively became involved in the routine operation of medical and social services, which continuously expanded. By 1998, for example, Médecins du Monde's syringe exchange programmes accounted for 49 per cent of the injecting equipment distributed across the whole country. AIDES runs twelve smaller programmes and provides 17 per cent of the injecting equipment. These interventions, which were first conceived as ways of highlighting the shortcomings of existing provision and testing the feasibility of new approaches, have therefore piloted new kinds of collaboration between the public and the non-profit private sectors.

Community approach, material assistance and peer participation

The operation of many of these new programmes is underpinned by principles of 'closeness'. The idea that organisations should wait for clients to come and ask for help has been abandoned. Building relationships with target groups and offering help unconditionally has become the order of the day. Outreach work, working in the evening or during the night, and having flexible admission routines all aim to facilitate accessibility. Drop-in centres have been established close to drug-dealing areas, and mobile units provide services close to where they are needed. The origins of such approaches can be found in the Amsterdam methadone buses or in various forms of community outreach work. However, similar approaches have been utilised by mobile clinics offering social and medical services to other marginalised populations. Since 1993, SAMU Social has been conducting night rounds to provide help and assistance to the homeless. First initiated in Paris, this programme has since been expanded to other French cities. Bus-based programmes also provide condoms, material assistance, peer and professional support to sex workers.

The functioning of these programmes is based on flexible procedures. There is no need for appointments, no forms to fill in, anonymity is guaranteed, and drug users are accepted. The relationship between staff and clients is characterised by openness and respect for individual autonomy: letting clients stay, go and come back and forth without asking any questions or requests is standard procedure (ARCADES, 1994; Gourmelon, 1997). New programmes not only provide counselling, support, condoms, injecting equipment and drug maintenance treatment, but also take care of material needs for food, hygiene (showers, washing machines, etc.), places to rest – what the Swiss call 'survival assistance'. It is easy to see the difference between this approach and that formerly used in drug treatment settings. The latter made the provision of help conditional on users' behaviour, asking drug users not to be high on drugs when attending services, to come for fixed appointments, to make clear requests for help, and to accept several interviews and psychological consultations before receiving practical support and treatment. It should be noted, however, that to date injecting rooms are not allowed in France and that drug use within service settings is not tolerated as it is in parts of The Netherlands, Germany, Switzerland and Australia.

The active participation of users or ex-users is also part of the new culture of these programmes. The aim has been to recruit peers and to use their networks of relations, their ability to make contact and their knowledge of drug users' community codes and language to promote safer practices, prevention messages and information. Projects may face problems when drug dealing, crime or simply drug use are present in the setting or its immediate vicinity, threatening the relationship between staff and clients, as well as between professionals and funding authorities. Programmes therefore have to seek a balance between the involvement of drug users and tolerance of activities closely related to drug use. Support projects for prostitutes and self-support drug users groups have sometimes failed to maintain such a balance and have had to close or face the threat of withdrawal of public funding (Anonymous, 1994; Toufik, 1997).

From public health to social integration

Harm reduction strategies in France seem already to have produced some positive outcomes. In particular, the medicalisation of services offered to drug users has improved the quality of care and, in drug treatment programmes, nurses and doctors now commonly work alongside psychologists and social workers. A large part of drug maintenance treatment now consists of buprenorphine prescription by GPs despite the persistence of discriminatory attitudes among the majority of GPs (Moatti *et al.*, 1998). Access to medical care for problems other than those directly related to drug abuse (such as physical illnesses, HIV and HCV infections) has become a priority. New organisations have been set up to improve accessibility to medical care by building formal networks between general practice, hospital departments and drug treatment settings.

A decrease in HIV-related risk behaviours, new infections and fatal overdoses among drug users has been documented (OFDT, 1999). Attitudes of the French general population towards drug users have become more accepting: drug users are now seen as sick persons rather than criminal offenders by the majority of respondents in public opinion polls, and they are acknowledged as having the right of 'access to the best possible medical care'. Openly coercive strategies are also widely rejected (Baudier and Arènes, 1997). Public health goals have therefore offered a rationale for a kind of political and social compromise which seeks to reconcile harm reduction with prohibition on injecting drug use. As Nadelmann (1993) has put it:

> The public health model, intended to curb morbidity and mortality, seems to provide a kind of neutral ideological line and parameters in connection with the development of drug policy measures.
>
> (Nadelmann, 1993: 158)

The history of drug policy and the fight against AIDS in France has been one of delays and drama leading to many deaths and much avoidable human suffering. But the lessons learned may be relevant to other countries, even those who were more successful initially in HIV transmission among drug users. In the near future, public health will have to deal with increasing problems as a result of social exclusion, and will need to broaden its scope to join the more general fight for the social integration of the most vulnerable segments of society.

References

Actes de la rencontre Franco-européenne sur la prévention du sida et les usagers de drogue (1994) 8–10 février, Paris: CRIPS.

Aeberhard, P. (1993) 'Sida, santé et droits de l'Homme', *Les Temps Modernes* 567: 264–269.

Anonymous (1994) *Prospective SIDA 2010. Le Sida en France. Etat des connaissances en 1994*, Ministère des Affaires Sociales, de la Santé et de la Ville, ANRS.

ARCADES (1994) *Travail de rue, actions de proximité, échange de seringues, accès aux services sanitaires et sociaux auprès des usagers de drogue de Seine-Saint-Denis. Bilan d'activité 1994.*

Baudier, F. and Arènes, J. (1997) *Baromètre Santé, adultes 95/96* Vanves: Editions CFES.

Benninghoff, F., Gervasoni, J. P., Spencer, B. and Dubois-Arber, F. (1998) 'Caractéristiques de la clientèle des structures à bas seuil d'accès pour toxicomanes mettant à disposition du matériel d'injection stérile en Suisse', *Revue d'Epidémiologie et de Santé Publique* 46(3): 205–217.

Bergeron, H. (1996) *Soigner la toxicomanie. Les dispositifs de soins entre idéologie et action*, Paris: L'Harmattan.

Berridge, V. (1994) 'Harm minimisation and public health: an historical perspective', in N. Heather *et al.* (eds) *Psychoactive Drugs and Harm Reduction: From Faith to Science*, London: Whurr.

Booth, R. E. and Watters, J. K. (1994) 'How effective are risk-reduction interventions targeting injecting drug users?', *AIDS* 8: 1515–1524.

Boullenger, N. (1994) 'Une expérience d'ethnographie d'intervention', in A. Ogien and P. Mignon (eds) *La Demande sociale de drogues*, Paris: DGLDT-Documentation Française.

Caballero, F. (sous la direction de) (1992) *Drogues et droits de l'homme en France*, Paris: Les empêcheurs de penser en rond.

Camus, A. and Dodier, N. (1994) *L'Intérêt pour les patients à l'entrée de l'hôpital. Enquête sociologique sur un service d'urgence médicale*, Paris: CERMES.

Carpentier, J. (1994) *La Toxicomanie à l'héroïne en médecine générale*, Paris: Ellipses.

Carrieri, P. *et al.* (1999) 'Access to antiretroviral treatment among French HIV-infected IDUs: the influence of continued drug use', *Journal of Epidemiology and Community Health* 53: 4–8.

Castel, R. (1995) *Les Métamorphoses de la question sociale. Une chronique du salariat*, Paris: Fayard.

Charles-Nicolas, A. (1989) *Sida et toxicomanie. Répondre*, Paris: Frison-Roche.

Coppel, A. (1996). 'Toxicomanie, sida et réduction des risques en France', *Communications* 62: 75–108.

Coppel, A., Bragiotti, L. and de Vincenzi, I. (1990) *Recherche-action prostitution et santé publique. Rapport final*, Paris: CESES.

Curtet, F. and Davidson, F. (1979) 'Le devenir des toxicomanes', *Annales Médico-Psychologiques* 9: 889–897.

Des Jarlais, D. C. (1990) 'Stages in the response of drug abuse treatment system to the AIDS epidemic in New York', *Journal of Drug Issues* 20(2): 330–347.

——(1995) 'Regulating controversial programs for unpopular people: methadone maintenance and syringe exchange programs', *American Journal of Public Health* 85: 1577–1584.

Drucker, E. (1993) 'Prohibition aux Etats-Unis', *Les Temps Modernes* 567: 143–150.

Drucker, E., Lurie, P., Wodak, A. and Alcabes, P. (1998) 'Measuring harm reduction: the effects of needle and syringe exchange programs and methadone maintenance on the ecology of HIV', *AIDS* 12: S217–S230.

Dumesnil, S., Grandfils, N., Le Fur, P., Grignon, M., Ordonneau, C. and Sermet, C. (1998) *Santé, soins et protection sociale en 1996. Enquête sur la santé et la protection sociale. France 1997*, Paris: CREDES.

Emmanuelli, J., Lert, F. and Valenciano, M. (1999) 'Evaluation of harm reduction policy in France through an information system on sales of sterile injection equipment to intravenous drug users', *Xth International Conference on the reduction of drug related harm, Geneva, 20–25 March*.

Friedman, E. R., Des Jarlais, D. C. and Sterk, C. E. (1990) 'AIDS and the social relations of intravenous drug users', *The Milbank Quarterly* 68 (Suppl. 1): 85–110.

Goedert, J. J., Pizza, G. and Gritti, F. M. (1995) 'Mortality among drug users in the AIDS era', *International Journal of Epidemiology* 85(11): 1514–1520.

Gourmelon, N. (1997) *Les boutiques ou dispositifs 'bas seuil': une nouvelle approche des toxicomanes en tant de sida*, Paris: Ministère du Travail et des Affaires Sociales, Association de recherche en sociologie.

Guerrieri, R. and Pinell, P. (1984) 'Expérience des drogués et positions institutionnelles: le cas de l'hôpital Marmottan', *Sciences Sociales et Santé* 2(3–4): 39–65.

Haut Comité de la Santé Publique (1998) *La santé des Français*, Paris: La Découverte.

Hirsch, F. (1991) *AIDES: Solidaires*, Paris: Editions du Cerf.

Hurley, S. F., Jolley, D. J. and Kaldor, M. (1997) 'Effectiveness of needle exchange programmes for HIV prevention of HIV infection', *The Lancet* 349: 1797–1800.

Legrain, S. (1995) 'La personne âgée à l'hôpital universitaire: des adaptations nécessaires', Mémoire de DEA, Université Paris VII.

Lert, F. (1998) 'Méthadone. Substitution ou traitement de la dépendance à l'héroïne. Questions en Santé Publique', in Alain Ehrenberg (ed.) *Drogues et médicaments psychotropes. Le trouble des frontières*, Paris: Esprit.

Lert, F. and Marne, M. (1992) 'Hospital care for drug users with AIDS or HIV infection in France', *AIDS Care* 4: 333–338.

Lert, F. and Lert, H. (1998) 'La stratégie de réduction des risques en actes. Une étude de cas en Ile-de-France', INSERM U88, Saint-Maurice.

Marks, A. (1994) 'Le vent du nord et le soleil', *Toxicomanies, sida. Droits de l'Homme et déviances, SOS Drogue International-DGLDT, 11–13 octobre,* Paris: Unesco, pp. 206–212.

Maxence, J. L. (1991) *La Métaprévention au temps du Sida*, Paris: Le nouvel Athanor.

Mino, A. and Arsever, S. (1996) *J'accuse les mensonges qui tuent les drogués*, Paris: Calmann-Lévy.

Moatti, J.-P., Souville, M., Escaffre, N. and Obadia, Y. (1998) 'French general practitioners attitudes toward maintenance drug abuse treatment with buprenorphine', *Addiction* 93(10): 1567–1575.

Morin, M., Obadia, Y. and Moatti, J.-P. (1997) *La médecine générale face au sida*, Paris: INSERM.

Moutin, P. and Briole, G. (1984) *Après la drogue. Les devenirs des toxicomanes*, Toulouse: Privat.

Nadelmann, E. (1993) 'Réflexions sérieuses sur quelques alternatives à la prohibition', *Les Temps Modernes* 567: 152–184.

Obadia, I., Feroni, I., Perrin, V., Vlahov, D. and Moatti, J.-P. (1999) 'Syringe vending machines for IDUs', *American Journal of Public Health*, in press.

Observatoire Français des Drogues et des Toxicomanies (1999) *Drogues et Toxicomanies. Indicateurs et tendances, édition 1999*.

Orti, R., Domingon, A. and Munoz, A. (1996) 'Mortality trends in a cohort of opiate addicts, Catalonia, Spain', *International Journal of Epidemiology* 25: 545–553.

Paugam, S. (ed.) (1996) *L'Exclusion: L'état des savoirs*, Paris: La Découverte.

Rapport de la commission de réflexion sur la drogue et la toxicomanie, Pr Roger Henrion (1995), Paris: Ministère des Affaires Sociales de la Santé et de la Ville, Documentation Française.

Stimson, G. V. (1996) 'Has the United Kingdom averted an epidemic of HIV1 infection among drug injectors?', *Addiction* 91(8): 1085–1099.

Stimson, G. V., Hunter G. M. and Donoghoe, M. C. (1996) 'HIV1 prevalence in community wide samples of injecting drug users in London, 1990–3', *AIDS* 10: 657–666.

Tonnelet, G. (1994) 'Droits de l'homme, démocratie, citoyenneté, toxicomanes, sida et soins', in *Toxicomanie, Sida. Droits de l'homme et déviances, SOS Drogue International-DGLDT, 11–13 octobre*, Paris: Unesco, pp. 237–244.

Toufik, A. (1997) 'Continuité et rupture dans l'histoire de l'auto-support des usagers de drogue en Europe', *Prévenir* 32: 127–150.

Tremblay, R. (1994) (Untitled), in Toxicomanie, *Sida. Droits de l'homme, et Déviances, SOS Drogue International-DGLDT, 11–13 October*, Paris: Unesco, pp. 230–233.

Van Haastrecht, H. J. A., Van Ameijden, E. J. C. and Van den Hoek, J. A. R. (1996) 'Predictors of mortality in the Amsterdam cohort of Human Immunodeficiency Virus (HIV)-positive and HIV negative drug users', *American Journal of Epidemiology* 143(4): 380–391.

Part IV

Accounting for the epidemic

15 The normalisation of AIDS policies in Europe

Patterns, path dependency and innovation

Monika Steffen

The institutionalisation of public health management and administration first took place in the late nineteenth and the early twentieth century when the control of tuberculosis and sexually transmitted diseases gave rise to the legal elaboration of medico-administrative methods, including the identification and compulsory treatment of the 'carriers' of disease. The application of these methods to AIDS was immediately controversial and was therefore finally rejected. Bypassing established public health procedures constituted the heart of the so-called 'AIDS exceptionalism' (Bayer, 1991). The mobilisation initiated by the gay communities against homophobia and the conservative social order provided the intellectual ground on which this exceptionalism developed. The horror scenario, so widely forecast in the early years of the epidemic, did not occur. On the contrary, in western democracies where individual freedom is recognised as an unquestionable part of citizenship, the epidemic was seen as offering a potential threat to the entire social system. AIDS policies became organised around a 'solidarity with the victims' in line with the fundamental principles of health in the European welfare states.

With the passage of time, AIDS has become more of an 'ordinary' issue in health policy, demanding concrete choices in specific circumstances. In industrialised countries, 'exceptionalist' approaches have weakened as the epidemic has come under control. Medical progress and the implementation of effective prevention strategies were driving forces and visible signs of this move from exceptionalism to mainstream policies. The global trend towards normalisation, however, does not explain national differences in policy content, implementation and outcomes. Furthermore, the commonly held view according to which AIDS needed to be treated as an entirely new issue should be questioned. History offers many examples showing how controversies around AIDS have their counterparts in earlier policies and developments. The international literature also shows differences in the amount of interest given to the normalisation of AIDS policies. In the English-language literature, the topic was of particular concern between

1988 and 1992. Questions about normalisation have been less frequently addressed in continental Europe but almost entirely ignored in France. These differences reflect the state of health policy research in the respective countries.

This chapter examines factors shaping the development of AIDS policies in several European countries: France, the UK, Italy and Germany. It focuses on three main policy areas, sexuality, drug abuse and blood transfusions and products, which previously had few links. The comparison seeks to show how systems of public health management, set in a broad national context, especially the institutional characteristics of the health policy system and the welfare system, have evolved in each country. First, the relevant literature will be reviewed in order to isolate the historical and political factors that contributed to the shaping of AIDS policies and controversies. This will offer a backcloth for the analysis of the national and sectorial policy systems that have determined concrete processes of policy making and implementation. Finally, innovations introduced in public health management will be examined. Although triggered in many cases by AIDS, these are part of the general changes affecting health policies, on national as well as international levels.

The burden of history and the medical mainstream

Systematic historical comparisons conducted by Fee and Fox (1988) have showed that debates about public authority versus individual freedom, so central to AIDS exceptionalism, were not new. The terms of the debate, however, were changed in the case of AIDS. They were modified through the participation of newcomers, unfamiliar with public health issues and management.

Porter and Porter (1988) offer an analysis of the emergence of the debate between state authority and individual freedom in the UK, and its evolution throughout the entire nineteenth century. The debate recurred with every new public health issue up to and including 1945–1946, when the UK inaugurated modern media-style campaigns on venereal disease. In the nineteenth century, the legitimacy of state authorities to limit individual liberty in order to protect public health was opposed by both the medical constituency and radical libertarians. They were joined by liberal economists convinced of the counterproductivity of any kind of state intervention. Ideological confrontations, however, had little influence on final policy choices. The 'subtle art of the administratively possible' proved central to public health legislation and the gradual acceptance of limits on individual liberty (Porter and Porter 1988: 98). These authors also identify two situations in which restrictions on individual liberty, through screening, contact tracing and the isolation of infected people, were accepted. These were situations characterised by lack of autonomy and danger to others. The first case is illustrated by the mid nineteenth-century legislation on lunacy which was intended to protect the individual from unjustified confinement at the will of his or her family, and to control private establishments accommodating the mentally ill. The legislation was applied when a person became incapable of free will. The second case is illustrated by legislation on venereal disease and by statutory provisions to protect others from harm originating from mental disturbance. It was applied when a person posed an obvious danger to the health of others.

Towards the end of the nineteenth century, debates were dominated by technical questions concerning the health of the community. Army and navy doctors called for authoritarian and systematic controls which they believed would be effective on the grounds of the army's experience, whereas clinicians defended the confidential personal relationship with the patient. The arguments of the clinicians were backed by defenders of civil rights and by the women's emancipation movement. Confinement, it was argued, should be decided on a case-by-case basis and on the local evaluation of risk (Porter and Porter, 1988: 107). The Local Government Act of 1875 and the Notification of Disease Act of 1889 vested in medical officers of health the authority to record cases of infectious disease and to order the confinement of patients if they constituted a 'nuisance to others'. The issue of venereal diseases was re-examined between 1913 and 1916 by Parliament and a Royal Commission. Previous legislation was considered a failure and was therefore eliminated from future policy agendas. The debates following the First World War inaugurated the UK approach of voluntary testing and free treatment. The new policy aiming at ensuring the active co-operation of infected persons was implemented through the new regulations on Local Government Boards (1916) and a new Venereal Diseases Act (1917). The latter provided for free care in specialised clinics where confidentiality and anonymity were guaranteed. At the end of the Second World War, when the incidence of venereal disease rose again, compulsory reporting was again argued for, this time by medical officers in charge of other infectious diseases, but they remained a minority voice. The medical profession as a whole largely supported an educational approach which led, as early as 1945 and 1946, to the first UK mass media campaign promoting condom use.

The success of fighting AIDS in the UK, where HIV incidence remained far lower than in France, Italy and Spain, was therefore rooted in previous policy choices and tools. Pragmatic campaigns, illustrated by explicit messages like 'Stick to one partner; if you can't, use a condom', were to a large extent linked to the achievements and lessons of the past, a legacy of history. The much criticised demand of the British Medical Association (BMA), in July 1987, for the systematic HIV screening of patients without their formal consent was also in line with this history. The BMA expressed the need to protect health professionals against the risk of infection at work, and in the UK, the protection of others from harm to their health was considered a public commitment. However, the BMA finally withdrew its demand and opted instead to support training programmes on occupational health.

The liberal UK tradition contrasts sharply with the Swedish case where the management of HIV/AIDS includes compulsory HIV testing, the identification of disease 'carriers' and contact tracing, a policy rooted in the Swedish history of public health management (Henrikson and Ytterberg, 1992). In 1915, Sweden had adopted legislation on venereal disease that included compulsory detention, prosecution for knowingly spreading infection and making marriage illegal for a patient until he or she was cured (*The Lancet*, 1942). All of these examples suggest that public health controversies and approaches to public health management have strong national and historical roots.

Of course, trends can be identified across countries, and in most developed countries the history of the AIDS epidemic can be described, as for the USA, as a steady move towards the 'medical mainstream' (Bayer, 1989, 1991). The 'exceptional treatment' of AIDS that characterised the first decade of the epidemic made specific resource allocation possible as well as the revision of public health regulations, and was initially linked to the presence of gay activists in the emerging AIDS policy community. Their major policy goal aimed at the protection of privacy and anonymity, and they argued strongly against screening, partner tracing and notification. More conventional public health techniques were thus set aside as a result of a political compromise with the most central risk group whose participation was necessary in order to promote safer sexual behaviour. There was 'no alternative but to negotiate' (Bayer, 1991: 1502). This compromise was challenged in the second phase of the epidemic by medical progress with respect to therapy and by the changing dynamics of the epidemic. The epidemic came subsequently to be viewed as a problem of care for the chronically ill rather than a fatal plague, more analogous to cancer than cholera (Fee and Fox, 1992)

Despite these global trends towards chronic disease management and routine medical management, the most exhaustive and systematic international comparison of AIDS policies showed the persistence of national variations (Kirp and Bayer, 1992). This was true both during the initial phase when political responses and activists outside government still constituted the driving force, as well as during the second phase when professionals and bureaucrats took over again (Kirp and Bayer, 1992: 364–370). Altman (1988) has linked such differences to variations in 'political culture', but has restricted the application of this concept to attitudes towards homosexuality, and to the degree of organisation of gay communities. He has noted that AIDS brought 'issues essential to the gay movement into the mainstream of the political agenda', a victory which he explained by growing interest-group politics in western democracies (Altman, 1988: 313).

Political culture, welfare states and policy systems

Public policy specialists have developed a more precise and operational approach to political culture and its influence on public health management.

Fox *et al.* (1989) have drawn specific attention to the role of institutions, the mechanisms for achieving consensus, and the degree of confidence that citizens have in their public administration. In their comparative study of AIDS policies in the USA, Sweden and the UK, they describe 'the triumph of professionalism'. They distinguished four stages in the process. First, governments were facing an unpredictable problem that forced them to cope with uncertainty, moral ambiguities and unknown long-term consequences. Second, confronted with popular pressure to act, governments took advice from medical experts and made decisions based on the values of the medical profession and public health experts. Third, an elite consensus was adopted to treat the epidemic as a technical matter, which invalidated perceptions of social and political risk. Fourth, interest groups in the health sector pressed for resources for AIDS research, prevention and care and for new drug policies, which firmly established AIDS as a classical public health problem with long-term commitments.

AIDS became shaped into an ordinary public health issue during its passage through institutional channels and the political decision-making processes (Day and Klein, 1989). The process varied, however, between countries with AIDS highlighting the shortcomings in health systems (Fox, 1988) as well as institutional mechanisms of adaptation and readjustment. In Europe, the key factor explaining social and political solidarity with HIV-positive people links to European welfare systems and traditions. The most notable exception concerning AIDS compared with other pathologies and health risks was substantial resource allocation in Europe despite neo-liberal politics and cost containment in health care expenditure as the main goal of official health policy. It was only in the early 1990s that the growth of AIDS budgets slowed as the epidemic came under control in Germany, the UK and Scandinavia. In France, however, where the number of people infected remained much higher, resource allocation has been maintained. Ongoing reforms of the French health insurance system, which emphasised cost control in all medical sectors and services, did not apply to AIDS expenditure, which has remained the only item unconstrained by budget ceilings.

Establishing a link between national responses to AIDS issues and welfare state systems seems, however, to contradict the international literature on the latter subject. AIDS policy responses such as, for example, the public/private mix in service delivery (Cattacin and Panchaud, 1997) do not correspond to the typologies of European welfare systems. This discrepancy needs explanation, as it results from the fact that the fight against the epidemic depends on policy responses from weakly established sectors situated *at the periphery of the welfare state.* Safer sex behaviour depends mainly on community-based intervention and social control systems outside the state, notably peer groups and interpersonal networks (van Campenhoudt *et al.*, 1997). The safety of blood transfusions, risk reduction for drug users and health education are in the hands of professional groups and often fragmented administrations. Only the UK National Health Service provides a comprehensive and government-linked institutional framework. Furthermore, chronic disease, public health and prevention are traditionally the stepchildren of health policies. The rooting of AIDS policies within complex, overlapping and marginal policy networks calls for comparisons of micropolicy at national as well as sectoral levels.

National normalisation patterns

Each of the four countries that are systematically compared here – France, the UK, Italy and Germany (Steffen, 1996) – had a similar commitment to solidarity with people affected by the epidemic and to the educational and participative approach advocated by early AIDS experts. The outcomes of policy interventions differed radically, however, with current HIV prevalence being three to four times higher in France and Italy than in the UK and Germany. How can such striking discrepancies occur in neighbouring countries sharing a common level of economic, social and cultural development? The arguments developed in this section focus on variations in national policy responses. In each country, the capacity effectively to implement general AIDS control strategies depended on existing institutions and policy tools, mechanisms for innovation, the social and political acceptability of the proposed measures, and the effective involvement of the beneficiaries. While an initial alliance between clinicians, gay activists and public health experts existed in each country, respective roles and access to decision making were different. In Germany and the UK, the government responded positively to the AIDS issue, while in France and Italy politicians refused to be involved. Basic characteristics of the political system, such as mechanisms of consensus building and the levels of decentralisation, influenced policy implementation and outcomes.

In France, the initial group of AIDS experts remained isolated since it was attached to the General Health Department, the weakest section of the health ministry. The medical elite shared the dominant attitude of minimising the AIDS problem. Condom promotion and the sale of needles, both previously forbidden by law, were delayed because of electoral politics. In the mid 1980s, an extremist right-wing party took up the subject and engaged in a campaign linking AIDS with immigration and delinquency, and demanding the quarantining of HIV 'carriers' (Bachelot and Lorane, 1988). The response of all major parties, intellectuals and the media was to 'defend liberty', which deflected attention from the public health risk. In 1987, in line with French centralism, the government decided to invest all authority for AIDS policy making in central government. The corresponding law aimed to protect the issue from the reach of the local extreme-right-wing politicians. Subsequently, this decision, largely approved of at the time by national politicians and the medical and intellectual elites, limited local initiatives. It also deprived AIDS policy of the legitimacy that elsewhere was provided by Parliament. From 1989 onwards, AIDS became an official policy priority with important resource allocation and the creation of specialised agencies entrusted with research, ethics and prevention. Policy conduct through *ad hoc* national agencies is a well-established French tradition.

Subsequent policy gave absolute priority to general prevention campaigns, emphasising the risk to everyone. Targeting was considered to be stigmatising. Prevention messages carefully distinguished condom promotion from AIDS, the first referring to sexuality, pleasure and joy, the second to solidarity with people with HIV. Forging a connection between sex and a fatal risk was considered counterproductive to the promotion of condom use. The French Agency for AIDS Prevention, created in 1989, was closed in 1994, after years of conflict with public authorities and the gay representatives both over their respective roles and the style and content of public campaigns. Its authority for prevention was relocated within the health ministry. The short and conflict-laden existence of the prevention agency illustrated the difficulties of developing large-scale prevention policies in the French context. AIDS provided a 'lens' through which to observe the structure of French policy systems and values. The weakness of public health authorities and the lack of government co-ordination became visible when the Department of Justice refused to release an official written order to stop blood collection in prisons. Hitherto, and despite the high health risks, blood donation from prisoners was considered a means of maintaining their links with society, a civil right and duty as well as a means of socialisation (IGASS/IGSJ, 1992). AIDS policies were reoriented towards more coherent public health goals only after the breakdown of the blood transfusion system and a major political scandal. Crisis is a common way of reform in the French health system (Jobert and Steffen, 1994).

In the UK, top executives within the National Health Service (NHS) pushed reluctant politicians into action. The 'exceptionalist' alliance between public health professionals, clinicians and gay men operated at grassroots level, with little space for gay advocacy at the top. Two parliamentary commissions and a cabinet committee legitimised policies conceived by the Department of Health. Public health experts who took up the challenge of AIDS could rely on the institutional strength of the NHS, which also resisted the neo-liberal ambitions of the Thatcher governments (Hayward and Klein, 1994). It provided the infrastructure for policy co-ordination and implementation. The domestic blood supply as well as drug injectors were thereby protected from HIV transmission. The UK case illustrates how a well-established institutional framework can, in the case of health protection, overcome political resistance and counter controversy.

In Germany, politicians played an active role in parallel with the AIDS-specific alliance and the private organisations promoted by gay activists. The latter became accepted policy partners at national as well as local levels. Self-help organisations were already recognised as part of the subsidiarity principle, according to which problems are to be dealt with at the lowest possible level. Higher level public interventions are only called upon when problem solving at lower levels proves difficult. The use of the subsidiarity principle is particularly well documented in the fields of prevention, rehabilitation and support for the chronically ill (Igl, 1994). This explains the substantial role given to voluntary organisations in those fields. Furthermore, the decentralisation of German policy making had advantages when it came to responding to AIDS. Responsibility for health in Germany lies with the regions (*Länder*) which promoted AIDS-related innovation through their own administrations and structures. The Standing Conference of Health Ministers, a working forum of the regional health ministers and top executives, formulated major policy choices in favour of beneficiary participation in policy development and implementation, improvements in social support and solidarity, and risk reduction for drug users. The health ministers pushed the AIDS issue through the federal decision-making system against the opposition of Bavarian ultra-conservatives. Political consensus was consolidated and legitimised through the federal parliament. Policy changes, particularly in the field of injecting drug use (IDU), were accompanied by legal action in the courts which arbitrated on disputed legislation and over the status of pilot projects. The ready translation of political into legal controversy constitutes part of the German political culture.

In Italy, a group of medical professors finally succeeded in the late 1980s in pushing the reluctant Christian Democrat government into action, against the influence of the Church, which was firmly opposed to public campaigns related to sexuality. Previously, public health administrators and professionals had initiated the systematic screening of drug users, prisoners and hospital patients. The epidemiological profile, which revealed an IDU-related epidemic, led the authorities further to ignore gay activists and sex education. The medical elite imposed its approach based on voluntary testing and education against demands for systematic screening from other administrations and health professionals, and against moral claims from religious authorities. The National AIDS Commission, dominated by medical professors, developed a comprehensive AIDS law which was passed in 1990. This gave legal support to the liberal and medical approach, provided public funding for AIDS, and created co-ordination structures with the private sector. The legal text was considered to offer the finest example of a coherent and complete approach to the management of a specific health problem.

Yet, almost total failure occurred during implementation. AIDS policy making at the national level, conducted largely by doctors, was in contradiction with the regionalisation of health planning and the prerogatives of local politicians and institutions. Moreover, the medical orientation of the policy ignored the important part that private associations, often linked to the Catholic Church, played in the management of drug addiction. These discrepancies provoked opposition from nearly all the agencies charged with health policy implementation. Effective AIDS-related interventions only occurred at local level where favourable conditions existed for policy co-ordination. In northern towns, like Bologna and Modena, public authorities and private agencies collaborated actively to respond to their own local AIDS and IDU priorities (Cattacin *et al.*, 1996).

Gay representatives played an innovative role in each of the four countries. In Germany, which provided the most sustained example of gay participation in public policy making, this inclusion of gay men was linked to the general German model of participative co-management and consensus policies (Lehmbruch, 1994). This model is particularly developed in the health field (Alber, 1994). In the case of AIDS, common policy goals were designated and defined as public health management. Gay identity and related issues, such as gay marriage or teaching about homosexuality as part of sex education in schools (Rosenbrock, 1997), remained outside the scope of these common goals and interests. The overall outcome, equal partnership in health policy making but no concessions to *Schwulenpolitik* (gay politics), has been described by Rosenbrock (1994) as 'normalisation (both) forwards and backwards'.

In the UK, gay participation was in line with the previous traditions of volunteerism. It also corresponded with reforms within the NHS aimed at reducing state responsibility for the delivery of social services. Gay associations thereby became instruments of public policy, acting as relays to the gay community. In Italy, homosexuality has always been ignored. Yet, the first prevention campaigns were launched by gay activists, early and rather effectively, within local networks. Struggles to achieve broader recognition failed (Steffen, 1996: 28–29). France was the only country where specifically gay demands entered the political agenda. In recent controversies over projects aimed at extending some of the legal benefits of marriage to gay couples, supporters as well as opponents refer to the need for 'equal treatment', a fundamental principle of French political culture.

Normalisation dynamics through new policies

In all four countries, AIDS has contributed to the renewal of public policies in the field of sexuality, drug abuse and blood transfusion. The introduction of public health goals and risk reduction strategies into these policies depended mainly on co-ordination and innovation inside those sectors with professionals playing a central role. The main problem has been to readjust priorities and restructure institutional dispositions, often against strong corporatist resistance. Furthermore, much uncertainty has existed over the necessity and the extent of political decision making and public intervention. This legitimacy and necessity was most evident in the case of reforms concerning the blood transfusion sector and drug policies, although this gave rise to much controversy in France and Germany. The necessity for public intervention was more questionable in the field of sexual behaviour since safer sex could be learned without state intervention.

However, educational strategies proved easier to promote in countries where sexuality was no longer considered a social issue subject to ideological debate, but a responsibility of educational authorities, both private and public. Here, it was possible to mobilise available professional competence and institutional resources to focus on health risks and the prevention of sexually transmittable disease. The difficulties proved most significant in Italy and France, but for opposite reasons. In Italy, AIDS policies raised almost no public controversy (Moss, 1990). Sex education in schools, although part of the official anti-AIDS programme, was only weakly developed. The shortcomings provoked no notable protest. The low level of interest which public opinion showed in the matter can be seen as an illustration of the 'importance of intermediate social levels (family, clans, local networks) in the Italian context where the two extreme ends of social organisation, the individual and the political institutions, appear nearly deprived of autonomous value' (Regonini and Giuliani, 1994: 135).

In contrast, France has a long tradition of state regulation over all aspects of social life, including sexuality. Prohibition prevailed until the early 1960s, on contraception and abortion as well as on sexual education. From the mid 1960s onwards, several laws have been passed favouring sexual freedom. Legislation has moved towards an endorsement of a model of 'sexuality without procreation and without norms' (Mossuz-Lavau, 1991). The final stage was the abolition of laws on homosexuality in the early 1980s. The rapid change from state regulation to the absence of collective norms and values, combined with the weak position of public health experts, provided uncertain grounds for effective AIDS prevention.

In the blood transfusion system, prevention from infection needed a two-fold approach, dependent equally on public authorities and transfusion professionals: the control of technological risk (e.g. via the industrial production of clotting factors) on the one hand, and a strict selection of blood donors on the other. Contrary to the general belief of French professionals and authorities, the public plasma manufacturing sector did not do any better in protecting people with haemophilia than did private international industry. While governments were criticised in the UK and Italy for lack of national self-sufficiency in plasma, and in Germany for insufficient control over the pharmaceutical industry, in France criticism centred on the public monopoly and the lack of legal protection for patients (Steffen, 1999).

A striking lack of risk awareness characterised the French response. France accounted for 60 per cent of all HIV infections in transfusion recipients in the twelve countries of the European Union. The organisation and functioning of the French blood sector had led to the overuse of transfusions in hospitals to blood collections in prisons (IGASS/IGSJ, 1992) and to appalling shortcomings in donor screening. The strong ideology of the altruistic blood donor and his or her moral integrity made it difficult to apply public health procedures with the required urgency. Voluntary donation of blood and its potent symbolism originated from the Resistance and the Liberation Army. Blood giving was akin to an act of national solidarity (Hermitte, 1996). The lasting political influence of blood-donor associations (Setbon, 1993), and general opposition to questions about private life did not allow the already weak public health department to impose its views, neither on the health minister nor on the closed community of blood professionals. In the other three countries, on the other hand, the blood transfusion service was not charged with comparable symbolic values and corporatist resistances, and could react more effectively to warnings about the new risk.

AIDS prevention had to struggle its way through very different drug abuse policies. Risk reduction demanded contact with drug users, through needle exchange, street intervention and methadone drug maintenance treatment (DMT). Repressive policies that had driven addicts underground had to be abandoned. The UK and Italy had a liberal legislative framework but developed policy responses with very different results. In December 1998, there were 1024 cases of AIDS related to IDU in the UK compared with 26,400 cases in Italy, although it has been estimated that 75 per cent of Italian injecting drug users have been reached by regular AIDS prevention messages, compared with only 40 per cent in the UK (Montagnier Report, 1993, annex 5.1.2).

The UK was the first of the four countries to initiate a coherent policy of health risk reduction centred on needle exchange. The ground was prepared by social harm reduction strategies already under way when AIDS occurred, promoted by volunteer associations and supported by professionals (Berridge, 1993). In Italy, the focus remained on social integration and support for drug users, which explains the wide network of therapeutic communities providing residential facilities and professional training and activities. Health risk reduction strategies were implemented only when deaths from AIDS could no longer be ignored. Furthermore, public and private institutions taking care of drug users supported different approaches, centred on abstinence in Church-linked institutions, and on the provision of clean needles, condoms and, if budgets allowed, methadone DMT in others. The two-fold line entailed contradictory messages, a circumstance which is known to be counterproductive in prevention (van Campenhoudt *et al.*, 1997).

France and Germany shared a similar repressive drug policy. However, important practical changes were developed in Germany from 1988 onwards. The initial impulse came from the Health Ministers' Conference, and from field professionals. Needle and syringe exchange programmes, street work and methadone programmes were first launched in *Länder* governed by left-wing parties. In the early 1990s, they were extended to cover most regions except those controlled by ultra-conservative politicians. Growing local and regional changes modified power balances at national level and weakened medical opposition to methadone. Controversies came to an end when the health insurance system decided to consider injecting drug users 'normal patients', entitled to all available medication.

In France, risk reduction strategies were blocked by three obstacles: a general AIDS policy that rejected the targeting of specific groups, the unwillingness of politicians of all parties to modify drug policies for electoral reasons, and the refusal by drug professionals to accept the 'medicalisation' of their field, fearing that they would lose their autonomy and become subject to medical authority. Practical changes have only come about since 1994, after a timid shift in national policy following the 'contaminated blood scandal'. Cattacin and his colleagues, who have compared HIV/drug management in cities from six European countries, observed the continuing influence of the previous policy in France. In Lyons, changes remained very limited compared with other European cities, because the people and agencies involved were still the same as in the 1970s when drug services were established with the overall aim of abstinence (Cattacin *et al.*, 1996: 137). The contrast between Germany and France indicates that the development of risk reduction strategies depended less on law than on the institutional framework and professionals. Conservative professional and political attitudes in France, and lack of political interest in Italy, were not counterbalanced by institutional factors as in Germany and the UK.

Normalisation through innovation

History seldom repeats itself. Lasting innovations have arisen from AIDS, with far-reaching consequences. Some of them resulted directly from AIDS, such as the inclusion of homosexuality in medical issues. Often however, AIDS favoured more rapid progress of previous tendencies towards change. The shock of the epidemic helped to overcome previous resistance to overdue changes. The best example of this is provided by the profound reform of the French blood transfusion system. Here, various AIDS-linked innovations supported moves towards the greater protection of patients, including legal guarantees.

With AIDS, the participation of beneficiaries has extended beyond the traditional limits of patients' associations dominated by doctors (Steffen, 1997). Gay mobilisation was an autonomous process and allowed the introduction of non-medical dimensions of illness into policy considerations. The struggle of people with haemophilia for compensation and access to safe blood products succeeded only after they had shaken off medical dependency and turned towards political mobilisation and legal support. These victories had a price. People with haemophilia thereby became ordinary consumers and gay organisations instruments of public policies. AIDS prevention undoubtedly favoured the social acceptance of homosexuality (Rosenbrock, 1997). The recognition of a specific gay identity, however, has remained dependent on the cultural evolution of gender roles, individualisation and models of family life (Bochow, 1997). Sex education as a whole has been recognised as part of public policy. Although in most countries it has remained a weak part of school programmes, its legitimacy had been reinforced. In Germany, research and teaching on sex education are now being developed in universities and the new academic field has developed on the basis of knowledge and experience acquired from AIDS (Sielert, 1995).

The growing public/private mix that developed in the AIDS field led to the provision of a wide range of new social services, henceforth considered a necessary part of health and medical care: group-specific prevention and information, mutual and psychosocial support, legal assistance and counselling. At the same time, AIDS contributed to the development of more comprehensive medical service structures. The care of AIDS patients has fostered better co-ordination between ambulatory and hospital-based services, a particularly difficult problem in France. Hospital infections have become a new issue with the development of antibiotic-resistant pathogens and accurate long-term tracing in the blood and organ donation systems. Legal innovation resulting from compensation for people with haemophilia has led to sustainable changes in the regimes of responsibility and the reinforcement of the control of pharmaceuticals. The current extension of standard treatment protocols for AIDS patients has contributed to the rationalisation of prescription practice and the distribution of medicine.

The participation of beneficiaries, the recognition of the social dimensions of health and illness, improvements in control over medical services and the legal protection of patients all contribute to breaking the traditional monopoly of the medical profession over health issues. Those AIDS-born innovations are major steps towards the erection of more coherent systems of public health management. AIDS has contributed to the upgrading of public health in many countries. In France, a new policy concept was developed in the aftermath of the contaminated blood scandal – that of 'health security' (*sécurité sanitaire*), and a series of reforms were implemented, reorganising the previously neglected public health sector. Will the medical progress introduced by the new combination therapies undo these policy achievements and lower the innovative capacity brought in by AIDS, as many insiders fear (Dannecker, 1997)? The massive distribution of expensive medication will certainly pose challenges for systems of AIDS management. The downside of generous resource allocation will probably be closer epidemiological monitoring. In the future, AIDS activists will have to share their privileged influence with the main actors in health policies, in particular with health insurance funds and international funding agencies.

Normalisation describes the integration of the AIDS issue into existing agendas, priorities and networks of public policies, in particular health and welfare policies. The process endows the newly introduced policies with long-term sustainability. Normalisation is a dynamic process, combining the path dependency of health policy and AIDS-rooted innovations. It has proved to be more complex and laden with conflicts in countries that were poorly equipped for public health management and, therefore, opposed to the recognition and the practical treatment of the new public health risks. Far-reaching consequences can be expected, particularly in these countries, because the epidemic contributes to the consolidation of the poorly established parts of the public health sector. This calls into question elements of the political culture, like the boundary between what can be considered public and private rights or responsibilities. Collective norms have had to undergo changes, which explains the existence of political controversy in many countries.

References

Alber, J. (1994) 'Le système de santé en RFA: mode de régulation et évolution', in B. Jobert and M. Steffen (eds) *Les Politiques de santé en France et en Allemagne*, Paris: Espace Social Européen, Observatoire Européen des Politiques Sociales.

Altman, D. (1988) 'Legitimation through disaster: AIDS and the gay movement', in E. Fee and D. Fox (eds) *AIDS, The Burden of History*, London: University of California Press.

Bachelot, F. and Lorane, P. (1988) *Une Société au rique du Sida*, Paris: Éditions Albatros.

Bayer, R. (1989) *Private Acts, Social Consequences: AIDS and the Politics of Public Health*, New Brunswick, NJ: Rutgers University Press (reprint with a new Afterword).

——(1991) 'Public health policy and the AIDS epidemic. An end to HIV exceptionalism?', *New England Journal of Medicine* 324: 1500–1504.

Berridge, V. (1993) 'AIDS and British drug policy: continuity or change', in V. Berridge and P. Strong (eds) *AIDS and Contemporary History*, Cambridge: Cambridge University Press.

Bochow, M. (1997) 'Hat AIDS die soziale Situation schwuler Mäner verändert?', in D. Grumbach (ed.) *Was heisst hier schwul? Politik und Identitäten im Wandel*, Hamburg: Männerschwarm Skript.

Cattacin, S. and Panchaud, C. (in collaboration with Véronique Tattini) (1997) *Les Politiques de Lutte contre le VIH/SIDA en Europe de l'Ouest. Du risk à la normalisation*, Paris: L'Harmattan.

Cattacin, S., Lucas, B. and Vetter, S. (1996) *Modèle des politiques en matières de drogue, une comparaison de six réalités européennes*, Paris: L'Harmattan.

Dannecker, M. (1997) 'Nouvelles thérapies et banalisation du Sida', *AIDS INFO Docu Schweiz, Reihe DIALOG AIDS*, Vol. IV, Berne, pp. 51–56.

Day, P. and Klein, R. (1989) 'Interpreting the unexpected: the case of AIDS policy making in Britain', *Journal of Public Policy* 9(3): 337–353.

Fee, E. and Fox, D. (eds) (1988) *AIDS, The Burden of History*, London: University of California Press.

——(1992) *AIDS, The Making of a Chronic Disease*, London: University of California Press.

Fox, D. (1988) 'AIDS and the American health polity: the history and prospects of a crisis of authority', in E. Fee and D. Fox (eds) *AIDS, The Burden of History*, London: University of California Press.

Fox, D., Day, P. and Klein, R. (1989) 'The power of professionalism: policies for AIDS in Britain, Sweden, and the United States', *Daedalus* 118(2): 93–112.

Hayward, J. and Klein, R. (1994) 'Grande-Bretagne: de la gestion publique à la gestion privée du déclin économique', in B. Jobert (ed.) *Le Tournant Néo-libéral en Europe*, Paris: L'Harmattan.

Henrikson, B. and Ytterberg, H. (1992) 'Sweden: the power of the moral(istic) Left', in D. L. Kirp and R. Bayer (eds) *AIDS in the Industrialized Democracies: Passions, Politics and Policies*, New Brunswick, NJ: Rutgers University Press.

Hermitte, M. A. (1996) *Le sang et le droit. Essai sur la transfusion sanguine*, Paris: Seuil.

IGASS/IGSJ (joint report) (1992) *Rapport d'enquète sur les collectes de sang en milieu pénitentiaire. Observations et Annexes*, Report IGAS No. SA 07 92 119, No. IGSJ RMT 12 92, Paris: Ministry of Health, Ministry of Justice.

Igl, G. (1994) 'La rencontre du médical et du social en RFA', in B. Jobert and M. Steffen (eds) *Les Politiques de santé en France et en Allemagne*, Paris: Observatoire Européen des Politiques Sociales, Espace Social Européen.

Jobert, B. and Steffen, M. (eds) (1994) *Les Politiques de Santé en France et en Allemagne*, Paris: Espace Social Européen, Observatoire Européen des Politiques Sociales.

Kirp, D. L. and Bayer, R. (eds) (1992) *AIDS in the Industrialised Democracies: Passions, Politics and Policies*, New Brunswick, NJ: Rutgers University Press.

The Lancet (1942) 'Medical Society for the Study of the Venereal Diseases', 1: 561–562.

Lehmbruch, G. (1994) 'RFA: Le cadre institutionnel et les incertitudes des strategies néo-liberales', in B. Jobert (ed.) *Le Tournant Néo-libéral en Europe*, Paris: L'Harmattan.

Montagnier Report (1993) *Rapport à Monsieur le Premier ministre sur le Sida*, Ministère des Affairs Sociale, de la Santé et de la Ville, Ministère délégué à la Santé, Paris.

Moss, D. (1990) 'AIDS in Italy: emergency in slow motion', in B. A. Misztal and D. Moss (eds) *Action on Aids, National Policies in Comparative Perspective*, Westport, CT: Greenwood Press.

Mossuz-Lavau, J. (1991) *Les Lois de l'amour. Les politiques de la sexuality en France (1950–1990)*, Paris: Payot.

Porter, E. and Porter, R. (1988) 'The enforcement of health: The British debate', in E. Fee and D. Fox (eds) *AIDS, The Burden of History*, London: University of California Press.

Regonini, G. and Giuliani, M. (1994) 'Italie: au-dela d'une démocratie consensuelle?', in B. Jobert (ed.) *Le Tournant Néo-liberal en Europe*, Paris: L'Harmattan.

Rosenbrock, R. (1994) 'Die Normalisierung von Aids – teils nach vorne, teils zurück', in D. Kirp and R. Bayer (eds) *Strategien gegen Aids. Ein internationaler Politikvergleich*, Berlin: Sigma.

——(1997) 'AIDS-Politik, Gesundheitspolitik und Schwulenpolitik', Paper presentated at the Conference 'Verqueere Wissenschaft? 100 Jahre Wissenschaftlich-humanitäres Komitee', Humboldt Universität zu Berlin, 20 July 1997.

Setbon, M. (1993) *Pouvoirs contre Sida. De la transfusion sanguine au dépistage: décisions et pratiques en France, Grande-Bretagne et Suède*, Paris: Seuil.

Sielert, U. (1995) 'Prävention: Erfahrung, Mythen und Möglichkeiten', *Dokumentation der Fachtagung vom 13–15 Juni 1994*, Landesinstitut für Schule und Weiterbildung, Soest.

Steffen, M. (1996) *The Fight against AIDS. An International Public Policy Comparison Between Four European Countries: France, Great Britain, Germany, Italy*, Grenoble: Presses Universitaires de Grenoble.

——(1997) 'La Santé: les bénéficiaires en dehors des réformes', in P. Warin (ed.) *Quelle modernisation des services publics? Les usagers au coeur des réformes*, Paris: La Decouverte.

——(1999) 'The nation's blood: medicine, justice and the state in France', in E. Feldman and R. Bayer (eds) *Blood Feuds: Aids, Blood, and the Politics of Medical Disaster*, Oxford: Oxford University Press.

van Campenhoudt, L. *et al.* (1997) *Sexual Interactions and HIV Risk. New Conceptual Perspectives in European Research*, London: Taylor & Francis.

16 UK HIV testing practice

By how much might the infection diagnosis rate increase through normalisation?

Christine Ann McGarrigle and
Owen Noel Gill

Given the continuing transmission of HIV infection in Europe, preventing new infections and alleviating the effects of infections that have already occurred are major public health priorities. Testing blood donations for HIV has an established role in preventing transmission of the virus. In other areas of prevention it is less clear whether more HIV testing would affect HIV transmission substantially.

The effectiveness of HIV testing for prevention in the USA has been demonstrated in a recent randomised controlled trial, which showed a reduction in sexually transmitted disease (STD) incidence in those who received a negative HIV test result combined with risk reduction counselling (Kamb *et al.*, 1998). In Sweden HIV testing is an important part of the prevention policy and the government strongly recommends voluntary confidential testing. More people have been tested per million population than have been tested in any other European country, even though seroprevalence rates have remained low. There is a greater emphasis on the individual's 'responsibility to find out' their HIV status in countries such as Sweden compared with the UK where the individuals 'right not to know' their HIV status is widely respected.

HIV/AIDS prevention has involved policies perceived as different from the traditional infectious disease approach, with a greater emphasis on confidentiality and informed consent, so-called 'HIV/AIDS exceptionalism' (De Cock and Johnson, 1998; Bayer, 1991). 'Normalisation' has been described as 'treating HIV/AIDS more like other infectious diseases for which early diagnosis is necessary for appropriate therapeutic and preventative measures within the requirements of informed consent and confidentiality' (De Cock and Johnson, 1998). Normalisation of HIV testing, it is argued, would allow pre-test discussion and testing for HIV to take place within all disciplines of general medicine. If exceptionalism tends to raise the barrier to patients being encouraged to be tested, then normalisation should result in a lower threshold for provider initiation of testing and a large increase in testing as a consequence.

What might be the public health consequences of a substantial increase in HIV testing, assuming 'normalisation' might lead to more testing being offered? Available surveillance data should be examined to see what inferences can be drawn about test uptake in the population and how it has changed over time, before advocating HIV testing as an essential part of direct preventive measures.

What available surveillance data can tell us

Data from a range of national HIV surveillance systems for England and Wales were used. These included AIDS case reports, and laboratory reports of diagnosed HIV infections. A sentinel surveillance system of HIV tests at seventeen laboratories, which together provide primary HIV testing for over 40 per cent of the population, including data on both HIV-positive and HIV-negative tests, was also utilised. Data from unlinked anonymous surveys which monitor HIV prevalence in accessible population groups were also included. The data used include data from an unlinked anonymous survey of attenders at fifteen STD clinics who are being routinely tested for syphilis. This survey collects some demographic and risk behaviour data, including age group, sexual orientation, STD diagnosed at that attendance and whether the individual is known to be HIV infected. The residual blood sample collected at that clinic visit for syphilis serology is then tested for HIV, after it is unlinked from all personal identifiers. Data from an unlinked anonymous survey of injecting drug users attending needle exchanges and specialist drug agencies were also studied as were data from behavioural surveys.

AIDS case reporting is almost totally complete in the UK, and so AIDS case reports represent almost all HIV infections which have now developed AIDS. They do, however, reflect transmissions which occurred at least ten years previously and so are unable to give useful information on current HIV transmission. Diagnosed HIV infections reflect a more current picture of HIV infection, although they only represent those people who have chosen to have a voluntary HIV test, and so are subject to biases related to health-seeking behaviour and an individual's perception of risk. The sentinel survey of HIV tests gives a sample of those who are having voluntary HIV tests, both negative and positive, allowing the distribution of HIV testing within different exposure categories to be monitored over time. Unlinked anonymous surveys provide information on prevalence of HIV infection among groups in which many infections remain undiagnosed and therefore undetectable through surveillance systems based on routine clinical and laboratory diagnosis, thus giving the true prevalence of HIV in the population.

Together the data were used: (a) to estimate the proportion of those infected with HIV who probably have had major risk exposures for the infection; (b) to show trends in HIV testing over time; (c) to estimate how many of those at risk of HIV infection have been tested, when in the course of their infection those who were infected were tested, and whether having an HIV test was associated with reduced risk in both the infected and the uninfected; and (d) to assess the level and likely direction of change in HIV transmission due to sexual intercourse between men in recent years.

Distribution of diagnosed HIV infections in the UK

In all, 69 per cent of AIDS cases and 60 per cent of diagnosed HIV infections are attributed to sex between men (Table 16.1). A further 6 per cent of AIDS cases and 10 per cent of HIV infections are attributed to injecting drug use. Also, 17 per cent of AIDS cases and 22 per cent of HIV infections are attributed to heterosexual transmission, and 78 per cent and 74 per cent respectively of these are probably acquired abroad in areas where heterosexual transmission of HIV is endemic. If heterosexual exposure in Africa, Asia or Latin America including the Caribbean is also considered a high-risk exposure for HIV, then 94 per cent of the total diagnosed and reported HIV-infected persons in England and Wales and 97 per cent of persons with AIDS have had a high-risk exposure to HIV infection (Table 16.1).

Trends in HIV testing

Sentinel surveillance of HIV testing in seventeen public health laboratories shows that since 1991 the volume of HIV testing has been more or less constant. While the large numbers of those tested each quarter at 'no reported HIV risk' or at risk because of many heterosexual partners have fluctuated somewhat in response to national publicity of varying sorts, the much lower numbers tested who have been at high HIV risk have stayed constant over time. Amongst those having voluntary confidential HIV tests at the four London laboratories in 1994–1997, the greatest risk factor for

Table 16.1   AIDS cases and known HIV-infected persons: UK to end December 1997

How infection was probably acquired	United Kingdom	
	AIDS (%)	*Known HIV-infected persons (%)*
Sexual intercourse:		
between men	11,022 (69)	20,105 (60)
between men and women	2738 (17)	7292 (22)
Injecting drug use	1024 (6)	3305 (10)
Blood factor treatment	644 (4)	1349 (4)
Blood/tissue transfer	141 (1)	231 (1)
Mother to infant	304 (2)	544 (2)
Other/under investigation	155 (1)	938 (3)
Total	16,028 (100)	33,764 (100)

HIV infection was to have 'lived in or visited Africa': 16 per cent of this group was infected compared with 10 per cent of those at risk through sexual intercourse between men (Table 16.2). Between 1994 and 1997, 80,688 HIV tests of 'no reported risk' were undertaken at the laboratories, and 0.1 per cent of these were HIV positive, an indication of what untargeted HIV testing may yield. Between 1996 and 1997 the prevalence of HIV infection, by unlinked anonymous testing, in non-drug-injecting heterosexuals attending STD clinics in London and who were born in the UK was 0.49 per cent in men and 0.28 per cent in women (1 in 203 and 1 in 355 respectively), compared with 0.19 per cent in pregnant women (1 in 533) (Department of Health, 1998). Prevalence in non-drug-injecting heterosexual clinic attenders in London born in sub-Saharan Africa was 4.0 per cent in men and 5.7 per cent in women.

Proportion of prevalent HIV infections which have been diagnosed

Prior to the introduction of combination antiretroviral therapy in 1996, AIDS cases could be used to estimate the proportion of HIV infections diagnosed. Individuals with AIDS cases can be divided into two groups, comprising those who had an HIV test well in advance of their AIDS diagnosis and those who were not known to be infected until they developed an illness, followed shortly by the diagnosis of an AIDS indicator disease. As almost all AIDS cases in the UK will be diagnosed, the interval between first HIV test and AIDS diagnosis can be used to estimate the proportion of all persons currently infected with HIV without AIDS who have had a voluntary HIV test. It is assumed that the proportion of recent incident AIDS diagnoses, in whom the interval between their first HIV-positive test and AIDS diagnosis is relatively long, represents the proportion of all

Table 16.2   Sentinel surveillance of diagnostic HIV tests in England (seventeen laboratories: four in London, three elsewhere): first tests for HIV infection, 1994–1997 (data to September 1997)

Exposure category	Place	No. of first tests	No. HIV infected	% HIV infected
Homosexual/ bisexual males	London	3179	306	10
	Elsewhere	5894	266	5
Injecting drug use	Elsewhere	588	26	4
	London	3912	54	1
Lived in/visited Africa	London	1042	171	16
	Elsewhere	892	54	6

persons infected with HIV (without AIDS) who have had a voluntary HIV test (Hughes *et al.*, 1998). For homosexual and bisexual men and injecting drug users this proportion rose sharply from 1986 to 1989 from less then 10 per cent of all AIDS cases to 54 per cent and 62 per cent respectively, and more steadily thereafter until 1995. Only 40 per cent of the AIDS cases diagnosed in 1995–1996 in individuals who were infected heterosexually had a diagnosis interval of over nine months compared with two-thirds of those exposed through sexual intercourse between men and three-quarters of those exposed through drug injecting. All these proportions fell in 1997 as new therapies altered the 'natural history' of HIV infection and delayed progression to AIDS in HIV-infected persons aware of their infection, and thus able to benefit from therapy. This means that AIDS cases are no longer useful for estimating the proportion of HIV infections diagnosed.

The proportion of all HIV-infected individuals currently in the UK that have had their infection diagnosed clinically can be estimated from the unlinked anonymous prevalence monitoring programme. These estimates are obtained from the STD clinic survey, by the clinician filling out the survey form stating that the individual is known to be HIV positive, or if the individual has had an HIV test at that visit and the unlinked anonymous specimen tests HIV positive. For the survey of injecting drug users, the survey form asks if the individual has ever had an HIV test, and what the result was. If the corresponding unlinked anonymous specimen tests HIV positive in those who have had a previous positive HIV test, then the individual is taken to have had his or her HIV infection clinically diagnosed. In 1995–1996 the proportions of infections diagnosed clinically in each exposure category were broadly similar to the proportions seen using the HIV to AIDS diagnosis interval approach (Table 16.3), suggesting that the unlinked anonymous survey method may also be an accurate estimate of the proportion of prevalent HIV infections which are diagnosed. For HIV-infected homosexual and bisexual men attending London STD clinics the apparent proportion in whom HIV infection was clinically diagnosed declined from 76 per cent in 1993 to 59 per cent in 1996. This was probably as a result of HIV care shifting away from clinic sessions at which syphilis testing was offered routinely, a pattern that was not observed in heterosexuals attending the same clinics.

With the advent of effective measures to prevent mother-to-infant transmission, including the use of zidovudine in pregnancy for HIV-infected women, there is a strong case for these women to have their infection diagnosed well before they give birth. In England, especially in London, much needs to be done to improve the situation; less than a quarter of HIV-infected pregnant women in London in 1996 were aware of their infection (Nicoll *et al.*, 1998; Gibb *et al.*, 1997). Increased uptake of ante-natal HIV testing, however, is likely to have little impact on HIV transmission due to heterosexual exposure as most of these transmissions take place abroad (Paine *et al.*, 1997) and transmissions which take place within England and Wales probably mostly occur before a first pregnancy.

Table 16.3   Proportions of prevalent HIV infections which have been diagnosed by exposure category, England and Wales 1995–1996

Exposure category	Place	Method	
		HIV to AIDS diagnosis interval (%)*	HIV test history (%)**
Homo/bisexual	London & SE	70	62
	Rest	63	76
Heterosexual	London & SE	45	47
	Rest	36	34
Injecting drug use	London & SE	83	88
	Rest	66	93

* Percentage of AIDS cases diagnosed in 1995–1996 in whom the 'diagnosis' interval between first positive HIV test and AIDS diagnosis was over nine months.

** Percentage of HIV-infected persons recognised by unlinked anonymous testing who have probably had their HIV infection diagnosed clinically.

Is HIV testing associated with behaviour change?

Amongst the HIV infected the association between awareness of their infection and probable recent high-risk sexual behaviour can be examined within the unlinked anonymous survey of STD clinic attenders (Table 16.4). Recent high-risk sexual exposure is indicated by diagnosis of another condition at the current clinic attendance that was likely to have been acquired through unprotected sexual intercourse, defined as an acute STD, as opposed to other conditions such as recurrent viral STDs, or no specific STD diagnosis. STDs continue in gay men who are known to be HIV positive. In 1996–1997 43 per cent of the HIV-infected homosexual and bisexual men who were unaware of their HIV infection also had an acute STD as had 20 per cent of the larger number who knew they were HIV infected. While there is a suggestion that some STDs may be acquired through unprotected sex with a partner of concordant serostatus, not all of these will be acquired this way, and there is continuing evidence through behavioural studies that known HIV-positive gay men do have unsafe sex with partners of discordant or unknown serostatus (Nardone *et al.*, 1998). At the same time, of HIV-infected heterosexual men who were unaware of their HIV infection, 45 per cent also had an acute STD, as did a third of similar women (Table 16.4).

However, particular caution must be exercised when interpreting surveillance data on the associations between past voluntary, confidential HIV testing and various risk behaviours both in the infected and uninfected. Those who subsequently have a syphilis test at an STD clinic are unlikely to be representative of all HIV-infected homosexual and bisexual men who are aware of their infection and for this reason it may be inappropriate to compare them with clinic attenders who are unaware of their HIV infection. Nevertheless the acquisition of acute STDs by gay men who know they are

Table 16.4 Proportion of HIV-infected STD clinic attenders (having syphilis serology) with evidence of probable recent high-risk sexual behaviour (i.e. diagnosis of one or more of a variety of other conditions at the current clinic attendance that were likely to have been acquired through unprotected sexual intercourse), 1996 and 1997

Exposure category and knowledge of HIV infection before clinic visit	No. positive	% with acute STD
Homosexual or bisexual men:		
aware of infection	538	20
not aware	422	43
Heterosexual men:		
aware of infection	125	3
not aware	184	45
Heterosexual women:		
aware of infection	119	6
not aware	182	32
Other/unknown:		
aware of infection	45	4
not aware	17	24

HIV infected shows that knowledge of HIV infection status does not eliminate behaviour associated with continuing risk of HIV transmission. It would be interesting to know whether more and earlier HIV testing of gay men would reduce the number of them presenting to STD clinics with both HIV infection and acute STD but the data cannot address this critical issue. The observational data can only show that the extensive HIV testing and health promotion undertaken so far have not controlled HIV transmission nor eliminated risk behaviours amongst gay men.

Data on the association between risk behaviour and voluntary confidential HIV testing among those who are HIV negative is available from the voluntary unlinked anonymous saliva survey of injecting drug users. In 1996–1997, sharing of needles and syringes in the past month was the same (17 per cent) in HIV-negative drug-injecting persons who had had a voluntary confidential HIV test, as in those who had not had a voluntary confidential test (19 per cent, Table 16.5).

Table 16.5 Association between risk behaviour and HIV testing among HIV-negative injecting drug users, England and Wales 1996–1997: the sharing of needles and syringes by those who had injected in the last month

Voluntary confidential HIV testing	Not shared needles or syringes	Shared needles or syringes
Yes	1635 (83%)	333 (17%)
No	1551 (81%)	356 (19%)

Of those HIV-negative injecting drug users who had injected in the month prior to participation in the survey and who had had two or more sexual partners in the previous year, the frequency of reported condom usage was similarly low whether they had had a voluntary confidential HIV test or not (Table 16.6). Regular condom usage was higher by a small amount in drug users who were not currently injecting and who knew they were HIV negative compared with those who were unaware of their HIV status (Table 16.6). HIV prevalence is very high in this group and the majority of infections are diagnosed. However, the injecting and sexual behaviours of those who have had a negative HIV test are not different from those who have no HIV test, thus indicating that having an HIV test is not sufficient to change behaviour.

Equal caution is called for in interpreting the data on HIV testing and risk behaviours in injecting drug users. We did not collect data on whether the HIV status of those the drug user shared with was known, or the direction of the sharing (i.e. those HIV positive may just have received rather than passed on). Unlike the situation with gay men having syphilis tests, these drug users were sampled at needle exchange and other services at which their attendance was not a direct consequence of engaging in unsafe injecting. Although it is disappointing that a voluntary confidential HIV test was not associated with reduced needle sharing in those who had injected recently, it would be important to know whether an HIV test is associated with stopping injecting so that drug services are no longer availed of. Even answering this question, however, would not establish whether early HIV testing of persons who inject drugs can substantially reduce their lifetime risk of contracting HIV over and above the effect of existing health promotion efforts.

Table 16.6   Associations between risk behaviour and HIV testing among HIV-negative injecting drug users, England and Wales 1996–1997:

	Voluntary confidential HIV testing	*Condom use by those with 2 or more sexual partners* in the last year*		
		Always used condoms	*Sometimes used condoms*	*Never used condoms*
Injected in month prior to survey participation	Yes	161 (25%)	306 (48%)	173 (27%)
	No	122 (19%)	304 (47%)	219 (34%)
Not injected in month prior to survey participation	Yes	43 (23%)	94 (51%)	49 (26%)
	No	30 (14%)	116 (54%)	70 (32%)

* Vaginal or anal sex only.

Evidence of ongoing transmission

Despite relatively high levels of HIV testing, sustained in recent years, there are clear indications that the rate of transmission of HIV infection due to sexual intercourse between men probably increased during the 1990s (Table 16.7). There were more new diagnoses of HIV infections in this group in 1996 than in earlier years and these numbers continued in 1997. At the same time the incidence of gonorrhoea in homosexual and bisexual men has risen. At least 1 in 200 young gay men attending STD clinics in London is becoming infected each year so that by the age of 25, 3 per cent of this group have undiagnosed HIV infection.

Conclusion

At the present time in England and Wales HIV infection is overwhelmingly confined to behaviourally vulnerable minorities – gay men, injecting drug users and migrants from high-prevalence countries – and practically all HIV infection can be predicted by the presence of major risk factors. Most of the HIV infected have probably had their infection diagnosed clinically and transmission of HIV infection due to sexual intercourse between men is probably continuing at an appreciable rate despite widespread HIV testing.

There is generally easy access to voluntary confidential testing for those at greatest risk of HIV infection. Lack of awareness of their infection status in those who are HIV infected may be the outcome of either a considered decision not to be tested or relatively recent infection, or both. Those at

Table 16.7   Trends in indicators of continuing transmission of HIV and other sexually transmitted infections due to sexual intercourse between men

Indicator	Age group (years)	1992	1993	1994	1995	1996	1997
New diagnoses of HIV infections	15–19	18	23	14	19	20	17
	20–24	183	155	134	143	143	139
	25–29	364	359	361	372	403	320
	30	865	865	887	944	1107	938
	Median age	32	32	33	33	33	33
Prevalence of HIV infection as % (n), unlinked anonymous tests on specimens for syphilis tests	≤24 London	14% (471)	11% (406)	9% (555)	7% (800)	6% (652)	6% (561)
	≤24 Elsewhere	2% (289)	2% (411)	2% (376)	2% (332)	2% (361)	2% (350)
New episodes of gonorrhoea in homosexual men attending STD clinics		1326	1158	1332	1334	1650	1777

greatest risk who choose not to be tested are unlikely to change their minds until evidence in favour of early HIV diagnosis becomes more compelling.

It is fascinating that 'normalisation' of HIV testing has become a rallying cry at the same time as it is clear that HIV infection in Europe is likely to remain largely within marginalised groups in society. Normalisation of testing rests partially on the belief that HIV infection can be diagnosed before onward transmission takes place and that the rest of the population would be protected if all the infected could be diagnosed. Pursuing a policy of early testing may divert effort from strengthening primary prevention. People at higher risk of HIV infection generally choose to be tested when they feel ready or when they fall ill. The key issue is not why were they tested late, but rather why were they at risk in the first place.

Research is needed to establish the added value for primary prevention of early testing and the true benefit of early versus deferred combination antiretroviral therapy. Helpful insights may be obtained relatively easily through studying the prior HIV test behaviour and prior opportunities for HIV testing of newly diagnosed HIV-infected persons.

The unique features of HIV infection make it unlikely that an HIV test can ever or should ever be 'normalised'. There is an inexorable progression to early death in practically all those who are infected, although antiretroviral therapies are now successfully increasing survival, the mode of transmission threatens us all because any of us or our loved ones may be at risk sexually, and testing for the presence of the infection is highly accurate, simple to perform and relatively cheap. Rather than 'normalising' HIV testing within medical practice, effort should be directed towards improving the recognition of major risk factors for HIV infection and towards undertaking one-to-one health promotion with those at higher risk at every health care opportunity. Normalised HIV testing is associated with a diminished role for counselling. This is ironic just when a major study has shown the effectiveness of counselling at modifying sexual behaviour (Kamb *et al.*, 1998).

In high-risk groups, the barriers to HIV testing may not change through normalisation, as the proportion of HIV infections diagnosed is high already and nearly all infections are in these high-risk groups (including heterosexuals from high-prevalence areas). These groups have had prolonged access to, and a high uptake of, testing. The barrier to testing is not erected by providers, but by the high-risk individuals. The public health consequences of directing resources towards encouraging everyone to be tested, instead of concentrating on those at risk of HIV infection, may include a dilution of other prevention activities. Efforts should concentrate upon behavioural interventions for those at continuing high risk regardless of their HIV test history or HIV test result.

References

Bayer, R. (1991) 'Public health policy and the AIDS epidemic. An end to AIDS exceptionalism?', *New England Journal of Medicine* 324: 1500–1504.

De Cock, K. M. and Johnson, A. M. (1998) 'From exceptionalism to normalisation: a reappraisal of attitudes and practice around HIV testing', *British Medical Journal* 316: 290–293.

Department of Health (1998) *Annual Report of the Unlinked Anonymous Prevalence Monitoring Programme. Prevalence of HIV in England and Wales in 1997*, London: Department of Health.

Gibb, D. M., MacDonagh, S. E., Tookey, P., Duong, T., Nicoll, A., Goldberg, D. J., Hudson, C. N. N., Peckham, C. S. and Ades, A. E. (1997) 'Uptake of interventions to reduce mother to child transmission of HIV in the United Kingdom and Ireland', *AIDS* 11: F53–F58.

Hughes, G., Porter, K. and Gill, O. N. (1998) 'Indirect methods for estimating prevalent HIV infections: adults in England and Wales at the end of 1993', *Epidemiology of Infection* 121: 165–172.

Kamb, M. L. *et al.* (1998) 'Efficacy of risk-reduction counseling to prevent human deficiency virus and other sexually transmitted diseases. A randomised controlled trial', *Journal of the American Medical Association* 280: 1161–1167.

Nardone, A., Dodds, J. P., Mercey, D. E. and Johnson, A. M. (1998) 'Active surveillance of sexual behaviour among homosexual men in London', *Communicable Disease and Public Health* 1: 197–201.

Nicoll, A. *et al.* (1998) 'Epidemiology and detection of HIV-1 among pregnant women in the United Kingdom: results from national surveillance 1988–96', *British Medical Journal* 3: 253–258.

Paine, K., Nicoll, A., Evans, B., Molesworth, A., Mortimer, J. and Rogers, R. (1997) *HIV Infection in Lambeth, Southwark and Lewisham Attributed to Sexual Intercourse Between Men and Women*, London: Public Health Laboratory Service.

17 Modelling network structure

Implications for the spread and prevention of HIV infection

Mirjam Kretzschmar

Since the beginning of the AIDS epidemic in the early 1980s much effort has been devoted to designing mathematical models that can predict the further course of the epidemic. In the development of these models from simple compartmental to complex individual based network models, much insight has been gained. In particular, the importance of knowledge about sexual behaviour, sexual network structure and its relationship with the spread of sexually transmitted diseases (STDs) has been better recognised. This in turn has stimulated research in the behavioural sciences to obtain more detailed information about patterns of human sexual behaviour. Currently, a multitude of such data is available (e.g. ACSF investigators, 1992; Hubert *et al.*, 1998; Johnson *et al.*, 1994), alongside a rich variety of modelling approaches (e.g. Anderson and May, 1991; Kaplan and Brandeau, 1994).

This chapter offers an overview of issues pertaining to the modelling of sexual networks and their relevance to HIV prevention. The models considered are dynamic models that incorporate a description of the transmission process and relate this to epidemiological outcomes. These contrast with statistical modelling approaches such as the back-calculation method which has been designed to predict the number of HIV-infected persons on the basis of AIDS data (Downs *et al.*, 1997). In view of the simplifications that need to be made when describing a complex process such as transmission via sexual contact, one usually cannot expect a dynamic model to deliver quantitative predictions. While this may seem disappointing at first, the value of such models should not be underestimated.

A model can be viewed as an experimental situation in which some parameters are kept constant while others are varied. One can then study the effects of changes in parameters in the model population. In relation to HIV prevention, models provide a cheap and controllable means of testing different strategies and comparing their effectiveness. Even if it is not possible to make clear quantitative statements about the likely future effects of a specific intervention, it is nevertheless useful to know which approaches may be superior to others, and to have an understanding of why this is the case.

Infectious diseases modelling

In mathematical modelling, one tries to understand the relationship between the characteristics of a specific disease, patterns of contact in the population within which it is transmitted, and the resulting incidence and prevalence. These insights can be used to support the interpretation of epidemiological data, help decide which data are needed to assess an epidemiological situation, and design effective prevention measures.

Important parameters in describing a specific disease include the probability of transmission per contact (where a contact is defined as an event that potentially leads to transmission), the duration of the infectious period, the fraction of infected persons who are asymptomatic and infectious, and the recovery rate. Which of these parameters is incorporated into a model depends on the disease one wants to study, the level of detail that is needed to describe transmission properly, and the required outcome variables. In modelling HIV transmission, relevant parameters include the probability of transmission per contact or per partnership, the incubation time distribution, infectivity at various stages of infection, and disease-related mortality.

The definition of what constitutes a contact and what are the relevant contact patterns is determined by the transmission route of a disease. For HIV, different transmission routes are related to different contact networks. For transmission by sexual contact it is important in modelling to differentiate between transmission by homosexual and heterosexual contact. Furthermore, the number of sexual partners per time unit (e.g. per year), the duration of the sexual partnerships, the overlap of partnerships or their 'concurrency', and finally heterogeneity with respect to these variables in the population, are all determinants of the overall contact pattern. Similarly, for injecting drug use the contact structure is determined by the social contacts of drug users among whom the sharing of injecting equipment takes place. These can vary from anonymous contacts in shooting galleries to longer lasting relationships with friends and sexual partners. Where two different transmission routes exist, namely needle sharing and unprotected sexual contact, contact patterns are more complex.

Even before the AIDS pandemic had focused attention on sexual behaviour, it was recognised that heterogeneity in sexual behaviour plays an important role in determining patterns of STD transmission. In modelling prevention strategies for gonorrhoea, for example, Hethcote and Yorke (1984) introduced the concept of a 'core group', a small subgroup of the population with a very high rate of sexual partner change. With the advent of AIDS, the need for more detailed descriptions of sexual behaviour increased, and a number of modelling approaches were developed. In *mixing models*, the basic idea was to distinguish different activity levels in the population and to define a 'mixing matrix' describing the contact rates within and among subgroups of different sexual activity (see e.g. Anderson and May, 1991; Blythe and Castillo-Chavez, 1989; Jacquez *et al.*, 1989). It was then possible to investigate how mixing between subgroups determines epidemic spread, and how prevention focused on specific subgroups might affect incidence and prevalence.

A different approach to modelling has examined the influence of partnership duration on transmission. In mixing models, one implicitly assumes that every contact is with a new individual, and there are no longer lasting partnerships. In contrast, in so-called *pair formation models* (first introduced in the context of STDs by Dietz and Hadeler, 1988), the formation and separation of possibly long-lasting partnerships between pairs of individuals is taken into account. Although pair formation models are conceptually appealing, they have the disadvantage that the incorporation of more structure in the model, such as subgroups with different levels of sexual activity, or the possibility of having more than one partnership at a time, increases their overall complexity rapidly.

A further step towards a more detailed description of sexual behaviour occurs in *network models* (Anderson *et al.*, 1990; Blanchard *et al.*, 1990; Haraldsdottir *et al.*, 1992; Kretzschmar *et al.*, 1994, 1995). These try to capture the essential features of sexual networks by describing the population as a collection of individuals connected by links that represent sexual partnerships. In this way, phenomena such as concurrent partnerships and larger connected network components can be described. In contrast to mixing and pair formation models that are formulated in terms of differential equations, network models are inherently stochastic. Except in very simple cases, it is not possible to derive 'parameter value independent' results. Instead, it is necessary to run and analyse a large number of simulations and to apply statistical techniques as one would also use for analysing real data. The advantage here is that results are easily comparable with data obtained by sexual behaviour surveys.

Although these different modelling approaches were developed with the aim of describing sexual contact structure in a population, they can also be used to describe the transmission of disease via the sharing of injection equipment. Again, an important determinant of transmission here is heterogeneity in behaviour; that is, the existence of groups of the population with high-risk behaviour and their mixing patterns with the rest of the population with lower risk levels. It is also important to consider whether the sharing of needles takes place within long-lasting relationships (e.g. with friends or regular sexual partners) or more or less randomly as in shooting galleries. Third, if longer lasting relationships are the basis for risk behaviour and disease transmission, the key question is how best to describe the networks constituted by these contacts. Modelling techniques that have been developed for describing the spread of infection via sexual contacts, can – with appropriate adjustments – be used for modelling transmission via needle sharing.

Much discussion in HIV/AIDS has focused on its long incubation period and varying levels of infectiousness during that period. Using statistical models, Longini *et al.* (1989), and Hendriks *et al.* (1998) have estimated the time from infection to development of AIDS for homosexually active men and injecting drug users, respectively. For transmission dynamics the probability of transmission per contact in the various stages of infection is important. As Longini *et al.* (1989) and Jacquez *et al.* (1994) have argued convincingly, infectivity is high in the first acute phase of infection, low during the long asymptomatic phase, and higher again when the first symptoms of AIDS become manifest.

Contact structure and individual behaviour

For a long time in sexual behaviour surveys and in modelling, the focus was on variables that could be measured for every individual without taking his or her partners into account. These included the number of partners an individual had in the last year, or in his or her lifetime; sexual orientation; age; social status; and other demographic variables influencing partner choice.

In the modelling process, this approach leads to a 'matching problem'. For a given distribution of partners or specific partner preferences, one has to find a distribution of partnerships that satisfies these constraints. Often, the so-called proportionate mixing assumption is used. Here, it is assumed that partnerships are formed randomly and each individual is weighted according to his or her number of partnerships. Actual mixing patterns are subsequently determined by supply–demand dynamics in which it is assumed that individuals form partnerships with those that are available. This assumption makes many models analytically tractable.

Several authors have highlighted the shortcomings of the proportionate mixing assumption and a variety of other types of mixing have been proposed, ranging from 'preferred mixing' (Blythe and Castillo-Chavez, 1989), where individuals reserve a certain number of contacts for individuals within their activity class and distribute the rest randomly, to 'structured mixing' (Jacquez *et al.*, 1989) which is a combination of preferred mixing and mixing by demographic preferences. The terms 'assortative mixing' and 'disassortative mixing' have been used by some authors to describe mixing patterns ranging from 'having most contact within their own activity class' to 'mixing mainly with individuals of a different activity class' (Anderson and May, 1991). Common to all those approaches is the idea that an individual, when choosing a partner, has some notion of the sexual activity of the prospective partner. Another implicit assumption in many models is that individuals do not move between activity classes. Empirical research has shown, however, that individuals do in fact move in and out of high-activity groups, and that typical 'life histories' consist of various phases of high and low sexual activity (Reinking *et al.*, 1994).

Another simplifying assumption made in many models is that partnership duration is of negligible importance. Contacts are assumed to be instantaneous and every contact is assumed to be with a new partner. Although this assumption may be true for diseases such as influenza, it is not so for sexual partnerships during which many contacts between the same pair of individuals may occur, especially if partnerships are long lasting. A problem is that in sexual behaviour surveys there is often little or only global information about the duration of partnerships. Although the effects of concurrent partnerships have been investigated, in a model where partnership duration is not explicitly included, the model construction used is somewhat artificial (Watts and May, 1992).

Sexual networks: focusing on the partnership

A first step towards explicitly including partnership dynamics in models of STD transmission was taken by Dietz and Hadeler (1988) when they introduced pair formation models into epidemiology. In these models, the population is subdivided into singles and pairs, and disease transmission takes place between pairs of susceptible and infected persons. Partnerships are characterised by their duration, and are assumed to be monogamous. As a result, the behaviour described in those models is what is called 'sequential monogamy'.

The existence of longer-lasting partnerships together with sequential monogamy can, however, have important consequences for HIV transmission. If an HIV-infected person is highly infectious during the first few weeks of infection and has a much lower infectivity after that, the duration of partnerships can play a major role in determining whether the basic reproduction ratio R_0 is larger or smaller than 1,[1] and also in determining the rate of spread of the epidemic. The value of R_0 provides information about the speed with which an infectious disease can spread in a population, and the level of prevalence that will be attained in endemic equilibrium. Kretzschmar and Dietz (1998) have recently shown that in a population with an average partnership duration of forty days, it can be many years before HIV prevalence reaches detectable levels, while if one neglects partnership duration and considers a model with the same value of the basic reproduction ratio R_0, prevalence levels of 30 per cent can be attained after just a few years. This clearly shows that models that neglect partnership duration cannot be expected to make sound predictions about the epidemic among heterosexuals in Western European countries.

A major shortcoming of pair formation models lies in their assumption that individuals do not have more than one partner at a time, which is not true in the case of many 'core group' individuals. Generalising pair formation models to include concurrent partnerships is possible if one allows only incidental contacts alongside a steady partnership. This covers a large fraction of possible situations. If one wants to model situations in which individuals have more than one longer-lasting partnership simultaneously, restricting the situation to 'triangles' of three individuals connected by two partnerships can be handled (Dietz and Tudor, 1992). With more complex situations, computational problems rapidly arise.

Where there are concurrent partnerships, the contact structure of the population cannot be described as a collection of single and paired individuals. If individuals have more than one partner, their partners can also have more than one partner, and 'chains' of partnerships can exist. Here, groups of individuals are connected to one another by a path of partnerships along which the transmission of infection can take place. The first step towards modelling this situation is simple and the concepts derived from mathematical graph theory can be used to describe the contact pattern.

A graph consists of a set of vertices (points) that are connected by links (see Figure 17.1). In this framework, individuals are the vertices of the graph and the partnerships are the links. In more formal language, one defines a set $V = \{v_1, ..., v_n\}$, where n denotes the population size, and a set $E = \{(i, j) \mid v_i, v_j$ in V, ij is a link$\}$. The number of partners an individual has is described by its degree (i.e. the number of links connected to this particular vertex). The degree distribution is the distribution of the number of links per vertex. So far, this is just a reformulation in abstract terms of the sexual network. Now the key question is, what are the properties of the graph in terms of the degree distribution and other distributional properties that determine the spread of an infectious disease through the network?

A contact graph describes either partnerships accumulated over a time interval or partnerships at one moment in time. In the case of a cumulative graph, the degree distribution can be directly compared with data about the numbers of partners in a given time interval. In the latter case, data about

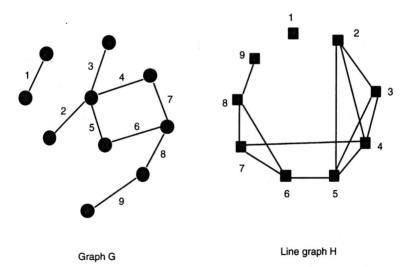

Graph G

Line graph H

Figure 17.1 On the left a graph G is shown with ten vertices and nine links. On the right the line graph H of the graph G is shown. The squares in H represent the links (numbered from 1 to 9) of G, the links in H represent vertices of G

the relational status of individuals at one moment in time are required. Although some relationship can be found between the size of the largest component of the cumulative graph and variables describing disease transmission (Kretzschmar *et al.*, 1995), the interpretation of these results is difficult, because in a cumulative graph information about the timing of partnerships is lost. The order of partnerships in time is, however, crucial for the spread of infection. If A has a partnership with B, and only becomes infected after having separated from B, then B is not at risk of being infected by A. This means that not all paths in a cumulative graph are possible transmission routes.

There are other difficulties in defining a network as the graph of all individuals and their partnerships at one point in time. Apart from the actual sexual encounters, when can we define a partnership as being ongoing? There may be partnerships that consist only of incidental contacts between the individuals concerned, without any plans for future contact. At the beginning of a relationship, partners' expectations may differ. Then there are partnerships that might be perceived as steady, but where sexual contact no longer takes place. These are of course irrelevant for disease transmission. So, when conducting a sexual survey the definition of when a partnership is ongoing may be difficult. In modelling, one usually assumes that while a partnership is ongoing there is some average frequency of sexual contact. This takes the form of either an average frequency of sexual contacts per individual distributed over the available partnerships, or an average frequency of sexual contacts per partnership.

Based on existing stochastic simulation models such as those developed by Blanchard *et al.* (1990), Peterson *et al.* (1990) and Kretzschmar *et al.* (1994), Altmann (1995) has recently developed a deterministic model based on the dynamics of pairs or dyads, which allows for the possibility of concurrent partnerships. In this model, partnerships are distributed at random in a homogeneous population (i.e. the degree distribution in the network approximates to a Poisson distribution). Although the model in its present form cannot deal with more complex degree distributions, it offers an interesting approach to developing analytically tractable models based on dyad dynamics.

Measuring network structure

In a model that included concurrent partnerships (Morris and Kretzschmar, 1995; Kretzschmar and Morris, 1996), it has been shown that the number of partners alone does not determine the course of the development of the epidemic. This particular model described a homogeneous population with a fixed average number of partnerships, but where there is a varying distribution of partnerships in the population. A situation where everybody had at most one partner at a time (sequential monogamy) was compared with a situation where partnerships were distributed randomly, which means that the number of partners per person was approximately Poisson distributed. The course of an epidemic starting from one infected individual differed greatly between these two situations. In the case of sequential monogamy, there was a slow epidemic growth, while with a random distribution of partners the epidemic grew explosively, even though the average number of partners per person did not differ.

The reason for those differences lies in the structure of the contact network. With sequential monogamy there are no concurrent partnerships, but if partnerships are randomly distributed many partnerships are concurrent. In a monogamous population, to pass on infection an individual has first to separate from his or her partner and start a new partnership (i.e. the rate of producing secondary infections is restricted by the average duration of partnerships). This is not the case if many partnerships are concurrent. Here, there may be only a short delay between the infection of an individual and the passing on of infection to the same individual's partner. The size of the largest connected component in the network is therefore correlated with the growth rate of the epidemic.

How can the level of concurrency in a population be determined, and does level of concurrency predict the course of the epidemic? To find a measure of concurrency, Kretzschmar and Morris (1996) took partnerships as the basic unit of the network and looked at how they were connected by individuals. In technical language here one looks at the line graph H of graph G. The line graph H has as vertices the links of the original graph G (see Figure 17.1). Two vertices of H are connected to each other if the respective links in G have a vertex of G in common. In other words, two partnerships are considered concurrent if there is an individual who participates in both of them. At the population level, concurrency can therefore be defined as the mean degree of the line graph H, or the mean number of partnerships that a partnership is concurrent to. In simulations it has been shown that the level of concurrency in a population, measured by the mean degree of the line graph, determines the course of the epidemic. The exponential growth rate of the epidemic in its initial phase increases with increasing concurrency in a linear fashion, if mixing by degree is proportionate (i.e. if there is no bias towards assortative or disassortative mixing).

If there is a tendency towards assortative or disassortative mixing, the situation becomes more complex. Increasing concurrency still leads to increasing epidemic growth rates and higher prevalence, but when mixing is assortative, growth rates increase faster than for disassortative mixing (Morris and Kretzschmar, 1995). This shows that the mean degree of the line graph is not sufficient as an only measure of network structure, and that higher moments of the degree distribution of the line graph play a role in determining the impact of concurrency.

Insights obtained in modelling concurrent partnerships can contribute to the discussion of reasons for the rapid spread of HIV in heterosexual populations of sub-Saharan Africa (Hudson, 1993). Besides the hypothesis that

concurrent STDs may facilitate HIV transmission, and beyond a consideration of 'core groups' and mobility patterns, the existence of long-term
concurrent partnerships provides another possible hypothesis for rapid
transmission (Morris and Kretzschmar, 1997). The possible impact of
concurrent partnerships on the beginning AIDS epidemic has recently been
investigated using data from a sexual behaviour survey in rural Uganda
(Morris and Kretzschmar, forthcoming).

Implications for prevention

Some specific examples will be used to demonstrate how modelling can
provide important insights for prevention. In Kretzschmar *et al.* (1996) a
network-based model was used to investigate the effectiveness of different
prevention strategies for gonorrhoea and genital infections with *Chlamydia
trachomatis* (CT). Spread of these infectious diseases was modelled on an
age-structured population with a highly sexually active 'core group'.
Members of this group could have casual partnerships as well as a steady
partner; all other individuals were posited to be monogamous. The prevention measures analysed were a simple form of contact tracing: namely, the
treatment of partners of symptomatically infected people, the screening of
various subgroups, and condom use. A striking outcome was the high effectiveness of contact tracing in reducing prevalence. Also, consistent condom
use by a part of the population proved effective in reducing prevalence.
Recently, the model has been used in combination with a cost-effectiveness
study to evaluate which groups of the population should be screened for CT
infection in order to avert long-term complications in infected women
(Kretzschmar *et al.*, forthcoming). A clear lesson is that prevention that
includes the partners of infected or targeted individuals (here, through
contact tracing or condom use) can be highly effective. If partners are
treated, or if a partnership is protected through consistent condom use, the
transmission of infection is effectively stopped, whereas if only the infected
individual is treated, the structure of the network remains unchanged and
transmission continues uninterrupted.

In a model of HIV transmission among injecting drug users, the importance of stable networks of relationships within which risk behaviour takes
place was investigated (Kretzschmar and Wiessing, 1998). A homogeneous
population was considered in which there were two types of risk contacts:
the first, through the sharing of injecting equipment with friends or partners
within long-lasting relationships; the other, through sharing in incidental
contacts with strangers. The spread of HIV was slowest in an intermediate
situation, in which the network of stable sharing relationships was dense
enough to make borrowing from strangers unnecessary. If borrowing in incidental contacts with strangers is the only possible way of obtaining injecting
equipment, the epidemic's spread is maximal. These results show the importance of a stable social environment for injecting drug users, but also

demonstrate how the spread of the epidemic depends on the structure of the needle-sharing network. In terms of prevention, one can conclude that it is not sufficient to educate injecting drug users to share less. It is also necessary to stress the importance of who they borrow from. Again it can be concluded that the frequency of risk behaviour is only one aspect of behaviour that should be targeted by prevention; another important aspect is the relationship within which risk behaviour takes place.

A prevention approach that targets not only individuals, but also their partner(s), is even more important for HIV than for other STDs, because effective prevention is as yet the only means we have to fight AIDS. It is increasingly recognised that an individual's behaviour cannot be understood outside the context of the partnership within which it takes place, and cannot be reduced to simple quantities such as the rate of partner change.

It is interesting that a shift of perspective from individuals to partnerships has also taken place in sociological research. Recently, Hubert *et al.* (1998) concluded that research in prevention against HIV has focused too much on the behaviour of individuals and has not taken sufficiently into account the influence of partnerships in determining behaviour.

Future research

Although much insight has been gained in the last two decades into human sexual behaviour and its influence on STD and HIV transmission, much still remains to be learned. Especially in developing a network-based approach to STDs and their prevention, existing tools have to be sharpened and theoretical insights have to be further developed (Morris, 1997).

A first step will be to modify existing sexual behaviour surveys so as to collect new data about networks of partnerships instead of individual sexual behaviour. Besides network studies such as those conducted by Haraldsdottir *et al.* (1992) and Woodhouse *et al.* (1994), a few individual-based surveys have tried to obtain more information about partnerships and the partners of individual respondents. It is, for example, possible to ask individuals to report on all their sexual partnerships in the last year with dates of first and last sexual contact, and whether the partnership is still ongoing, in order to get a more dynamic picture of onset and duration of sexual partnerships. However, more research is needed on the variables that can be asked about that lead to reasonably reliable answers.

A second key area of research concerns statistical methods for the estimation of model parameters from sexual surveys. Morris (1991) has introduced a log–linear framework for estimating parameters of the mixing matrix, and Hsu Schmitz and Castillo-Chavez (1994) have developed methods for the estimation of mixing matrices. Using different methods Blower (1993) and Garnett and Anderson (1993) have estimated rates of partner change in different activity classes in a UK sexual behaviour study. As yet, there are no standard methods for parameter estimation for other types of models.

Ghani *et al.* (1997), Altmann *et al.* (1994) and Rothenberg *et al.* (1995) among others have discussed the question of what are relevant quantities that determine the spread of an infection throughout a sexual network.

A promising approach involves the comparative analysis of different diseases that spread on the same network. This is likely to yield information about the key features of the underlying network if a modelling approach is applied to analyse the empirical data. An important area of research here may be the comparative analysis of HIV, HBV and HCV spread among heterosexual and injecting drug user populations. Not only are there different diseases with different transmission parameters involved, but also two interacting transmission routes. Additionally, the effectiveness of different prevention strategies may be different for different diseases (Kretzschmar *et al.*, 1996).

Finally, putting everything into the perspective of public health and health care systems, the cost-effectiveness of prevention strategies is becoming more important and future research is needed to tie cost-effectiveness analysis to epidemic modelling.

Note

1   The basic reproduction ratio is the number of secondary cases that one infected individual produces during his or her entire infectious period in a completely susceptible population.

References

ACSF investigators (1992) 'AIDS and sexual behaviour in France', *Nature* 360: 407–409.

Altmann, M. (1995) 'SIR epidemic model with dynamic partnerships', *Journal of Mathematical Biology* 33: 661–675.

Altmann, M., Wee, B. C., Willard, K., Peterson, D. and Gatewood, L. (1994) 'Network analytic methods for epidemiological risk assessment', *Statistics in Medicine* 13: 53–60.

Anderson, R. M. and May, R. M. (1991) *Infectious Diseases of Humans: Dynamics and Control*, Oxford: Oxford University Press.

Anderson, R. M., Gupta, S. and Ng, W. (1990) 'The significance of sexual partner contact networks for the transmission dynamics of HIV', *Journal of the Acquired Immunodeficiency Syndromes* 3: 417–29.

Blanchard, Ph., Bolz, G. F. and Krüger, T. (1990) 'Modeling AIDS epidemics or any venereal diseases on random graphs', in J. P. Gabriel *et al.* (eds) *Stochastic Processes in Epidemic Theory*, Lecture Notes in Biomathematics, Vol. 86: 104–117, Berlin: Springer.

Blower, S. M. (1993) 'Exploratory data analysis of three sexual behaviour surveys: implications for HIV-1 transmission in the UK', *Philosophical Transactions of the Royal Society* B 339: 33–51.

Blythe, S. P. and Castillo-Chavez, C. (1989) 'Like-with-like preference and sexual mixing models', *Mathematical Biosciences* 96: 221–238.

Dietz, K. and Hadeler, K. P. (1988) 'Epidemiological models for sexually transmitted diseases', *Journal of Mathematical Biology* 26: 1–25.

Dietz, K. and Tudor, D. (1992) 'Triangles in heterosexual HIV transmission', in N. P. Jewell *et al.* (eds) *AIDS Epidemiology: Methodological Issues*, Boston: Birkhauser.

Downs, A. M., Heisterkamp, S. H., Brunet, J. B. and Hamers, F. F. (1997) 'Reconstruction and prediction of the HIV/AIDS epidemic among adults in the European Union and in the low prevalence countries of central and eastern Europe', *AIDS* 11: 649–662.

Garnett, G. P. and Anderson, R. M. (1993) 'Contact tracing and the estimation of sexual mixing patterns: the epidemiology of gonococcal infections', *Sexually Transmitted Diseases* 20: 181–191.

Ghani, A. C., Swinton, J. and Garnett, G. P. (1997) 'The role of sexual partnership networks in the epidemiology of gonorrhoea', *Sexually Transmitted Diseases* 24: 45–56.

Haraldsdottir, S., Gupta, S. and Anderson, R. M. (1992) 'Preliminary studies of sexual networks in a male homosexual community in Iceland', *Journal of AIDS* 5: 374–381.

Hendriks, J. C. M., Satten, G. A., van Ameijden, E. J. C., van Druten, J. A. M., Coutinho, R. A. and van Griensven, G. J. P. (1998) 'The incubation period to AIDS in injecting drug users estimated from prevalent cohort data, accounting for death prior to an AIDS diagnosis', *AIDS* 12: 1537–1544.

Hethcote, H. W. and Yorke, J. A. (1984) *Gonorrhea Transmission Dynamics and Control*, Lecture Notes in Biomathematics, Vol. 56, Berlin: Springer.

Hsu Schmitz, S. F. and Castillo-Chavez, C. (1994) 'Parameter estimation in non-closed social networks related to the dynamics of sexually transmitted diseases', in E. H. Kaplan and M. Brandeau (eds) *Modeling the AIDS Epidemic: Planning, Policy, and Prediction*, New York: Raven Press.

Hubert, M. C., Bajos, N. and Sandfort, Th. G. M. (eds) (1998) *Sexual Behaviour and HIV/AIDS in Europe*, London: UCL Press.

Hudson, C. (1993) 'Concurrent partnerships could cause AIDS epidemics', *International Journal of STD and AIDS* 4: 349–353.

Jacquez, J. A., Simon, C. P. and Koopman, J. (1989) 'Structured mixing: heterogeneous mixing by the definition of activity groups', in C. Castillo-Chavez (ed.) *Mathematical and Statistical Approaches to AIDS Epidemiology*, Lecture Notes in Biomathematics, Vol. 83: 301–315, Berlin: Springer.

Jacquez, J. A., Koopman, J. S., Simon, C. P. and Longini Jr, I. M. (1994) 'Role of the primary infection in epidemics of HIV infection in gay cohorts', *Journal of Acquired Immunodeficiency Syndromes* 7: 1169–1184.

Johnson, A. M., Wadsworth, J., Wellings, K. and Field, J. (1994) *Sexual Attitudes and Lifestyles*, Oxford: Blackwell Scientific.

Kaplan, E. H. and Brandeau, M. (eds) (1994) *Modeling the AIDS Epidemic: Planning, Policy, and Prediction*, New York: Raven Press.

Kretzschmar, M. and Dietz, K. (1998) 'The effect of pair formation and variable infectivity on the spread of an infection without recovery', *Mathematical Biosciences* 148: 83–113.

Kretzschmar, M. and Morris, M. (1996) 'Measures of concurrency in networks and the spread of infectious disease', *Mathematical Biosciences* 133: 165–195.

Kretzschmar, M. and Wiessing, L. G. (1998) 'Modelling the spread of HIV in social networks of injecting drug users', *AIDS* 12: 801–811.

Kretzschmar, M., Reinking, D. P., Jager, J. C., Brouwers, H., and Zessen, G. van (1994) 'Network models: from paradigm to mathematical tool', in E. H. Kaplan and M. Brandeau (eds) *Modeling the AIDS Epidemic: Planning, Policy, and Prediction*, New York: Raven Press.

Kretzschmar, M., Jager, J. C., Reinking, D. P., Zessen, G. van and Brouwers, H. (1995) 'A network modelling approach for assessing the efficiency of prevention strategies', *Journal of Mathematical Sociology* 20: 351–374.

Kretzschmar, M., Duynhoven, Y. T. H. P. van and Severijnen, A. J. (1996) 'Modeling prevention strategies for gonorrhea and chlamydia using stochastic network simulations', *American Journal of Epidemiology* 144: 306–317.

Kretzschmar, M., Welte, R., Hoek, J. A. R. van den and Postma, M. J. (1999) 'A comparative model-based analysis of screening programs for *Chlamydia trachomatis* infections', to be published.

Longini Jr, I. M., Clark, W. S., Byers, R. H., Ward, J. W., Darrow, W. W., Lemp, G. F. and Hethcote, H. W. (1989) 'Statistical analysis of the stages of HIV infection using a Markov model', *Statistics in Medicine* 8: 831–843.

Morris, M. (1991) 'A log-linear modeling framework for selective mixing', *Mathematical Biosciences* 107: 349–377.

——(1997) 'Sexual networks and HIV', *AIDS* 11 (Suppl. A): S209–S216.

Morris, M. and Kretzschmar, M. (1995) 'Concurrent partnerships and transmission dynamics in networks', *Social Networks* 17: 299–318.

——1997) 'Concurrent partnerships and the spread of HIV', *AIDS* 11: 641–648.

——(1998) 'A micro-simulation study of the effect of concurrent partnerships on the spread of HIV in Uganda', to be published.

Peterson, D., Willard, K., Altmann, M., Gatewood, L., and Davidson, G. (1990) 'Monte Carlo simulation of HIV infection in an intravenous drug user community', *Journal of Acquired Immunodeficiency Syndrome* 3: 1086–1095.

Reinking, D. P., Zessen, G. van, Kretzschmar, M., Brouwers, H., Jager, J. C. and Stringer, P. (1994) 'Social transmission routes of HIV. A combined sexual network and life course perspective', *Patient Education and Counseling* 24: 289–297.

Rothenberg, R. B., Potterat, J. J., Woodhouse, D. E., Darrow, W. W., Muth, S. Q. and Klovdahl, A. S. (1995) 'Choosing a centrality measure: epidemiologic correlates in the Colorado Springs study of social networks', *Social Networks* 17: 273–297.

Watts, C. H. and May, R. M. (1992) 'The influence of concurrent partnerships on the dynamics of HIV/AIDS', *Mathematical Biosciences* 108: 89–104.

Woodhouse, D. E. *et al.* (1994) 'Mapping a social network of heterosexuals at high risk for HIV infection', *AIDS* 8: 1331–1336.

18 Understanding risk management

Towards an integration of
individual, interactive and social
levels

Geneviève Paicheler

It is a truism to say that the fear inspired by AIDS does not directly lead to preventive behaviour. Numerous KABP (Knowledge, Attitudes, Beliefs and Practices) studies have established no direct link between information and action (Peruga and Celentano, 1993). Many of these studies have been largely inspired by the Health Belief Model (Rosenstock, 1974), which has been widely criticised (e.g. Bloor, 1995a, 1995b; Fee and Krieger, 1993) and alternative approaches have been proposed. Instead of trying to impose preconceived models onto knowledge and practice, phenomenological approaches, which study how people integrate the threat of AIDS and what they actually do about it, should be adopted.

This chapter hypothesises that preventive behaviour is linked more to the perception of personal risk and therefore to socially constructed vulnerability than to knowledge or attitudes concerning illness. We will first examine how these notions have been formalised according to individualistic and psychosocial frames. These approaches conceptualise the process through which people come to adopt new behaviours as an educational process, imposed on individuals. They stress that individuals be equipped with the resources they lack, such as knowledge or new skills. Reflection on AIDS prevention to date has questioned this approach and has led to the adoption of more complex and global frameworks that focus on individuals' comprehension of the social and situational logic influencing their behaviours.

Risk: a polysemic notion

Understanding, or giving meaning to illness, is a fundamental social process amply described in the social sciences. Obviously, this process concerns AIDS, an illness that has become exemplary because it is both epidemic and lethal. Moreover, the public has to do more than simply assimilate necessary and sufficient information in order to practise appropriate preventive behaviour. Confronted with uncertainty and a plethora of information from diverse sources, lay people engage in an intense activity of sorting and interpretation as they are forced to situate themselves in terms of risk (Warwick *et al.*, 1988).

Risk offers a modern way of understanding pathological danger (Scott and Freeman, 1995) as an omnipresent and invasive sanitary threat to both populations and individuals (Armstrong, 1993). However, it does not provide a clear view of the danger involved nor a precise evaluation of it (Douglas and Wildavsky, 1982). A polysemic and contradictory notion (Hayes, 1992), the concept of risk applies to both external factors, over which no control is possible, and conditions considered under the control of individuals, such as pathogenic lifestyles. Furthermore, the concept of risk assumes a process that obeys laws based on a long series of observations from which it is paradoxically possible to isolate oneself individually.

For some authors, who assume that people exert full control over their conduct, self-control is a prerequisite for health (Greco, 1993). If people get ill, it is a result either of personal weakness or of free choice. Yet, empirical studies of risk taking often note the difficulties individuals face in having a clear vision of the alternatives, in assessing the probabilities of events and the consequences of action. In contrast, Douglas (1992) situates the problematic of risk in a cultural perspective. For her, risk is a modern way of contemplating danger by evaluating it in terms of probability, in a context of uncertainty. However, this ostensibly more scientific perspective does not prevent risk selection from being heavily influenced by moral criteria.

The individualistic vision of risk has been the object of numerous critiques (Bloor *et al.*, 1992). It underplays the social, cultural, moral and political dimensions of risk, especially as they relate to health (Lupton, 1993; Gabe, 1995). It assumes that if individuals or scientific evaluators make an incorrect evaluation about given risks, it is because the instruments of evaluation are flawed. Thus, objective and rational perception serves as a reference but, for lay people, risk is translated into the terms of subjective, lived experience. Accordingly, that one perceives risk at a societal level does not automatically imply that one feels personally at risk. However, understanding of personal risk, combined with the objective margin of action allowed by concrete situations, does shape how people manage the risk.

In all of the theories reviewed here, two notions are evident: vulnerability and control. This chapter will focus on the ways these notions are used in individualistic, or situational/interactional frames. The importance of vulnerability/control factors in the management of health risk was first demonstrated in the 1950s (Janis and Feshbach, 1953). If one assumes that a link exists between fear and perception of actual vulnerability, playing up this potentially powerful emotion can only lead to a change in behaviour if the feeling of vulnerability can be controlled by an endorsed action. If the fear is too strong, we will witness instead flight, denial or paralysing panic.

Individualistic theories

Some theories develop these vulnerability/control concepts according to the individualistic mode of confronting a problem, danger or risk (e.g. the Health Belief Model). Alternatively, they are integrated into a vision of personality or of permanent traits (e.g. via locus of control theory). These theories' individualistic dimension has been and still is an easy target for criticism. Nevertheless, it constitutes a fundamental and much esteemed way of thinking and acting in western societies.

The Health Belief Model

The Health Belief Model (HBM) was elaborated according to a logic of rationality and individual choice (Rosenstock, 1974). In this sense, it is close to models of the microeconomic strategy of maximising advantages and minimising costs. In order to understand the adoption of a health behaviour, one must consider two types of beliefs. The first concerns the extent of the health threat, while the second refers to the belief in efficiency of a particular behaviour in reducing this threat. In the case of AIDS, for example, belief in a threat to health depends on three factors: how much health is valued; specific beliefs about vulnerability (e.g. having sex without a condom can give one AIDS); and beliefs about the consequences or seriousness of the illness (AIDS is deadly). In order for the adoption of a behaviour to be linked to a reduction in the health threat (e.g. using condoms allows one to avoid AIDS), one must believe in the effectiveness of this preventive action. In addition, the costs of this new behaviour must not be greater than its benefits (while it is difficult to use condoms, this is preferable to getting AIDS).

This model has proved insufficient for explaining changes in behaviour, as well as the persistence of risky behaviours among individuals fully conscious that they endanger their own health. Because it is strictly situated on an individual level, this model necessarily underestimates the influence of social ties on individual decisions. Finally, the model tends to present decision making through a rather mechanistic schema of benefits maximisation. This individualistic dimension has been the subject of much criticism (Bloor, 1995a, 1995b; Fee and Krieger, 1993). Nevertheless, this model makes an important contribution by stressing the centrality of beliefs. Regardless of the reality of the pathogenic threat, its subjective reality depends on how it is perceived and integrated in a universe of beliefs. The model integrates two of our central concepts – vulnerability and control – in the form of belief in the efficacy of behaviour.

Locus of control

In the HBM, the individual is presented as a responsible, rational and free actor, motivated by the desire to live as long as possible in good health. This model is only pertinent if individuals have both real control over their life and a feeling of control. At the centre of the 'locus of control concept' is the feeling of individual control, conceived as a permanent trait of personality (Rotter, 1966). Those who have an internal locus of control think that they can act on the events affecting them. In contrast, individuals with an external locus of control think that external agents or uncontrollable circumstances are responsible for these events. Wallston and Wallston (1982) have developed a locus of control scale specific to health. This notion has implications for the adoption of preventive behaviour. 'External' individuals will be less likely to adopt health behaviour than 'internal' individuals, because only the latter accept personal responsibility for their own state of health.

Since individuals with an external locus of control are considered more impervious to prevention, the aim is to instil in them knowledge and feelings of self-control so that they will be able to adopt healthy behaviours. Nonetheless, the notion of locus of control is built in a social and cultural vacuum. Concurrently, those individuals with the greatest social deficits and shortfalls are shown to be the same people who are farthest from having integrated a correctly understood model of prevention.

The concept of locus of control is strongly marked by the Protestant ethic of 'where there's a will, there's a way'. Implicitly revering individuals with internal control, it does not account for the circumstances that lead to an external locus of control. Is it by accident that women, for instance, have become progressively more conscious of the external constraints weighing on them and their actions? Locus of control is treated as a collection of personality traits when the question could be better addressed by analysing which social situations and contexts allow people control or a feeling of control over their health.

Psychosocial theories

Compared with HBM, other psychosocial models such as the theory of reasoned action give greater emphasis to the normative values that influence individual decisions. They also conceptualise control as a collection of malleable traits acquired by practice and experience in a favourable social environment (self-efficacy). Such psychosocial theories strive to integrate social variables, such as norms and social support, in order to explain how individuals adopt preventive conducts and to inform preventive actions directed towards them.

Theory of reasoned action

Fishbein and Ajzen's (1975) model should allow for behavioural prediction because it postulates that people act according to their intentions. This assertion would be quite trivial were it not accompanied by a reflection on how intentions are determined by two series of factors: attitudes and social pressure. This theory assumes that attitudes are expressed in behaviour itself via two factors: expectations, and values linked to the anticipated outcome. When applied to AIDS prevention, the model predicts that people's risky as well as protective behaviours will, first of all, depend upon a variety of beliefs about the behaviour and its outcomes. The second factor acting on behaviour, social pressure, depends on both normative beliefs and the motivation to comply. The former refers to the opinion of others regarding what one should do in a particular situation and the value accorded to this opinion. Thus, individuals will be more likely to use a condom if they have the impression that using one has become the norm in their group, especially if identity with this group is strong and positive.

This theory has difficulties taking into account factors such as force of habit, routine behaviour, and the role of emotions like pleasure or fear which are so important in sexuality, and thus in the prevention of AIDS. However, some proponents of that theory recognise that an intention cannot be actualised through behaviour unless circumstances permit it, and that behaviour can occur without a clear and conscious intention having been formulated beforehand. In a study on an AIDS prevention behavioural intervention, Fishbein and his colleagues (1997) found a relatively low correlation between the intention to use a condom and effective condom use ($r = 0.54$ for men and 0.26 for women).

More positively, this model does account for the influence of social integration. So as not to be perceived as deviant and be rejected, individuals act in relation to what they think others expect from them. This social dimension is crucial. However, it only exists in the perception of individuals, rather than in external conditions and sanctions.

Personal effectiveness, social influence and situation

For Bandura (1992), two beliefs simultaneously influence behaviour: belief in the effectiveness of a particular behaviour for resolving a given problem, and the belief in self-efficacy or the feeling that one can obtain a desired objective by successfully adopting a particular behaviour. Being used to having control over social situations allows for the construction and reinforcement of personal efficacy. AIDS prevention demands that individuals exert influence over their own motivation and behaviour (Bandura, 1992). In order to provoke change, they must not only have reasons to control the risk but also the necessary means, resources and social support. They perceive their choices, mobilisation, perseverance and commitment to the action as results of their own capabilities. If they do not think they possess such capacities, they cannot manage risky situations, even if they know what to do. The feeling of inefficacy creates a gap between knowledge and self-preventive action. As Bandura (1992: 90) put it:

> The major problem is not teaching people safer sex guidelines, which is easily achievable, but equipping them with skills that enable them to put the guidelines consistently into practice in the face of counteracting influences. Difficulties arise in following safer sex practices because self-protection often conflicts with interpersonal pressures and sentiments. In these interpersonal situations, the sway of coercive threat, allure-ments, desire for social acceptance, social pressures, situational constraints, and fear of rejection and personal embarrassment can over-ride the influence of the best of informed judgment. The weaker the perceived self-efficacy, the more such social and affective factors can increase the likelihood of risky sexual behaviour.

Situational and social resources and mastery

Mastery or control cannot be treated only as individual characteristics or as latitude of decision. Mastery involves several dimensions. The first is intel-lectual mastery, or an understanding of the problem or danger that can be transposed into concrete action. It is always possible to comply with preven-tive recommendations without truly understanding them, but preventive conduct will be even more robust if people have an intellectual mastery of the given problem.

The second dimension is the ability to have mastery in an interaction, including possibilities of negotiation. AIDS prevention is not a problem that one can resolve alone, nor a decision that one can make by oneself. Each person's actions depend on the actions and reactions of their partner, on the hierarchy or balance of power in a relationship, and on each person's moti-vations and investment in prevention. This interaction will then undercut or confirm feelings of mastery.

It goes without saying that situations and possibilities for interaction are connected: interaction constitutes one of the constraints of a situation. It is determined by one's position in a social space structured by fundamental oppositions: masculine/feminine, active/passive, in love/indifferent, depen-dent/independent, etc. Situations may or may not reinforce the power relations between partners. Likewise, they may or may not enable intentions to be transformed into conduct.

A phenomenological approach to a theory of social action

The approaches that will be presented here do not assume that the tech-niques of 'prevention experts' are the only way to deal with a health risk.

Rather, they explore the actual ways in which people define risk for themselves and use personal resources to deal with it in their lives.

In his study of risk management among male sex workers in Glasgow, Bloor (1995a) developed a phenomenological analysis which, inspired by the work of Schutz (1970), integrated power relations into the transaction relation. He showed how, in order to master the situation, male sex workers had to strip away the ambiguity that would otherwise surround the encounter. Unsafe sex was associated with client control and safer sex denied clients the interactional initiative.

A phenomenological approach to a theory of social action focuses on unconsidered behaviour and on taken-for-granted understanding. Some risk behaviour may be calculative, but other risk activities may be undertaken on a routine basis, without prior calculation or even any perception of the availability of alternative possible actions. In the world of routine activities, there is no distinction to be made between interpretation and 'recipes of action'.

In novel situations, judgement may be suspended while the person inaugurates a 'subsidiary project' in order to arrive at a satisfactory interpretation. Topical relevances refer to the voluntary pursuit of an interpretation. Interpretative relevances are the limited range of elements in the individual's stock of knowledge to which the situation in question may be compared (with different degree of certitude: possibility, plausibility, probability). Motivational relevances will determine how far the search for an interpretation is pursued and the degree of certitude required. Having arrived at an interpretation, the person may consider which among several associated 'recipes for actions' to embark upon. Different recipes of action are attached to a given interpretation. Some recipes are performable in the situation and others not. Some may imply a certain risk.

This model therefore distinguishes between routine and on-the-spot risk management, the latter demanding an effort of interpretation and which is constrained by the situation and the interaction.

Perceptions of risk and actions: a circular approach

Since knowledge about AIDS transmission seems good in the general population, many observers are surprised that not more people practise behaviours, like safer sex, to minimise risk of contracting the disease. Yet, previous studies have shown that there is not a direct link between knowledge and behaviour. Descriptions based on people's concrete experiences are therefore needed. Through a qualitative research, based on sixty-one in-depth interviews conducted in France, my aim has been to describe how people understand the threat of AIDS, and how they face the risk of transmission in their sex lives (Paicheler, 1994, 1996).

In order to understand how people develop preventive actions, we must learn how information is interpreted and how knowledge is integrated so that individuals perceive general or personal risk. We must also specify the way in which people distinguish between aspects of risk perception and vulnerability; feelings of personal control, constructed on the basis of social experiences; characteristics of situations; and finally, the dynamics of action. The proposed risk management model accounts for these diverse factors in elucidating the great diversity of actions reported. This dynamic, non-linear model has been designed to capture both the impact of perceptive and cognitive elements on action, and vice versa.

The perception of personal risk is elaborated in terms of one's own feelings of vulnerability and the possibility of protection from danger. Douglas and Calvez' (1990) analysis distinguishes two categories of individual protection: the 'corporal envelope' and the 'social envelope'. A third category should be added to this analysis. When protection seems impossible and when people display a catastrophic view of danger, they are therefore at the highest level of vulnerability.

Managing the risk of sexual transmission of HIV varies depending on whether one is male or female, younger or older, and whether one lives in a world that is financially and professionally stable, or in which precariousness is an omnipresent threat. Actions reported during the interviews offer a very composite palette. Several factors converge to contribute to particular configurations at any given moment. These include representations of the body; identity; feelings of vulnerability, security or efficacy; position in a sexual trajectory; perception of risk; subjective distance from the illness; ethical orientations, etc. Knowledge probably also intervenes, but indirectly.

Individual and interactive strategies combine to compose a complex collection of risk management methods. On one hand, the diversity of actions depends on the perception of risk and the constraints and resources of the situation. On the other hand, the feeling of security that these strategies can ultimately provide can be linked to knowledge, but it is also associated with a vision of the world and of the self, and with a conception of one's self-efficacy.

The different kinds of risk management can be differentiated: preventive, centred around using a condom and necessarily interactive; protective, favouring individual forms of risk management like abstinence, selection of partners; or mixed, combining the use of a condom with other forms of protection depending on the situations, and interactive capacities.

Whatever actions are used to protect oneself from danger, people can derive a sense of security from the belief that their actions are sufficient and efficient, or they can decide that these do not allow them to control the risk. This feeling of security does not only depend on the actions performed. It is also associated with risk perception which is informed by feelings of personal or social vulnerability, in turn linked to earlier experiences. This perception conditions whether one feels one is controlling the risk. Yet actions are not only dependent on perceptions; they are also subordinated to the constraints and resources that characterise the specific situations in which they take place. Feelings of security, which can effect vulnerability and risk management, vary in strength depending on the intensity of the perception of risk and the possibilities that a given action will be more or less adequate. The components of risk management form a dynamic system in which all of the elements are in constant interaction (see Figure 18.1).

When facing a danger, people may perceive they are unable to escape from it and therefore they develop a catastrophic view of their situation: they are exposed to an unpredictable threat. They may perceive their own body as strongly protected or quite exposed to the outside threat as the virus entry routes are numerous and fuzzy. Also, they may perceive their community or their group as a good or bad shield against danger, and accordingly feel secured or unsecured by their social identity. It is the combination of three forms of perceived vulnerability in terms of catastrophe, bodily threat and social threat that allows for the comprehension of actions and their diversity, accounting for the effect of how much control people feel they exercise over themselves, others and the world. That which is controllable is obviously linked to that which is predictable. Prevention therefore relies on a dynamic of empowerment which occurs not only by integrating information, but also by being able to discern a controllable risk and managing it to the best of one's ability. The model presented here stresses context so as to allow for the articulation of risk perception and action. At the level of socio-cognitive processes, it suggests a complex perception of risk that is developed on several registers. It builds on the ideas contained in earlier models – vulnerability, control, self-efficacy – but, by drawing on concepts and findings from social psychology, sociology and anthropology, it provides

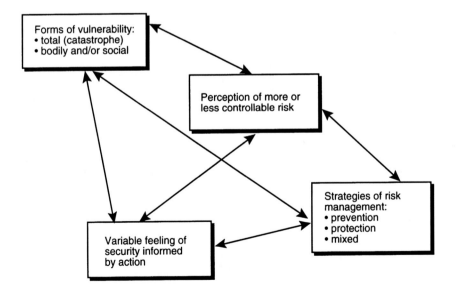

Figure 18.1 Components of risk management

a broader interpretation than one that is purely individualistic. Finally, it considers the links between risk perception and action, not in a linear perspective from cognition to action, but in an interactive way. Action, while dependent on processes of interpretation, engenders ways of perceiving risk and orienting feelings of vulnerability by enacting the possibility or impossibility of mastery.

The in-depth individual interview method of data collection, which only allows us to consider the impact of factors of interaction and context through the accounts of the people interviewed, limited our capacity to explore the adequacy of the model.

Women's heterosexual experiences provide a useful case for understanding when mastery of actions, interactions and situations might not allow for strategies of risk management that are consistent with intentions. Different women have more or less resources for getting their partners to use condoms. Relations of power between men and women are generally not to the advantage of the latter, which is why women sometimes adopt complex strategies in trying to manage risk.

While preventive recommendations often suggest that condom use be discussed and negotiated before a sexual act, it is not always possible to act on this advice. In fact, men and women usually find themselves in a situation of unequal control regarding the condom (Campbell, 1995; Carovano, 1991; Holland *et al.*, 1990; Kippax *et al.*, 1990; Krieger and Margo, 1990; Waldby *et al.*, 1993). Men can always use one without having to ask their partner, but, if men do not suggest it, women have to ask, and sometimes demand it. Based on our interviews, negotiation is sometimes conflictual and difficult, and women may legitimise condom use by arguing that it serves to prevent pregnancy. One option is to present the choice of either a sexual act with a condom or no sexual act. But, in fact, in these cases dependency and feeling of vulnerability are high, and risk is perceived as difficult to master. Actions are dependent on the partner and the margin of negotiation is reduced.

Let us take an example. For Thérèse (38 years), who is employed as a secretary and is single, and who considers herself 'the epitome of the non-informed', danger is both omnipresent and uncontrollable. AIDS is a real threat, a 'concern' that worries her, because she knows that she has taken risks in her 'very dispersed' sex life. She does not have the comfort of 'the confidence of a stable relationship'. 'We can know what precautions we should take, but that doesn't mean we can act on them. Things don't always work out without a hitch'. She says that she usually has condoms on her but 'sometimes, things happen too fast', and she does not always 'pay attention'. What bothers her most is that one has to use them 'at the very beginning', during the uncertain and undetermined moment of amorous conquest. Desire is thwarted when calculation and planning take over that which one would like to consider unpredictable or improvised.

It's definitely true that just being ready to anticipate in that way makes you less into it ... You have to think about those kinds of things calmly, but that almost leads you to renounce altogether.

In addition, condoms 'limit the romp', particularly fellatio: 'if it's with a condom, I won't do it'. Since the test has to be 'performed again every day', the only 'remedy' would be fidelity, but that is not compatible with her sexual activity, because she is not 'in a stable couple'. 'We're always ready to do without condoms', she says, reversing a common slogan. She hates to have to demand their use sometimes, which leads her to consider that her lovers do not practise prevention and that they 'could get stuff and then transmit it'. For her, danger is everywhere, among her probably imprudent lovers, in different contacts and diverse practices. She tries to hang on to categorisation that proves not very reassuring: 'as long as someone isn't a junkie or a homosexual, you think that he is already less at risk, but that's not true'. Since her lovers would only say 'what they want to say', so that she cannot trust them, she thinks she has to do all she can to use condoms or abstain, but does not really do this. 'In fact, the whole thing for me boils down to this: abstain or take the risk.'

Other examples of dependent feminine strategies can be found among women who are involved in serious relationships, doubt their partner's fidelity, but refuse to jeopardise their relationships by addressing this question directly. Note that more women doubt the fidelity of their partner than men, who tend to feel extremely protected when they are involved in serious relationships. Thus, 20-year-old Corrine drags her companion to a blood transfusion centre so as to assure herself of his serological status. Julie, a 38-year-old designer, is loyal to her apparently fickle companion. Because of this, she protects the familial peace by regularly checking her own serological status.

As we see, women may be receptive to arguments about prevention but they do not always have control over their partners. Interaction or negotiations around prevention are that much harder because they put a valued relationship in jeopardy. It is therefore easier to forgo entirely a relationship considered risky than to manage perfectly the uncertain risks that can emerge in a stable relationship. The danger of losing the partner or of damaging the relationship is therefore more present than the potentiality of AIDS transmission.

Conclusions

Because individualistic theories of risk management are too rationalist and exclusively cognitive, they cannot properly account for the link between knowledge and action which is mediated by perceptions of risk. Likewise, they fail to explain the internal dynamic of action whereby emotional, cognitive and social activity and interaction appear linked. Because of this deficiency and the need to untangle several complex behaviours, we have tried to develop new theories capable of accounting for this complexity. We have argued for the importance of transcending individualistic, mechanistic, reductive and predetermined models to develop a more phenomenological analysis of action. Risk perception and management depends more on the contexts and situations that provide resources to individuals than on knowledge or intrinsic individual characteristics. Moreover, the links between risk perception and action must be considered not in a linear perspective from cognition to action as is usually done, but in an interactive perspective. Action, while dependent on processes of interpretation and risk perception, may also engender new ways of perceiving risk. For instance, varying experiences with mastery, or lack thereof, can foster alternatively feelings of vulnerability or control. Such a global approach is necessary for conceiving prevention programmes based on a dynamic of empowerment.

Acknowledgements

The author's research described in this chapter was funded by the Agence Nationale de Recherche sur le Sida (ANRS) of France. Thanks to Abigail Cope Saguy for the translation of this chapter. Elements of this chapter have been published as 'Perception of HIV risk and preventative strategies: a dynamic analysis', *Health* 3(1): 47–70, and are reproduced here by permission of Sage Publications.

References

Armstrong, D. (1993) 'Public health spaces and the fabrication of identity', *Sociology* 27(2): 393–410.

Bandura, A. (1992) 'A social cognitive approach of the exercise of control over AIDS infection', in R. DiClemente (ed.) *Adolescents and AIDS: A Generation in Jeopardy*, London: Sage.

Bloor, M. (1995a) *The Sociology of HIV Transmission*, London: Sage.

——(1995b) 'A user's guide to contrasting theories of HIV-related risk behaviour', in J. Gabe (ed.) *Medicine, Health and Risk*, Oxford: Blackwell.

Bloor, M., McKeganey, N., Finlay, A. and Barnard, M. (1992) 'The inappropriateness of psycho-social models of risk behaviour to understanding HIV-related risk behaviour among Glasgow male prostitutes', *AIDS Care* 4: 131–137.

Campbell, C. A. (1995) 'Male gender roles and sexuality: implications for Women's AIDS risk and prevention', *Social Science and Medicine* 41(2): 197–210.

Carovano, K. (1991) 'More than mothers and whores: redefining the AIDS prevention needs of women', *International Journal of Health Services* 21(1): 131–142.

Douglas, M. (1992) *Risk and Blame*, London and New York: Routledge.

Douglas, M. and Calvez, M. (1990) 'The self as risk-taker: a cultural theory of contagion in relation to AIDS', *Sociological Review* 38(3): 445–464.

Douglas, M. and Wildavsky, A. (1982) *Risk and Culture*, Berkeley, CA: University of California Press.

Fee, E. and Krieger, N. (1993) 'Understanding AIDS: historical interpretations and the limits of biomedical individualism', *American Journal of Public Health* 83(10): 1477–1486.

Fishbein, M. and Ajzen, I. (1975) *Belief, Attitude, Intention and Behaviour: An Intro-duction to Theory and Research*, Reading, MA: Addison-Wesley.

Fishbein, M., Hennessy, M., Rhodes, F., Malotte, C. K., Kent, C., Hoxworth, T. and the Project RESPECT Study Group (1997) 'Estimating the intention-behaviour correlation for consistent condom use: results from a multi-site longitudinal study', Presentation at the 3rd International Conference 'AIDS Impact: Biopsy-chosocial Aspects of HIV Infection', Melbourne, Australia, June.

Gabe, J. (1995) 'Health, medicine and risk: the need for a sociological approach', in J. Gabe (ed.) *Medicine, Health and Risk*, Oxford: Blackwell.

Greco, M. (1993) 'Psychosomatic subjects and the "Duty of the Will": personal agency within medical rationality', *Economy and Society* 22(3): 357–372.

Hayes, M. V. (1992) 'On the epistemology of risk: language, logic and social science', *Social Science and Medicine* 35(4): 401–407.

Holland, J., Ramazanoglu, C., Scott, S., Sharpe, S. and Thomson, R. (1990) 'Sex, gender and power: young women's sexuality in the shadow of AIDS', *Sociology of Health and Illness* 12: 336–350.

Janis, I. L. and Feshbach, S. (1953) 'Effects of fear arousing communication', *Journal of Abnormal Psychology* 48: 78–92.

Kippax, S., Crawford, J., Waldby, C. and Benton, P. (1990) 'Women negotiating heterosex: implications for HIV prevention', *Women's Studies International Forum* 13: 533–542.

Krieger, N. and Margo, G. (1990) 'Women and AIDS', Introduction to 'Section on AIDS: the politics of survival', *International Journal of Health Services* 20(4): 583–588.

Lupton, D. (1993) 'Risk as moral danger: the social and political functions of risk discourse in public health', *International Journal of Health Services* 23(3): 425–435.

Paicheler, G. (1994) 'Le public face de la menace du sida. Vol. I: Interprétation des connaissances et prise de conscience du risque', Unpublished report, Paris: Agence Nationale de Recherche sur le Sida.

——(1996) 'Le public face de la menace du sida. Vol. II: Gorer le risque', Unpub-lished report, Paris: Agence Nationale de Recherche sur le Sida.

Peruga, A. and Celentano, D. D. (1993) 'Correlates of AIDS knowledge in samples of the general population', *Social Science and Medicine* 36(4): 509–524.

Rosenstock, I. M. (1974) 'The Health Belief Model and preventive health behaviour', *Health Education Monographs* 2: 354–386.

Rotter, J. B. (1966) 'Generalized expectancies for internal versus external control of reinforcement', *Psychological Monographs* 80(1): 609.

Schutz, A. (1970) *Reflections on the problem of relevance*, New Haven, CT: Yale University Press.

Scott, S. and Freeman, R. (1995) 'Prevention as a problem of modernity: the example of HIV and Aids', in J. Gabe (ed.) *Medicine, Health and Risk*, Oxford: Blackwell.

Waldby, C., Kippax, S. and Crawford, J. (1993) 'Research note: heterosexual men and "safe sex" practice', *Sociology of Health and Illness* 15(2): 246–256.

Wallston, K. A. and Wallston, B. S. (1982) 'Who is responsible for your health? The construct of health locus of control', in G. S. Sanders and J. Suis (eds) *Social Psychology of Health and Illness*, Hillsdale, NJ: Lawrence Erlbaum.

Warwick, I., Aggleton, P. and Homans, H. (1988) 'Constructing commonsense: young people's beliefs about AIDS', *Sociology of Health and Illness* 10(3): 213–233.

Index

Printed in the United Kingdom
by Lightning Source UK Ltd.
129269UK00003B/62/A